THE TRILLION
DOLLAR
REVOLUTION

THE TRILLION DOLLAR REVOLUTION

*How the Affordable Care Act
Transformed Politics, Law, and
Health Care in America*

EDITED BY

EZEKIEL J. EMANUEL
ABBE R. GLUCK

PublicAffairs
New York

PublicAffairs
Hachette Book Group
1290 Avenue of the Americas, New York, NY 10104
www.publicaffairsbooks.com
@Public_Affairs

Printed in the United States of America
First Edition: March 2020

Published by PublicAffairs, an imprint of Perseus Books, LLC, a subsidiary of Hachette Book Group, Inc. The PublicAffairs name and logo is a trademark of the Hachette Book Group.

The Hachette Speakers Bureau provides a wide range of authors for speaking events. To find out more, go to www.hachettespeakersbureau.com or call (866) 376-6591.

The publisher is not responsible for websites (or their content) that are not owned by the publisher.

Editorial production by Christine Marra, *Marra*thon Production Services. www.marrathoneditorial.org

Book design by Jane Raese
Set in 12-point Adobe Garamond

Library of Congress Cataloging-in-Publication Data has been applied for.

ISBN 978-1-5417-9779-6 (trade paperback), ISBN 978-1-5417-9777-2 (ebook)

LSC-C

10 9 8 7 6 5 4 3 2 1

To my grandchildren
Yonah, Anina, and Lincoln
As part of my effort to improve the American health care system—
and society—for you and your fellow citizens
—E. J. E.

To my children
Ollie, Ryan, and Ruthie
Proof that the future is bright, and advocates for
"the law about doctors and hospitals"
ever since they could speak
—A. R. G.

CONTENTS

THE TRILLION DOLLAR REVOLUTION

PREFACE

Sylvia Mathews Burwell

With President Barack Obama's signature on a Tuesday morning, March 23, 2010, the Patient Protection and Affordable Care Act (ACA) officially became one of the seminal laws impacting American health care.

It was the largest reform of the nation's health care system since Congress and President Lyndon Johnson created Medicaid and Medicare nearly half a century before. One could argue it was even larger, as the ACA made structural reforms to both of those programs as well as to the private health insurance market and the nation's health care delivery system. Alongside its scale and import, the ACA has also undoubtedly been one of the most controversial laws in modern American history.

As we approach the 10-year anniversary of its passage, it is fitting to look back at the past decade and capture the history of the law, its successes, and its challenges. As we embark on that retrospective, we should do so with a dose of humility. Assessing the full impact of the ACA ten years after its passage is important but probably incomplete.

The lessons we can learn from this law's passage and its implementation can illuminate much about American politics and policy, our health care system, and the ways that decisions made by policymakers affect the lives of the American people.

Sylvia Mathews Burwell is the president of American University in Washington, DC, and served as the 22nd secretary of the US Department of Health and Human Services (2014–2017) and director of the Office of Management and Budget (2013–2014).

How to begin an analysis of such a comprehensive and complex law? There are innumerable ways to measure and analyze our nation's health care system. But I have always found it most helpful to focus on the 3 questions that matter most to American patients and their families. First, is health care accessible? Second, is it affordable? And third, is it quality care?

Those 3 aspects—accessibility, affordability, and quality—and their impact on the health of the American people are the through-line of the history of the ACA and this book. And these aspects will guide policymakers as they consider future reforms to American health care.

From where I sit and the experiences I had as secretary of Health and Human Services, a few things are clear.

First, the ACA helped more Americans access health care. An estimated 20 million Americans gained coverage due to the ACA's Medicaid expansion, subsidies to afford private health insurance through the Health Insurance Marketplace, and various reforms to the health insurance market like allowing young adults to stay on their parents' health plan until they turn 26. These reforms led to the lowest uninsured rate in American history.

Many of those previously uninsured were the people who needed coverage the most. Cancer survivors, people with chronic conditions, and others who, in the past, were denied coverage because of a preexisting condition were finally protected by the ACA's ban on that practice.

In the years since, we have also uncovered abundant evidence that access to coverage translates into greater protection from financial risk, greater access to care, and, subsequently, better health. Housing stability also improved, as declines in evictions have been associated with the ACA's expansion of Medicaid.[1] Nationwide, from 2010 to 2016, there was a nearly 30% drop in the share of nonelderly adults skipping treatment or not filling a prescription due to cost.[2] The ACA's expansion of Medicaid is probably its most studied policy, and researchers have found it is improving access to care, financial security, and health outcomes, including reducing premature deaths.[3]

Second, the ACA led to significant progress on affordability. As already noted, the ACA helped more people pay for health care services. Among people gaining coverage, it has led to lower medical debt and greater access to credit.[4] As a result, feelings of financial strain caused by health care have also dropped.[5] By reforming Medicare payments and launching innovative payment models that have been imitated by many private payers, the ACA has contributed to slowing health care cost growth across the entire economy.[6] Nonetheless, issues like rising deductibles and the struggles of middle-class families to keep up with health care costs are still quite problematic and a key focus for policy-makers today and in the future.

Finally, the ACA massively improved the quality of coverage for people who are currently covered through the individual market, as plans are required to cover essential health benefits; through their employer, as plans are no longer allowed to create lifetime or annual limits on coverage; or through Medicare, as the ACA closed the "donut hole" in Medicare Part D and now covers preventive services. It also improved the quality of care by reducing re-admissions and hospital-acquired conditions. Yet the United States still has work to do, as we fall behind other major developed nations in many measures and must do more to address behavioral health crises and infant and maternal mortality.

Among these 3 measures—the accessibility, affordability, and quality of American health care—the Affordable Care Act has directly led to significant progress.

Although none of these achievements means our work on these issues is done, each should be seen in the broader context of an effort—nearly unprecedented in modern American history—to undermine and attack the law.

From the early resistance to a traditional technical-fixes bill to the litigation filed the first day the statute was enacted, resistance to the ACA only grew. Modern American history has other examples of resistance to expansions in coverage. In 1961 the American Medical Association hired a well-known actor to record an LP warning that, if the newly proposed "Medicare" program passed, "We are going to spend our sunset years telling our children and our children's children what it once was like in America when men were free."[7] But a couple of decades later, when that actor became president, Ronald Reagan would not only protect Medicare but would expand it himself, adding protections for the elderly and disabled against catastrophic health costs.[8]

Opponents of the ACA have yet to accept it as part of the health system. The sustained repeal efforts through legislation, litigation, and executive action at the state and federal levels have all too often distracted us from building on progress and have taken a toll on many of the law's provisions and, thereby, the Americans who depend on them. Today, continued efforts by the current administration and others to undermine the legislation have zeroed out the individual mandate, limited access to contraception, drastically limited the outreach efforts during open enrollment periods, and weakened the ACA in many other ways. Some Americans find coverage slipping out of reach, as a modest but all-too-real increase in the uninsured rate since 2016 demonstrates.[9]

Despite all of this, the law at 10 years has proven more resilient than expected. Many times throughout the past decade conventional wisdom considered the ACA finished. Through midterm elections, Supreme Court decisions, a presidential reelection, and an election in 2016 that saw the legislative and executive branches united around repeal, the ACA has nevertheless survived. In fact, it has only grown more popular.[10] The 2018 midterms, where health care was listed as voters' top priority, was in many ways a rejection of repeal.

How did the law survive? In 2017 the law faced an opposition united in its commitment to repeal the law—an opposition equipped with the legislative tools through reconciliation to do so with a simple majority in both houses, and—after years of a guaranteed, protective veto from the executive branch—there was a president ready to offer his signature.

It was in this precise moment that the through-line of the law in many ways became its lifeline. Access, affordability, and quality were not just abstract metrics; they had real, tangible impacts on Americans' lives, and the uncertainty of repeal, the opacity of the process, and the warning signs from nonpartisan analysts like the Congressional Budget Office motivated a remarkable grassroots effort.

The lived examples of the ACA's progress motivated organizations and constituents as they appealed to their legislators to slow the process down and consider alternative routes to improving American health care.

By the slimmest of margins, the ACA survived and today remains the law of the land.

DESPITE THE PROGRESS of the ACA, there is more to do as we mark ten years. Policymakers and politicians continue to debate how to make progress on affordability, access, and coverage. The questions of repeal are also still with us. Currently there is yet another federal case, *Texas v. Azar*, in which 18 state attorneys general and the Trump administration Department of Justice argue that the entire ACA should be struck down.[11] We are, yet again, at a crossroads on health care.

In the midst of it all are countless Americans who have engaged with this journey in Washington and around the country—from legislative chambers to hospital corridors—to make our health care more affordable, more accessible, and higher quality and to refuse to go backward because they know that health care in America is personal.

What, then, is the legacy of the ACA? In short, it was a historic legislative achievement and a seminal step in American health policy. It led to great progress on access and some on affordability and quality. And yet there is still more to do.

The insights in the following chapters, gathered by Ezekiel J. Emanuel and Abbe R. Gluck, outline the journey and provide a rich context. The pages of *The Trillion Dollar Revolution: How the Affordable Care Act Transformed Politics, Law, and Health Care in America,* filled with stories and perspectives of those who were deeply involved at every step of the way, will illuminate the path we have taken so that we can more clearly see the path ahead. For it is through this kind of reflection that we can celebrate our progress and better understand the challenges that remain in our nation's health care system. Tempered with the humility of hindsight, we can take on the unfinished business of building a health care system worthy of our great nation and worthy of the American people who rely on it.

INTRODUCTION

Ezekiel J. Emanuel and Abbe R. Gluck

"This is a big fu@&ing deal."

—Vice President Joseph Biden whispering to President Obama during the ACA's signing ceremony, March 23, 2010

"ObamaCare is a broken mess."

—President Donald Trump, tweet, October 13, 2017

The Affordable Care Act (ACA) is arguably the most important health care legislation in US history—but it is much more than that.

The ACA has reached far beyond health care and into the corners of American politics, law, and the economy as well. It profoundly influenced our elections. Opposition to the ACA galvanized the Republicans and helped them recapture the House in 2010. But after multiple failed repeal efforts, the ACA then helped the Democrats take the House back in 2018.

The law has been subject to continuous litigation since the moment it passed. It has gone to the Supreme Court 5 times thus far and set new constitutional precedents on the reach of Congress's power. It also has yielded important lessons about how American laws are implemented,

Ezekiel J. Emanuel, MD, PhD, is the vice provost for Global Initiatives, Diane and Robert Levy University Professor, and codirector of the Healthcare Transformation Institute at the University of Pennsylvania. He was a special assistant in the Office of Management and Budget in the Obama administration (2009–2011).

Abbe R. Gluck, JD, is professor of law and founding faculty director of the Solomon Center for Health Law and Policy at Yale Law School and professor of internal medicine at Yale Medical School.

including how much federal law can or should rely on states or the private market.

At the same time, the ACA has transformed the health care economy. It has fostered dramatic health care market consolidation, upended the way the insurance industry does business, and helped to change the daily practice of medicine and how services are paid for. It is a $1 trillion investment in universal coverage, delivery reform, and cost containment, only part of which has been successful thus far. But it also has allowed millions of new Americans to obtain insurance and measurably improved the population's health.

Perhaps most fundamentally, the ACA seems to have shifted the baseline of what Americans understand to be the goals of their health care system. Ten years into the ACA's lifespan, an alternative that would undo a substantial part of the law's coverage gains no longer appears acceptable to the public. In thus changing our expectations, the ACA has paved the way for future health reforms that may extend even farther.

So is the ACA a "big fu@&ing deal" or "a broken mess"? Is it neither? Or both?

The ACA is much more ambitious than its comparable predecessor acts. Its most obvious predecessors—the Medicare and Medicaid legislation of 1965—were laws that expanded health coverage to two specific populations: the elderly and certain categories of low-income individuals. Those statutes never aspired to universal coverage—a health care system that would provide access to all Americans—rich and poor, old and young, employed or not, healthy or sick. Nor did they make fundamental changes to private health insurance or attempt to control costs or improve quality.

In contrast, the ACA targets every part of the health care system. Paradoxically, it makes these sweeping changes through an incremental strategy—a strategy that the politics of the moment required. The ACA does not wipe the slate clean or eliminate the private health care system, but instead it builds on what came before. For better or perhaps for worse, the ACA accepts the sprawling and fragmented complexity of the US health care system but seeks to make it more inclusive, more generous, more effective, and less expensive.

To say these changes are controversial is a massive understatement. The ACA has been the most attacked and—as it turned out—the most resilient piece of social welfare legislation Congress has ever passed. The law was challenged in court minutes after it was enacted and then partially gutted by the Supreme Court before its main provisions even took effect. The challenges continue to come—both in the courts and from a presidential administration that considers the ACA a "broken mess" in need of abolition. The very states that asked to implement the ACA rebelled against it from the start. Congress has tried more than 60 times to repeal it. But the law has survived—and gained in popularity in the process.

Ten years in, it is time for a critical analysis of the ACA. The authors of the essays in this volume examine the ACA's goals and its arc of policy and politics. They look at the legal battles the ACA survived and how these battles changed American law. They examine the ACA's impact on the health care system and economy and consider how its decade in existence will influence the health care agenda for the 2020s.

Enactment

During the 2008 presidential primaries and election, health care was a major issue, maybe second only to—and intertwined with—the economic recovery from the Great Recession. The election seemed to confirm the nation's desire for health care reform. Barack Obama was elected by a 52.9% to 45.7% margin over John McCain, and Democrats picked up 21 seats in the House and secured (with independents) a filibuster-proof 60 votes in the Senate. Obama put health care at the top of his agenda, overruling members of his team who thought he needed to focus first on Wall Street, and he created the first-ever position of White House health care czar.

Any piece of major legislation contains policy tradeoffs and political ramifications. On policy, there were many choices and many things that could not be achieved even within the Democratic Party. There were also sharp memories of President Clinton's failed attempt at health reform in 1993–1994 and a determination not to repeat previous mistakes.

Ultimately, an incremental approach won the day. The fragmentation of the health care system between varied public programs and private insurance companies would not be swept away and a new system built from the ground up. Coverage would remain split among the different insurance programs but would be expanded in every existing category: Medicaid would be converted from a program that covered only certain categories of people (like pregnant women) to an income-linked entitlement for all lower-income Americans; Medicare saw expanded benefits, particularly in preventative care and pharmaceutical payment; the employer-sponsored health care system (which at the time covered 50% of Americans), with the tax exclusion that supports it, was retained with additional consumer protections and benefits; uninsured Americans—those with incomes from 100% to 400% of the federal poverty level (just over $100,000 for a family of 4)—were to receive subsidies to help them buy private insurance in newly created marketplaces.

There were also two fateful decisions made about the structure of the insurance marketplaces. In an effort to appeal to Republicans, the Senate made the insurance marketplaces state based rather than, as the House wanted, national. This added to the ACA's administrative complexity—but ultimately it was not sufficient in itself to attract the votes of any Republican senators. Similarly, in an effort to appease conservative Democrats, especially Joseph Lieberman of Connecticut (by then an Independent), the plan to include a public option—a government-operated insurance offering that utilized Medicare payment rates—was dropped.

Many of the pivotal choices on coverage were made largely for fiscal reasons. The president wanted a bill that met 3 key financing criteria: (1) the total cost of the ACA should not exceed $1 trillion over 10 years, (2) half the money to pay for the ACA should come from savings in government health programs and half should come from new revenue, and (3) the law should be self-funded and not deficit financed—if anything, the ACA should pay down the national debt (which it did).

These financing decisions shaped the structure of the reforms. Because Medicaid was less expensive than purchasing private insurance in the exchanges, it was preferable to expand Medicaid to households at up to 138% of the federal poverty level (FPL) rather than covering all the uninsured through the insurance exchanges. Because of the high cost of subsidies, they were phased out at 400% of the FPL with a steep cliff rather than at higher income levels.

Complementing these new coverage provisions, the ACA also imposed new national rules that dramatically change the way the private health insurance industry does business. Insurers can no longer "risk underwrite"—reject customers or charge them substantially more or rescind their plans due to their poor health, preexisting conditions, or other individual characteristics. In addition, insurers can no longer impose annual or lifetime caps. Other key new policies include the requirement that all ACA exchange plans must offer 10 essential health benefits and that, even outside the exchanges, many preventative services (like vaccines and cancer screening) must be covered without deductibles or co-pays. Coverage of children up to age 26 on their parents' health plan is another popular new benefit.

There was no shortage of criticism. One consistent theme was that the ACA was 90% about coverage and did little to improve quality or cost. It is true that 3 of the ACA's 10 titles do focus on insurance access and coverage—the private insurance reforms in Title I, the Medicaid expansion in Title II, and new provisions about long-term care in Title VIII that ultimately were not implemented because they could not meet fiscal targets of being self-financing. Title III also includes significant reforms to Medicare to reduce co-pays and make pharmaceuticals more affordable. But the ACA contains many other pages directed to improve quality. For example, the law had incentives and penalties to reduce hospital readmissions and hospital-acquired conditions and to require public reporting on performance. Some key reforms did take the form of only limited programs, such as new programmatic incentives to improve integration and coordination across physicians and demonstration projects to move away from payment for each treatment—fee-for-service—to payment for holistic episodes of care—bundled payments. These pilot projects were strategic, aiming to effect broader system-wide transformation. The establishment of integrated medical practices called accountable care organizations (ACOs) is another important example of the effort to reform the delivery system and thereby improve quality and reduce costs.

Important new centers and funds were also created, including the Prevention and Public Health Fund; the Center for Medicare and Medicaid Innovation, a novel organization within CMS given the opportunity to experiment with various approaches to improving quality and reducing costs; and the Patient-Centered Outcomes Research Institute, an organization charged with investigating the clinical and comparative effectiveness of different medical treatments. There are myriad other provisions, including provisions to facilitate a generic market in biologic drugs, to reauthorize the Indian Health Service, and to enhance the medical workforce, nutrition, and more. Taken together, these new programs and incentives mark an extensive—if not comprehensive—effort to transform and improve almost every aspect of the American health care system.

Political considerations of course shaped the bill. Because of President Obama's inclination to appeal to Republicans and forge broad coalitions to address problems and because Senator Max Baucus, as Senate Finance Committee chair, believed he could achieve a bipartisan agreement, the ACA rests on a market-oriented structure. Indeed, its foundation adopts some conservative proposals: it was the Heritage Foundation that popularized the concept of an individual mandate—the requirement that nearly everyone hold health insurance or face a financial penalty—combined with subsidies and a facilitated marketplace where individuals could purchase private insurance. That concept was adopted by the Massachusetts Republican governor (later GOP presidential nominee) Mitt Romney. (Income-linked government subsidies to enable the purchase of private health insurance has been a Republican idea dating to the 1940s.)

In the end, despite many efforts to create bipartisan legislation, it became clear that Republicans would unanimously oppose the bill. Beginning in August 2009, that position was reinforced by a series of voluble and disruptive town hall meetings that propelled to national prominence the conservative, no-compromise, Tea Party movement.

Many factors made passage possible, including some key moments of serendipity. Many political veterans, such as Obama chief of staff Rahm Emanuel, had learned the lessons of the earlier, Clinton-era failures. The administration brought in the major health care interest groups early and offered them what they needed, including omitting controversial pharmaceutical pricing regulations, to get them on board. President Obama helped give the bill needed momentum when he urged its enactment before a rare joint session of Congress on September 9, 2009. That speech also provided an example of the deep-seated anger the ACA provoked. For the first time ever in a presidential speech to a joint session of Congress, a member of Congress publicly heckled the president. Representative Joe Wilson (R-SC) shouted, "You lie!" during the address. That insult emboldened wavering Democrats to remain supportive of the law.

House Speaker Nancy Pelosi played a pivotal role. First, she ensured there would be only one bill coming out of the 3 House committees with jurisdiction over health care reform. And even more significantly, once the victory of Scott Brown in the Massachusetts Senate race to replace Senator Kennedy deprived the Democrats of a filibuster-proof 60 Senate votes to revisit any House revision of the ACA, Pelosi rallied the House Democratic members to essentially accept the Senate bill. Pelosi's actions were an estimable feat of effective politicking that convinced the House to abandon its own bill—which had some significant differences—and made the ultimately successful vote possible.

The ACA was enacted into law on March 23, 2010. *National Federation of Independent Business v. Sebelius*, the challenge to the ACA that threw the early stages of implementation into uncertainty and would eventually reach the US Supreme Court, was filed the same day.[1]

Goals

Much has been written about the details of the ACA's trajectory through Congress and its enactment politics. This book largely picks up where those accounts leave off. But to set the stage, **Timothy Stoltzfus Jost** and **John E. McDonough** analyze the problems that plagued the health care system in 2008 on the eve of the ACA's drafting and explain how specific provisions in the ACA seek to address those problems. They also highlight what the ACA did not do, including failing to make significant advances in drug pricing and replacing "a fragmented, exasperating health system balkanized by public and private financing and delivery."

Peter R. Orszag and **Rahul Rekhi** delve deeper into the policy tradeoffs incorporated into the ACA, especially around cost and quality. They suggest that many of the efforts—even if small and tentative—at cost control and quality improvement may have contributed positively to the slowdown in health care expenditures and "fundamentally altered the national conversation around health care expenditures among provider and insurer executives and in boardrooms."

Joseph Antos and **James Capretta** offer a perspective of where they believe the ACA went right and wrong. Republicans have had a hard time articulating a coherent alternative to the ACA. The scores of efforts to "repeal and replace" failed, and the party faced additional challenges as it became clear that the public would not tolerate rolling back some of the ACA's key benefits. Antos and Capretta present an alternative vision that is grounded more squarely in market principles focused on cost containment and emphasizing the need for consumer choice. It is interesting to note that, despite their disagreements with some of the policies behind the ACA, Antos and Capretta nevertheless embrace the new reality that, after a decade of the ACA, the goal of any new reform must include giving every American health coverage.

The Policy and Politics of Implementation

The ACA seems nearly inseparable from the last decade of politics— and the politics around the ACA affected both health policy and the broader electoral landscape.

The Obama administration faced political, policy, and technical challenges from the moment the law was signed. **Kathleen Sebelius**, who was the secretary of the Department of Health and Human Services (HHS) for the first 4 years of the ACA's life, and **Nancy-Ann DeParle**, the first health care czar, detail what it was like to implement the law in the face of unexpected state resistance, legal onslaught, disastrous technology failures, and a Congress that refused to give HHS the money it needed to implement and administer the massive new law.

Joel Ario, the first director of the HHS Office of Health Insurance Exchanges, then explains the specific challenges the Obama administration faced in trying to convince Republican-controlled states to run their own exchanges. Even though Republicans in the Senate were the ones who had pushed for a state-based model, the extreme political polarization around the ACA that followed enactment made resistance to ACA implementation, including exchange implementation, a Republican Party loyalty litmus test. The exchange implementation struggle illustrates across several dimensions the challenge of designing a law to achieve the right balance between federal standards and local control and flexibility.

The political environment evolved alongside implementation and shook electoral politics for the better part of the decade. **Jonathan Cohn** and former House Republican majority leader **Eric Cantor** each offer a perspective on the political arc. Cohn tracks the changing fortunes of Democrats and Republicans around the ACA from the 2010 midterm election to the 2018 election, and the failure of repeal and replace, which, he concludes, ultimately revealed a shift in public opinion about the importance of universal coverage that, while tentative, is "meaningful . . . a signal that, for all of its well-documented flaws, the ACA has provided the public with something that it truly values and does not want to give up."

Cantor laments a lack of sincere interest in bipartisan negotiations over the ACA and, in the House—where he was the Republican Party's majority leader—the absence of Republican input in the process of drafting the law. Like Cohn, he details the initial momentum for repeal and replace and then how the process began, as Cantor puts it, "to backfire" against the Party. Cantor also makes a very significant point about how the ACA has catalyzed a profound shift of the policy baseline: "after Obamacare's enactment, the test for an alternative was a comparison of coverage numbers." A Republican alternative would need to provide insurance coverage for substantially the same proportion of the population as the ACA—a difficult goal for a party that has traditionally focused on cost. Cantor calls for future bipartisan work on bending the cost curve as a way to move past the political gridlock on health reform.

Law and Governance

In the words of **Paul Clement**, the former US solicitor general under President Bush who argued against the ACA in the Supreme Court, the ACA's 10 years of constant litigation have been "outsized in every respect." The ACA has been to the Supreme Court 5 times over the course of the decade. Still, another case that threatens the entire existence of the ACA is working its way through the lower courts, and yet more challenges are likely ahead. These cases are about a lot more than health care: their impact extends to constitutional law, religious liberty, American federalism, and more. Clement and President Obama's own solicitor general, **Donald B. Verrilli**, who defended the ACA in the Supreme Court 3 times, each offers a perspective.

Both remark on the intensity of the stakes of the first constitutional challenge, *National Federation of Independent Business v. Sebelius*, and the unprecedented attention the case received. In the end, although Verrilli was unable to overcome Clement's argument that the ACA's insurance mandate was an unconstitutional attempt to "regulate inactivity" under the Commerce Clause, Verrilli nevertheless prevailed on the key argument that most of the ACA could be saved as a valid exercise of Congress's taxing power.

Unexpectedly, the Medicaid expansion was a major casualty. The Court held that the design of the expansion was unconstitutionally coercive—that states had no real choice but to accept it. This surprise holding had significant implications for both ACA implementation and the structure of state-federal programs beyond health care.

And yet, as Verrilli recalls, the Court's decision to uphold most of the ACA meant "many on the right refused to accept *NFIB* as legitimate." Another high-stakes existential challenge—*King v. Burwell*— soon followed, this one based not on the Constitution but on a likely mistake in the ACA's text that could have proved fatal to the viability of the insurance exchanges. This time Verrilli's victory was definitive. Verrilli recalls that many, including him, thought *King* "would, finally, put an end to the legal battle over the ACA's legitimacy. We were wrong again."

Clement details how ACA opponents then moved to "more targeted challenges to specific provisions of the ACA," many of which have fared "substantially better" than the broader challenges. These included religious objectors' challenges to the ACA's contraception mandate and a case heard by the Supreme Court in December 2019, addressing some $12 billion in payments the ACA promised to insurers but which were cut off by the Republican-controlled Congress. Finally, as Verrilli and Clement each recount, now pending in the lower courts is a third major constitutional and statutory challenge that again amounts to an existential threat to the entire ACA. Thus far, Verrilli concludes, "the ACA has managed to survive as sustained an assault in the courts as has ever been brought against an Act of Congress."

Different battles played out in the states. **Abbe R. Gluck** and **Nicole Huberfeld** detail how the ACA's vision of health care "federalism"—its allocation of responsibility between the federal government and the states—was flipped on its head soon after enactment when, instead of state-run exchanges and a universal Medicaid expansion, there was state resistance to exchanges and the Court's optional version of Medicaid expansion. The Obama administration played a long game, however—offering Medicaid concessions and creative exchange structures to bring opposing states on board and even giving them political cover to publicly resist the ACA while privately cooperating with it. At the same time, the very choices that the ACA's federalism puts to the states—whether to expand Medicaid, whether to run an exchange—made the ACA and its core value of coverage the stuff of everyday newspaper articles, state government elections, and even state ballot initiatives. Paradoxically, this sustained public attention on health care, Gluck and Huberfeld point out, helped to elevate and entrench the law and its goals. In another paradox, the state's role in the ACA has proved an unexpected and powerful defense against the hostile Trump administration. And yet, for all its political benefits, the authors conclude, it is not clear that federalism has actually improved health care outcomes.

Nicholas Bagley tells the story of presidential power under the ACA, focusing on its excesses. A law of the ACA's scale necessarily delegates an enormous amount of implementation authority to the executive branch. An atmosphere of historic political gridlock may further incentivize future presidents frustrated with Congress to stretch the limits of executive power in ways that have serious negative long-term consequences for the rule of law. Notably, Bagley sees this risk in the actions that both President Obama and President Trump took with respect to the ACA but also concludes that the two presidents "committed very different legal sins." On the one hand, President Obama, he writes, "cut corners" to implement the law "in the face of congressional resistance." President Trump, on the other hand, "exploited his position as the head of the executive branch to mount an unconstitutional campaign to sabotage the very law that he is charged with faithfully executing."

Assessing Impact

What were the ACA's direct effects on the health care system? Did it improve coverage? Did the ACA lower costs or improve quality?

One thing that is clear is that while the ACA did not achieve universal coverage, it did significantly improve health coverage. **Katherine Baicker** and **Benjamin D. Sommers** explain that more than 20 million Americans received health coverage who were uninsured before the ACA and that the uninsurance rate declined to 10% of the American population. They assess the evidence, concluding that expansion of coverage improved the health of the population, including better access to primary care and medications, improved diagnosis of chronic conditions, and, as some studies suggest, reduced deaths from conditions, including heart disease. But even as 12 million Americans received insurance through the exchanges, those figures have been lower than predicted. Baicker and Sommers explore multiple reasons for the depressed exchange enrollment. Instead, Medicaid has been the centerpiece of the ACA's coverage expansion. Sixteen million gained Medicaid coverage, including an additional 2 million in nonexpansion states. Medicaid now covers more than 75 million people, and expansion states have experienced improved hospital finances, reduced racial and ethnic disparities in coverage, and improved affordability of care.

There is also some evidence that quality of health care has improved. **Ezekiel J. Emanuel** and **Amol S. Navathe** present data suggesting a modest decline in avoidable readmissions as well as evidence that the headline-grabbing claim that the readmission policy increased 30-day mortality is likely incorrect. They note that payment changes and reforms to the delivery system have not produced substantial improvements but also have not increased costs or worsened quality. Hence, the picture is more mixed. In addition, Emanuel and Navathe review the myriad demonstration projects related to payment reform launched by the ACA's new Center for Medicare and Medicaid Innovation (CMMI) and report that both ACOs and bundled payments for surgical procedures seem to be associated with very modest declines in costs and perhaps slight improvements in quality. They conclude that with no evidence these programs raise costs or lower quality, continued experimentation to find more impactful alternative payment models that consistently reduce costs is justified.

Cost, however, remains a highly controversial topic. It is clear that health care costs have risen less than the US Congressional Budget Office had expected at the time the ACA was enacted. **Carrie H. Colla** and **Jonathan Skinner** note that per capita spending in Medicaid has been flat for decades and flattened in Medicare coincident with the Great Recession. They document that there was a "great pause" in commercial insurance spending between 2010 and 2013. Colla and Skinner argue that while the "ACA has not been entirely successful at bending the cost curve," this pause in cost growth may have "laid the foundation for a shift away from the uncoordinated fee-for-service payment systems and toward a future environment of alternative payment contracts, global budgets, scaled-back reimbursement rates, and public pricing options."

Another important trend in the delivery system has been consolidation—the growth of bigger insurance companies, ever-larger hospital systems, and increasing purchases by hospitals of physician groups and other components of the delivery system. Exploring this post-ACA consolidation, **Leemore S. Dafny** emphasizes that although "consolidation has occurred in virtually every corner of the health care industry," causal connections between the ACA and the "merger floodgates open[ing]" are difficult to substantiate. Similarly, she writes, insurer mergers have led to higher group premiums and less competition. She reminds us that the ACA "sought to harness the power of markets." Now, we need to "mitigate trends that would undermine it."

The practice of medicine has changed dramatically over the ACA's decade too, but **David Blumenthal**, **Melinda K. Abrams**, **Corinne Lewis**, and **Shanoor Seervai** conclude that it is difficult to draw a direct linkage between the ACA and these changes in the medical profession. Expanding coverage and ACOs were undoubtedly important in changing and improving the practice of medicine. But other changes may reshape the medical profession more. They explain that, most notably, the HITECH Act—which was part of the last decade but came from the Recovery Act, not the ACA itself—expanded electronic health records and significantly changed physician practice, as has the digital revolution in health care in general, which they conclude will "likely dwarf any effects of the ACA."

Blumenthal and colleagues also note payment changes introduced after the ACA. They suggest that the changes introduced by the Medicare Access and Chip Reauthorization Act of 2015 (MACRA), which was enacted 5 years after the ACA and replaced the fee-for-service physician reimbursement system with a new framework that encouraged value-based compensation, will "likely affect more physicians more directly with respect to both compensation and reporting requirements than the totality of the ACA's provisions."

The Future

What comes next? And what does the ACA teach us about how to approach health care in the future?

Over the last decade the exorbitant price of prescription drugs has become a public obsession. As **Rachel E. Sachs** and **Steven D. Pearson** explain, the pharmaceutical industry escaped the ACA "largely unscathed." Going forward, however, confronting drug pricing seems unavoidable. Sachs and Pearson delineate 3 areas for special focus: (1) they advocate capping out-of-pocket costs related to drugs for Medicare beneficiaries, (2) they propose specific changes to eliminate perverse incentives in the drug supply chain, and (3) they believe the United States should look to the examples of other countries and institute value-based payment for drugs—paying on the basis of the cost effectiveness and the health benefits (the clinical effectiveness) of the drug.

Sara Rosenbaum then looks to the future of health justice. She describes the ACA as "the most significant advance in more than half a century" for health equality but also notes that the ACA still leaves significant gaps. She explores the major equality advances: Medicaid expansion, the ACA's expansion of community health centers, and the ACA's new and important antidiscrimination provisions, which Rosenbaum argues "better reflect evolving social and cultural norms regarding the types of people and health needs meriting special legal protections against discrimination and exclusion." Yet she argues there is more to do, including devising a pathway to affordable coverage for undocumented immigrants, shoring up the ACA's new civil rights protections in the face of attack from the Trump administration, and, most importantly, addressing the large coverage gap in states that have not expanded Medicaid. Rosenbaum concludes by suggesting a radical structural change to Medicaid: a new federalism model, similar to the one the ACA uses for the exchanges, that would require the federal government to step in and cover the population if the states refuse to do so.

A different perspective comes from **Rahm Emanuel**, who was President Obama's chief of staff through the ACA's enactment and would have embraced a different model of reform from the one the president ultimately chose. Emanuel notes that while health care reform may be good policy, it is inherently difficult politics. It has to be done at the right time, he writes, in a bipartisan manner, and yet it never produces immediate political benefits for the party sponsoring change. Emanuel would have addressed the economy and financial reform before turning to health care reform. He also would have moved more incrementally than did President Obama, seeking to expand coverage for small businesses and families as an attainable first step. Even so, Emanuel gives the Obama administration's accomplishments in the ACA an "A grade" for what it achieved with respect to coverage. He is less sanguine about the political story and, in particular, the enduring impact on the ACA's legitimacy from its failure to obtain any Republican votes in support. Going forward, Emanuel urges incremental reform instead of Medicare for All, which he sees as a political liability for the Democrats. He urges expanding Medicare coverage to politically sympathetic groups such as Americans aged 50 to 64.

Jacob Hacker is more optimistic. Rejected as too progressive during the ACA debate, the public option is now embraced by many Democrats as a middle-of-the-road option. Hacker is one of the original proponents of the public option and explores what he views as a changing political environment that makes various new coverage proposals seem more politically viable. Like Emanuel, Hacker worries that Medicare for All may be too much too fast. Ultimately, Hacker suggests that a reasonable compromise approach would be to maintain the employer-sponsored insurance system (with stronger protections against high out-of-pocket costs and network inadequacy) but merge Medicaid, the exchanges, and other individuals into Medicare, which should be made available as an option for all. Policy designers, he argues, must counter-act the perception that any part-way approach will stall progress toward universal coverage by "hardwiring" momentum for eventual universal coverage into any new program.

Conclusion

At the end of a decade it is becoming increasingly clear that the ACA has indeed been an outsized and historic achievement. It has had a substantial impact on the US health care system and, therefore, on 18% of the US economy. It has expanded coverage for more than 20 million Americans. It created exchanges and a mechanism for people to obtain subsidies to buy private insurance. It changed eligibility for Medicaid in 36 states, the District of Columbia, and counting. It led to at least a temporary slowdown in health care costs and lower than expected national health expenditures. It introduced and expanded non-fee-for-service payment models, reduced readmissions, and more.

But its impact extends well beyond health care. The ACA has changed the country's politics, law, and governance. It crystalized anger in conservative segments of the population that fueled Republican elec-tion victories and then backlashes that returned Democrats to power. It also generated new constitutional understandings of Congress's au-thority to regulate commerce and state implementation of federal law. It legitimized certain employer religious objections to covering health benefits. Finally, it has empowered the executive branch to use its ex-tensive authority to implement—and sometimes circumvent—the ACA's commands, with broader implications for the rule of law.

As monumental as it is, the ACA also leaves important gaps. It never even tried to address the health care system's complexity and fragmen-tation—and very likely exacerbated it. It has fallen short in achieving universal coverage, transforming health care delivery, and significantly bending the cost curve. And it did not touch drug prices.

None of this means the ACA is a "broken mess," however. In fact, it may not have been ambitious enough. As the chapters detail, political, fiscal, and legal considerations put practical limits on how much change could be accomplished at once—and the ACA did change more at once than any major health care legislation in American history.

Perhaps, most importantly, the ACA has changed the public's views and expectations. Its protections, coverage aims, and vision for a changing health care system have created a new understanding of what the American health care system should be. And its historic resilience through unprecedented challenge has proven that it is not disappearing—or receding—in importance. In fact, it may just be the beginning.

That is a "big fu@&ing deal."

Part I

GOALS

CHAPTER I

THE PATH TO THE AFFORDABLE CARE ACT

Timothy Stoltzfus Jost and John E. McDonough

The Affordable Care Act (also known as Obamacare, or the ACA) is a living, 5-star case study of US health policymaking. Its story is multi-layered and dynamic and touches all the health care system's compelling dimensions: historical, financial, legal, statutory, economic, sociological, personal, political, and so much more.

This chapter aims to lay a foundation for this volume's exploration of the ACA's multiple dimensions over its 10 years by addressing 4 questions:

1. What were the main problems that the ACA was enacted to address?
2. What key elements of the 2009–2010 legislative process to passage remain important today?
3. What components of the original ACA statute matter the most 10 years later?
4. What are key elements of US health reform left undone?

Timothy Stoltzfus Jost, JD, is an emeritus professor at the Washington and Lee University School of Law and a contributing editor at *Health Affairs*.

John E. McDonough, DrPH, MPA, is a professor of practice at the Harvard TH Chan School of Public Health and served as a senior adviser on National Health Reform to the US Senate HELP Committee (2008–2010).

The Problems That Motivated the ACA

By any measure the ACA is a consequential law. It is the only federal
health law in US history that merits the term "comprehensive" because
it is the only one that seeks, by intent, to improve broad system performance on all 3 essential components of health policy: access, quality,
and costs. Even the landmark 1965 law that established Medicare and
Medicaid only addressed access by providing health insurance to most
Americans over age 65. ACA crafters sought to address these 3 challenges because of the system's documented and well-recognized shortcomings. We consider access first and then cost and quality in tandem.

Access

Eight days after the November 4, 2008, election that elevated Barack
Obama to the presidency, Senator Max Baucus of Montana, chair of
the US Senate's powerful Finance Committee, released a white paper
to set the stage for an anticipated health reform legislative process.[1] His
paper described in detail the problems facing American health care,
along with proposals for legislative solutions. Many of the solutions
Baucus offered became part of the final ACA.

The white paper identified significant problems concerning access
to health insurance and the high cost and poor quality of Americans'
medical care. Access problems were a top priority, with 45.7 million
Americans—15.3% of the nation's population—lacking health insurance in 2007, up from 38.4 million in 2000. By 2009, while Congress
debated reform, the number had climbed to 50.7 million, or 16.7% of
the population.[2] Every other advanced industrial nation had already
achieved near-universal health insurance coverage for its citizens, providing access to care and protection from catastrophic financial risks.[3]

Since its inception in the 1930s, US health insurance has been mostly
job related. Though most Americans who worked for larger employers or for higher-wage smaller employers received insurance through
their jobs, most uninsured (8 out of 10 in 2007) came from low- and
lower-middle-income working families whose employers did not offer
health insurance to them or offered it at unaffordable rates.[4] Disproportionate numbers of uninsured Americans worked for small businesses, always a larger source of uninsured than major companies, and

their coverage had steadily dropped over decades.[5] Many part-time, seasonal, and low-income workers were not offered coverage or could not afford their share of the premium. The 2008 recession worsened the situation, as millions of Americans lost jobs and health insurance as well.

Although individuals and families who were ineligible for public or employer-based coverage could try to buy insurance from their state's individual (nongroup) market, such coverage was often unaffordable or unavailable. The federal tax code subsidizes employer-sponsored insurance (ESI) because premiums are exempt from income and payroll taxes, but individual market-policy holders had received no such consideration.[6] The experience of shopping for individual coverage was also byzantine, as insurance products came in multiple and confusing forms with no intelligible way to compare products effectively.

Coverage disparities were not solely economic. African Americans and Hispanics were far more likely to be uninsured than whites. Nonwhites, making up about ⅓ of all Americans, represented more than half of the US uninsured population. Younger adults were overrepresented in the uninsured population because of their lower incomes and better health status. Older adults between ages 55 and 65—more likely to have preexisting medical conditions, including many with disabilities whose ailments did not meet the Medicare disability threshold—often found coverage unavailable or unaffordable. Geographic disparities resulted in southern and poorer states experiencing far higher numbers of uninsured than northern states.

Moreover, in 2009, in 45 of the 50 US states, insurers evaluated individual policy applicants based on their medical histories, a practice called "medical underwriting." Those with preexisting health issues, such as mental health problems or pregnancy, were denied coverage or charged unaffordable rates, while coverage of their preexisting conditions was often excluded. This triggered many claims denials and often coverage rescissions—when insurers attributed treatment costs to a preexisting condition.

The 1996 federal Health Insurance Portability and Accountability Act (HIPAA) had offered relief for some. That law banned preexisting condition exclusions for people with employer-sponsored coverage who maintained continuous coverage for at least 18 months with no break over 63 days. It prohibited medical underwriting in employer groups. But HIPAA offered little for those with preexisting conditions seeking individual coverage. People with preexisting health conditions often could not leave their job-related coverage or the jobs through which they got that coverage. "Job lock" kept many working at undesirable jobs even when their talents could have been used to launch new businesses or when they might have retired early from jobs that had worn them out.

Other expensive problems plagued insurance consumers. Many health plans imposed annual and/or lifetime benefit limits, exposing those with high-cost conditions to financial ruin. Individual market coverage often imposed high deductibles, co-insurance, and/or co-payments, leaving medical care unaffordable even for the insured. Since the early 2000s, "underinsurance" had been tracked as a growing problem, while medical bankruptcies were common for insured and uninsured alike.

Public programs—primarily Medicare and Medicaid—covered most of the elderly, some persons with disabilities, low-income children, and pregnant women. The Children's Health Insurance Program (CHIP), enacted in 1996, expanded coverage for lower-middle-income children in the late 1990s and early 2000s; however, because it was not an entitlement like Medicare and Medicaid, CHIP became a recurring political football. In most states Medicaid was unavailable for adults without dependent children, no matter how poor they were, and was only available for the poorest parents of covered children.

As far back as the 1980s some progressive states began using federal Medicaid and state dollars to expand coverage to varied categories of uninsured lower-income adults and children, adding fuel to the adage, "If you've seen one state Medicaid program, you've seen one Medicaid program." Importantly, Massachusetts enacted a near-universal coverage law in 2006, expanding subsidized insurance eligibility to all low- and lower-middle-income adults while imposing a mandate on individuals to purchase insurance or face a tax penalty. The bipartisan support for the law drew national attention to a potential breakthrough reform model, especially as the law was successfully implemented in 2007 and 2008.

The Cost and Quality of Care

If Democrats and Republicans agree on anything in health-reform debates, the goal of higher-quality care at lower cost might be it. In 2009 the United States spent $2.5 trillion on health care, 17.6% of its gross domestic product and $8,086 per capita. No other nation came close to this level of spending. That same year average per capita health spending for OECD (Organisation for Economic Co-operation and Development) countries was about $3,200, only 9.6% of GDP.[7] US health spending was high in the early 2000s and grew rapidly in that decade, continuing a trend that reached back into the previous century, particularly with Medicare and Medicaid's creation in 1965, and accelerating more rapidly beginning in the 1980s in President Ronald Reagan's era.[8]

This cost burden was felt widely.[9] Payments for medical care were among the largest and fastest-growing categories of public and private spending. By 2009 the federal government accounted for 27% of health care costs, while state governments accounted for 17%. Government paid for health care directly and also forfeited revenue from generous tax exclusions for employer-sponsored insurance.[10] Health care imposed substantial burdens on private business, accounting for 21% of all health care spending in 2009. Much health care cost—18.5%—was borne directly by private individuals and households through insurance premiums and cost sharing by those who paid for items and services not covered by insurance and by uninsured individuals who paid out of pocket for services.[11]

Numerous studies warned that the high cost paid for US medical care did not ensure high quality care. Most notably, the Institute of Medicine's 2001 landmark study of US health system quality began: "The American health care delivery system is in need of fundamental change. . . . Quality problems are everywhere, affecting many patients. Between the health care we have and the care we could have lies not just a gap, but a chasm."[12]

Medical care providers received the same payment for each medical service regardless of outcome and regardless of whether the service was appropriate, while useful and accessible quality information was lacking. Health policy experts had long identified the system's dominant fee-for-service (FFS) payment model as incentivizing excess provision of visits, tests, images, and other high-technology services rather than positive and higher-quality patient outcomes. FFS was viewed as discouraging collaborative and integrated care because providers were paid independently rather than rewarded for working together. Providers lacked incentives to move patients to more appropriate and less-costly settings. Slow or nonadoption of health information technology and electronic health records hampered care coordination.[13]

Baucus's white paper also focused on high and unnecessary costs from fraud, waste, and abuse, citing a conclusion by the US Congressional Budget Office (CBO) that up to one-third of health care spending had no positive effect on outcomes.[14] Lack of information on the comparative effectiveness of treatments, technologies, and procedures impeded both cost control and quality improvement. The absence of payment transparency by drug and device companies to physicians and other providers raised concerns about biased provider decision making.

Pharmaceutical and medical device prices were high and rapidly climbing, as brand-name drug manufacturers used their market power to stifle generic competition. The federal government—the largest pharmaceutical purchaser—was prohibited by law from using its market clout to negotiate with drug makers to slow the growing costs.

In addition, Baucus's report concluded that Medicare overpaid for many services and whole programs. Part C, or Medicare Advantage (MA), which pays private insurers to deliver Medicare services, often using provider networks, had been reengineered in the federal 2003 Medicare Modernization Act to the financial benefit of its participating insurers. They were substantially overpaid in comparison with traditional Medicare.

The system was ripe for reform in other ways as well. Experts concluded that the United States had medical professional shortages, especially for primary care providers and key professional categories such as mental health, and that many physician services could be offered efficiently by other professionals such as nurse practitioners and physician assistants. Little support existed to address Americans' long-term care needs beyond Medicaid, which only helped those with low incomes, including impoverished middle-income individuals who exhausted their assets paying for care out of pocket. Services and support for long-term care were mostly provided in institutional settings such as nursing homes, even when community-based care could be cheaper and more comfortable. A legislative pathway was needed so that the US Food and Drug Administration could approve the marketing and sale of biosimilar biologic drugs. The Indian Health Service also badly needed reform, resources, and reauthorization of a statute that had expired in 2001. These were just for starters.

Beyond these deficiencies were key public health and health system performance indicators such as infant mortality, life expectancy, incidence of overweight and obesity, gun-related injuries, racial and ethnic disparities, and other key measures by which the United States lagged badly compared with other advanced nations. Spending by far the most on a health care system offering low value and poor outcomes is an invitation for comprehensive health system reform. Public officials from both parties and officials in the new Obama administration were well aware of these shortcomings.

Key Markers on the Path to Passage

Comprehensive accounts of the ACA's path to enactment have been provided in other narratives.[15] Ten years out, some events and dynamics from that period appear vitally important to understanding the law and its perpetually unfolding, postenactment process. Here we identify those features of the ACA's legislative process.

Ten dates were critical in the process to passage:

June 16, 2008: Senator Max Baucus (D-MT) and Charles Grassley (R-IA) cohosted the "Prepare to Launch: Health Reform Summit" at the US Library of Congress, showing early bipartisan commitment to comprehensive health system reform.

November 4, 2008: Barack Obama was elected president—and inaugurated on January 20, 2009—with a public commitment to achieve universal health care in his first term.

November 12, 2008: Senate Finance Chairman Max Baucus released his health reform white paper.

February–March 2009: Republican and conservative activists found their footing with the emergence of the Tea Party movement against the Democratic-Obama agenda, including health reform.

April 28, 2009: Republican senator Arlen Specter (PA) announced he would switch to Democrat. Combined with the win of Al Franken in a tight Minnesota recount, Senate Democrats reached the 60-vote threshold by early July, enabling them to pass regular legislation with no Republican support; they maintained the 60-vote margin for 7 crucial months.

September 9, 2009: President Obama addressed a Joint Session of Congress to promote health reform and committed to a $900 billion, 10-year ceiling on the legislation's cost; Representative Joe Wilson (R-SC) shouted "You lie" when the president stated that undocumented immigrants would not receive benefits under his plan.[16]

November 7, 2009: The US House of Representatives approved the Affordable Health Care for America Act (AHCA) by a 220–215 vote.

December 24, 2009: The US Senate approved the Patient Protection and Affordable Care Act (PPACA) by a 60–39 vote.

January 19, 2010: Republican Scott Brown won the US Senate seat to replace the late Senator Edward Kennedy (D-MA), denying Senate Democrats their 60th vote for final passage; within weeks House Speaker Nancy Pelosi began a daunting push for clean passage of the Senate-passed PPACA by the House of Representatives because, absent 60 votes, a House-revised bill could not pass the Senate.

March 23, 2010: President Barack Obama signed the PPACA into law, followed one week later, on March 30, with his signing of the Health Care and Education Reconciliation Act (HCERA), which made changes to PPACA desired by the House and amenable to budget reconciliation rules that allowed expedited Senate approval with only 51 votes to close debate; PPACA and HCERA together became referred to as the Affordable Care Act, or the ACA.

Why Did Bi-Partisan Health Reform Not Happen?

The ACA's process to passage included 2 significant time periods. In the first, ending in the summer of 2009, health reform drew widespread support from across the political and stakeholder spectrums. In the second, intense and bitter partisan conflict prevailed through final passage—and beyond.

Early on, led by Iowa's Republican senator Charles Grassley, some influential Republican senators, including Orrin Hatch (R-UT) and Olympia Snowe (R-ME), openly embraced working with Democrats on reform, though interest among Republican House members was negligible. Although many senators expressed interest in using Massachusetts's 2006 reform law as the template, Baucus and Grassley viewed their 2003 bipartisan achievement in passing a law creating an outpatient drug benefit in Medicare as the better model.

At the same time, as early as the presidential transition period, Senate and House Minority Leaders Mitch McConnell (R-KT) and John Boehner (R-OH) began to express public and private determination to oppose all key Democratic priorities, including health reform. In early 2009 Obama's popularity silenced many Republican voices. By February and March 2009 conservative and Republican activists began finding their voices through the newly established Tea Party movement as a popular base against Obama's and Democratic Congressional plans.

While the Tea Party had some chilling effect on moderate congressional Democrats, its major impact was on Republicans, who were guaranteed conservative opposition at their next reelection if they supported the Democrats' agenda, especially on health reform. By June 2009 Republican support began to evaporate, especially as Democratic committee chairs released drafts of their health reform bills. Sides were taken.

Why Was a So-Called Public Option Not Included?

Many progressive, left-leaning Democrats wanted to include a Medicare fee-for-service health insurance option in all 51 of the newly created health insurance exchanges to compete with private insurers. Many who preferred a Canadian-style, single-payer health insurance system as their first priority compromised from that position, certain they could win the "public option" and hoping it would evolve into a pathway to single-payer.

Support for the public option was strong in the House, which included a version in their final bill. In his first legislative draft for Senate consideration, released in November 2009, merging versions of the health reform legislation approved by the Senate Finance and by the Senate Health, Education, Labor, and Pensions Committees, Senate Majority Leader Harry Reid (D-NV) included a public option. His message to pro–public option activists was that they needed to ensure unified Democratic support—60 votes—or else see the provision removed in the final draft.

Senator Ben Nelson (D-NB), a staunch ally of the insurance industry, said no. Senator Joseph Lieberman, who had switched parties from Democrat to Independent and represented Connecticut—a major insurance state—also could not be convinced. By early December 2009 Leader Reid had no choice if he wanted his legislation to win 60 votes; he deleted the public option from the final draft. In its place the ACA included an ultimately unsuccessful program to establish multistate plans administered through the federal Office of Personnel Management. Even with 60 Democratic Senate votes, the public option was too controversial among Democrats to win adoption in 2009.

How Did Key Stakeholders Line Up in the Legislative Process?

In the ACA process every stakeholder has a story. The macro story involved the White House's and Senate Democrats' desire to win support from certain important stakeholders who had opposed or sat out the 1993–1994 Clinton health reform process. Although the insurance industry initially participated in reform discussions, by later 2009 and 2010 the health insurance industry, along with key business organizations such as the US Chamber of Commerce, vigorously opposed the Democrats' legislation. In support were the American Medical Association (AMA) and other physician groups, major US hospital organizations such as the American Hospital Association, the pharmaceutical industry, much of organized labor, and organized patient and consumer voices.

The major switch for the Democrats involved the pharmaceutical sector, whose leadership wanted a different outcome from that of 1994, when their industry was key in defeating the Clinton plan. Many criticized a June 2009 deal involving the drug industry, the Obama administration, and Baucus. In that agreement the industry promised public support for the legislation plus $80 billion in 10-year financial concessions to help finance the law in exchange for commitments to not include matters opposed by the industry, especially price negotiations and reimportation of drugs from Canada. In truth, those items never would have survived the ACA legislative process, while overt drug industry opposition likely would have resulted in the legislation's defeat.

Hospital and physician organizations also had been neutral or hostile in the Clinton era. This time key hospital associations agreed to support the legislation and to accept substantial 10-year financial concessions ($155 billion) to help finance it, believing that long-term gains would far exceed their losses. The AMA also supported the legislation and was not required to offer financial concessions; although AMA leaders obtained neither promised relief from major cuts in Medicare physician reimbursement imposed by prior laws nor malpractice reform, they did gain additional paying patients and continued to support the bill.

While insurance industry leaders objected to many elements of the ACA's health insurance reforms, they had deal-breaking objections to Democrats claiming $120 billion in payment reductions from Medicare Advantage (Part C), an important and growing line of business for private insurers. Beginning in the summer and early fall of 2009, insurers became full public opponents and began funneling a reported $86.2 million in funding to the US Chamber of Commerce to pay for anti-ACA advertising that accused Democrats of harming small businesses.

What Animated Such Intense Republican Hostility to the ACA?

Republicans had ample ideological grounds on which to oppose the Democrats' legislation. They saw the ACA as the heavy hand of the federal government inserting itself into the process and product of state insurance markets and regulation. In so doing, the ACA weakened states in the federal-state relationship called "federalism," an important value for many Republicans. Also, many Republicans and conservatives believe that the primary cause of the explosive growth of US medical care costs since the 1965 creation of Medicare and Medicaid was excessive government spending and overregulation; undeniably, the ACA spends more public money and increases health-sector regulation. Republicans also asserted—and Democrats denied—that the law restricts patient choice of providers, health plans, and more. In short, the ACA was too much big government.

Other conservative charges against the law were patently false. The ACA did not create "death panels" of government bureaucrats to make life-or-death medical decisions for Medicare patients. The ACA did not increase the federal deficit; in fact, the ACA reduced it.[17] The ACA did not destroy the Medicare Advantage program. The ACA does not permit the use of federal funds to pay for abortion. The ACA does not permit undocumented immigrants to obtain publicly subsidized insurance.

Both parties agreed that the ACA creates and raises taxes, a core Republican concern: on high-income wage earners; on drug, insurance, and medical device companies; on clients of tanning salons; and more. Slightly less than half of the 10-year cost of the ACA is financed through tax-related sections contained in Title IX of the law.[18]

Final passage of the ACA in the US House and Senate did not attract a single Republican vote in 2009 and 2010. Of note, 2 other costly health-reform bills have become law in this century, the 2003 Medicare Modernization Act (MMA) and the 2015 Medicare Access and CHIP Reauthorization Act (MACRA). Both were financed primarily by increasing the federal debt, not with taxes. Both passed with overwhelming Republican support.

Why Did the Law Lack Effective Controls on Spending?

Federal government price controls were politically unachievable in the US Senate or House in 2009 and 2010. So a search began to identify politically salable delivery-system reforms, including initiatives that might lower costs while improving quality and efficiency (though the US CBO estimated little or no savings from them). Most of these are contained in ACA Title III. Both Democrats and Republicans have supported these reforms. Currently, no one advocates moving back to fee-for-service, and no one has advanced an alternative idea—apart from single-payer—moving forward.

Following are some of the key initiatives in the ACA:

- Creation of the Center for Medicare and Medicaid Innovation (CMMI) to house reforms.
- Development of new accountable care organizations (ACOs) in Medicare Parts A and B to move toward value-based provider payments.
- Establishing a Bundled Care program to pay some Medicare providers a single fee for an episode of care's total cost.
- Penalizing acute-care hospitals with high rates of preventable readmissions and hospital-acquired conditions or injuries.
- Implementing systems for Health Information Technology (HIT) in all hospital and physician practices (included in the earlier 2009 American Recovery and Reinvestment Act or "Stimulus Act" and further expanded by the ACA).
- Expanding and strengthening Patient Centered Medical Homes to improve primary care.

Key Elements of the Patient Protection and Affordable Care Act of 2010

The ACA's 952 pages contain 10 titles and more than 450 distinct sections, many of which amend multiple sections of other laws. Of the ACA's 10 titles, 4 are most significant: Title I regulates and expands access to private health insurance; Title II expands Medicaid coverage for low-income persons and families; Title III reforms Medicare and implements the law's medical delivery-system innovations, as noted above; and Title IX creates and raises taxes to pay for about half the law's 10-year costs.

Title I

Title I addresses the ACA's primary goal—to expand access to affordable and high-quality health insurance and care. (Title II shares this goal by expanding Medicaid.) Key Title I elements are fourfold: (1) to reform the practices of private—mostly individual—health insurance, (2) to establish a mandate on individual Americans to purchase or have health insurance or to pay an annual tax penalty, (3) to create a new system of public subsidies to make insurance more affordable for many of those whose only option is the individual market, and (4) to develop state-based or federal health insurance exchanges (or marketplaces) to provide consumers with an easier way to purchase coverage.

Title I establishes new legal protections for all American health insurance consumers, especially those whose only option is individual coverage. It outlaws the practice of "medical underwriting" by prohibiting insurers from determining coverage eligibility or premiums based on an applicant's health status, thereby protecting individuals with preexisting conditions. Title I requires insurers in the individual and small-group markets to only consider age (maximum 3:1 ratio), tobacco use (maximum 1.5-to-1 ratio), geographic location, family composition, and plan characteristics in setting premiums.[19] Premiums based on gender, occupation, or other individual characteristics are prohibited.

The ACA requires insurers to consider claims from all their enrollees in a state as one risk pool (or as separate pools for individuals and small groups) to determine rates. In contrast with pre-ACA, the law rewards insurers for accepting applicants with preexisting conditions. This includes a risk-adjustment tool that requires insurers in the individual and small-group markets that draw less-costly enrollees to contribute to excess costs of insurers drawing costlier-than-average enrollees. To ensure that healthier and younger persons participate (a goal that helpfully broadens the risk pool), the ACA included an individual mandate, imposing a tax on uninsured individuals deemed financially able to purchase coverage. The ACA also includes an employer responsibility provision that imposes a company-wide penalty on larger employers who do not offer all their full-time employees at least minimum coverage if one or more employees receive ACA premium tax credits.

Title I also provides federal subsidies for people who cannot afford the cost of health insurance and who do not qualify for Medicaid. It offers advance premium tax credits for citizens and lawful aliens with incomes between 100% and 400% of the federal poverty level (FPL) to purchase coverage through new insurance exchanges, designed as one-stop markets for individual insurance purchase and operated by states unless they decline to do so; the federal government operates exchanges for states choosing not to run their own. Tax credits decline as household income increases. SHOP exchanges were created for small businesses to purchase insurance. Title I also requires that individual and small-group insurance cover 10 essential health benefits, including services often excluded before 2014, such as maternity, behavioral health, and prescription drug benefits.

Title I includes other reforms as well. It mandates coverage without cost sharing or co-pays for almost all plans (not just those on the exchanges) for clinical preventive services such as cancer screening and vaccines, establishes appeals of adverse health-plan decisions, requires insurers to spend at least 80% to 85% of premium revenues on medical claims rather than administrative costs (medical loss ratios), and mandates that insurers provide uniform summaries of benefits and coverage in easily comparable formats. It prohibits discrimination on the basis of race, color, national origin, sex, age, or disability in health programs by entities or activities funded or administered by HHS and insurers participating in exchanges.

While some Title I reforms were implemented in 2010 and 2011, major changes—including key insurance market reforms, coverage and cost-sharing subsidies, individual mandate enforcement, and exchanges—took effect on January 1, 2014.

Title II

Title II includes a mandatory expansion of Medicaid programs in all 50 states (and the District of Columbia) to any citizen needing health insurance with a household income below 138% of the federal poverty line. This has become the largest coverage expansion in the law. It also became the biggest surprise in ACA implementation, as discussed later in this volume, when the US Supreme Court ruled in June 2012 that Medicaid expansion must be optional, not mandatory, for states, even though states pay no more than 10% of the cost of the ACA expansion group.[20]

Beyond eligibility expansion, Title II contains administrative reforms intended to make Medicaid a more national program with consistent eligibility and enrollment standards. Some states historically used their administrative authority to make it as difficult as possible for Medicaid applicants to get in or stay in the program. The ACA established greater uniformity to make it easier for eligible applicants to enroll and to stay enrolled in the program.

Title III

Title III deals with Medicare and the ACA's broader quality- and system-transformation agenda, discussed above. It enhances low-income subsidies for many Medicare beneficiaries and gradually eliminates an important gap that had existed in prescription coverage through the Part D drug program. Before the ACA, Part D covered drug costs up to a certain level and then ceased paying until catastrophic expenditure levels were reached, resulting in a so-called coverage donut hole. Title III also mandates payment cuts to hospitals and Medicare Advantage insurers to drive productivity improvements and to finance about half of the 10-year cost of the law.

As noted above, Title III uses a variety of approaches to incentivize health system transformation. The heart of these reforms is the new Center for Medicare and Medicaid Innovation (CMMI), created to implement new national programs to accelerate the transformation from FFS payment to paying-for-value. Most prominently, this title established an ACO program and a bundled-payments initiative as alternatives to FFS in Medicare Parts A and B.

Title IV

Title IV focuses on public and population health, reflecting the belief that health promotion and disease prevention can improve quality of life and reduce costs. Of most significance, it created a Prevention and Public Health Fund with a guaranteed funding commitment of $15 billion between 2010 and 2019, which has since become a frequent target for cuts and elimination by Republicans. It expands Medicare coverage without cost sharing for clinical preventive services such as screenings for breast and colorectal cancer, cardiovascular disease, and diabetes. Title IV also requires large employers to provide nursing mothers with break time and privacy, mandates nutritional/calorie menu labeling for chain restaurants and vending machines, and establishes school-based health center programs.

Title V

Title V addresses health care workforce challenges and included a number of student loan, loan repayment, and training programs to help develop an expanded health care workforce—especially for primary care—to treat the newly insured under the ACA.[21] The Title's most prominent initiative, establishing a National Healthcare Workforce Commission, was never implemented because of Republican opposition to appropriating funds for its operation.

Title VI

Title VI authorizes new programs to combat health care fraud and to increase health-sector transparency. It also enacts the Physician Payments Sunshine Act, which requires drug, medical device, medical supply, and biologics manufacturers to report transfers of value (i.e., gifts, honoraria) to physicians and others. The reports are made available to the public on a federal website called Open Payments.[22]

Title VI also mandates background checks plus dementia and patient-abuse prevention training for nursing home employees as well as enacts the Elder Justice Act to address elder abuse, neglect, and exploitation. Finally, it establishes the Patient-Centered Outcomes Research Institute (PCORI) to study clinical cost effectiveness.

Title VII

Title VII directs the US Food and Drug Administration to establish a regulatory pathway to permit biosimilar biopharmaceutical drugs (or follow-on biologics) into the US pharmaceutical market to instill competition for expensive biopharmaceutical products. Biosimilar products began appearing in the US market in 2015.

Title VIII

Title VIII created a voluntary, national, long-term-care insurance program called the CLASS Act (Community Living Assistance Services and Supports) to provide cash support for individuals who are permanently or temporarily disabled, including elderly and nonelderly disabled persons needing such support—an important policy change for American society. The Title included an actuarial soundness requirement.

On January 1, 2013, President Obama, along with Senate and House leaders, agreed to repeal the CLASS Act, concluding it could not be financially self-sustaining. This is the only title of the ACA that has been repealed in toto.

Title IX

Title IX, as noted, creates new taxes and mandatory payments that, together with Title III's Medicare payment cuts, were designed to fully finance the ACA and not increase the federal deficit. New taxes were imposed on higher-income households (over $200,000 on individuals and $250,000 on families), health insurers, medical device manufacturers, tanning salons, branded pharmaceuticals, and high-cost employer-sponsored plans. At the time of the ACA's final 2010 passage, the CBO projected that the law would decrease the federal debt by $124 billion between 2010 and 2019.[23]

Title X

Title X is the so-called manager's amendment (the bill manager in this case was Senate Majority Leader Harry Reid [D-NV]). It was added in December 2009 to incorporate various changes, corrections, and compromises made among 60 Democratic senators, each of whose vote was indispensable for final passage in the Senate. It makes numerous changes to the other 9 titles and also creates a pregnant and parenting teens program, authorizes medical malpractice demonstration projects, provides medical malpractice coverage for free clinics, funds community health centers and the National Health Services Corps, and incorporates extensive amendments to the Indian Health Services Act.[24]

The Health Care and Education Reconciliation Act (HCERA), enacted one week after the PPACA's first 10 titles, includes compromises agreed to between House and Senate Democratic majorities in March 2010 to reach the legislative finish line. Among many provisions, it increases Title I's premium tax credits, cost-sharing reduction payments, and the employer mandate penalty. It further cuts Title III's Medicare Advantage payments to insurers and formally authorizes closing the Medicare drug program's donut hole coverage gap discussed above. It imposes (and delays) a tax on high-cost employer (Cadillac tax) health plans as well as several other new taxes.

What the ACA Leaves Undone

The ACA is noteworthy for what is does and for what it does not do.

The ACA leaves in place a fragmented, exasperating health system balkanized by public and private financing and delivery. As a key political strategy to get the law passed, President Obama and congressional Democrats intentionally pursued minimally invasive reform to avoid interfering with system parts considered functional. A vital lesson learned from the 1993–1994 Clinton health reform calamity was to avoid fixing things the public did not perceive as broken.

The ACA does not create any new public health insurance program, relying instead on expanding Medicaid and creating tax credits for income-eligible individuals to purchase private insurance. Nor does the law create any public option on the exchanges as an alternative to private health insurance. The ACA avoids federal price regulation in favor of experimental delivery-system reform approaches. It neither gives the federal government authority to regulate or negotiate drug prices nor does it authorize drug reimportation. Direct intervention in provider payments is limited to Medicare, where the federal government has long set payments and payment rules.

Although the ACA expanded federal authority over health insurance, it favors state over federal regulation, reflecting the policy preferences of moderate Democratic senators who had major influence in drafting the act.[25] The ACA leaves state professional licensure and scope-of-practice laws untouched, an area suited to address cost reductions.[26]

Other problems were also avoided or left unaddressed. Premium tax credits, available to legal aliens, were deemed unavailable to as many as 12 million undocumented immigrants. Beyond establishing demonstration projects, the law neglected medical liability reform. Though the ACA enacted a large excise tax on high-premium employer-sponsored insurance (not yet implemented), it left in place generous employer tax subsidies, a major driver of health care inflation. Except for the short-lived CLASS Act (Title VIII), the ACA ignored long-term care beyond extending Medicaid community care options. The ACA retained federal funding prohibitions on abortion coverage (except in cases of rape, incest, or physical threat to the mother's life), extending them to premium tax credits, though not banning abortion coverage in individual markets.

Other challenges were only partially addressed. While the ACA increased access to health insurance for millions of uninsured Americans, the tax credits phase out quickly at higher middle incomes, and cost-sharing assistance phases out even sooner and was blocked from further implementation in 2017 by the Trump administration. Overall consumer cost sharing is capped in all health plans, but too many Americans are still vulnerable to sizable deductibles and coinsurance.

In sum, the law made major reforms to health care delivery and finance, addressing access, cost, and quality. Its reach is far greater than commonly understood. Yet although the ACA revolutionized many parts of the US health care system, it did not revolutionize the system itself. Many significant core problems that motivated Congress to enact the Affordable Care Act remain unaddressed. Much more waits to be done.

CHAPTER 2

POLICY DESIGN
Tensions and Tradeoffs

Peter R. Orszag and Rahul Rekhi

Introduction

In February 2009, after having enacted stimulus legislation to attenuate the recession associated with the Great Financial Crisis, then newly elected President Barack Obama laid out a vision for "transforming and modernizing America's health care system" as part of his inaugural budget.[1] That document set aside a reserve fund of over $630 billion for health care reform. It also articulated 8 governing principles for the effort: (1) "protect families' financial health," (2) "make health coverage affordable," (3) "aim for universality [of coverage]," (4) "provide portability of coverage," (5) "guarantee choice," (6) "invest in prevention and wellness," (7) "improve patient safety and quality care," and (8) "maintain long-term fiscal sustainability." Ultimately enshrined into law a year later in the president's signature domestic policy accomplishment, these principles speak to the scope and ambition of the legislation we now know as the Affordable Care Act (ACA).

The principles also reflect complex design tensions and tradeoffs. Some were constraints long familiar to students of economics or pub-

Peter R. Orszag, PhD, is CEO of Financial Advisory at Lazard Freres & Co. LLC and served as the director of the Office of Management and Budget (2009–2010) and director of the Congressional Budget Office (2007–2008).

Rahul Rekhi, MSc, is vice president in Financial Advisory at Lazard Freres & Co. LLC and previously was a staff economist on the Council of Economic Advisers (2015–2017).

lic policy: the presence of fiscal limitations (principle 8), for instance, on the scope of coverage expansion (principle 3), spending on prevention (principle 6), and reducing cost burdens on families (principle 1). Other tradeoffs were fundamentally philosophical or even political: whether to administer coverage expansion through a public insurance entity or through private insurers and, in either case, whether to preserve existing coverage options. Moreover, the desire to enact sweeping, progressive reforms that could stand the test of time was bound by the practical limitations of knowledge at drafting, such as limited public data on commercial health insurance spending and the inherent unpredictability of Supreme Court review. The uncertainty inherent in comprehensive reform at the federal level was substantial: How would employers respond to new incentives? How would providers respond? Opponents' assertions—that employers would drop their plans wholesale and waiting lines for doctors would rise substantially—received significant media attention in part because of this uncertainty. Put simply, the playbook for (1) the first nationwide coverage expansion for nonelderly adults since the creation of Medicaid in 1965 and (2) contemplating major changes to the health care delivery system was, out of necessity, long on concepts and short on the tried and tested.

Overlying these tensions and tradeoffs was the worst financial crisis since the Great Depression. According to the National Bureau of Economic Research, the Great Recession reached its trough in June 2009; economic conditions invariably left their mark on the ACA's development. The historic federal spending associated with recovery measures, like the $800 billion "stimulus" legislation in 2009, as well as the shortfall in tax revenues triggered by the economic slowdown tightened existing fiscal constraints on the bill. Economic conditions also militated in favor of legislation that would minimize disruptions to care and coverage, including to employer-sponsored insurance. Conventional wisdom suggested that major reform had to be undertaken early in President Obama's term or else it would not happen at all. The crisis exacerbated this timing constraint while also limiting the bandwidth of policymakers and President Obama, creating a political window perceived to be closing in its wake.

Overall—and especially in the face of these challenges and tradeoffs—the ACA should be viewed as the most successful social policy legislation since the Great Society, a legacy chronicled extensively throughout this volume and elsewhere. It contained several key decisions, including to retain employer-sponsored insurance, to expand coverage through a mix of public and private insurance mechanisms, and to couple coverage expansion with deficit reduction measures and delivery-system reforms. These choices, even in hindsight, were the right ones. The passage of time has suggested the ACA was inadequate in some dimensions. For instance, it is probably correct that the subsidies to consumers for buying insurance should have been larger and provided for higher incomes—for instance, to 500% of the federal poverty level (FPL). But in other dimensions the ACA has far outperformed even the best hopes. For example, the ACA outperformed predictions in both restraining health costs and in not causing the collapse of Medicare Advantage.

Nevertheless, the decade since the ACA's passage affords a privileged opportunity to reexamine its tradeoffs through the lens of hindsight. We do so here with the goal of shedding light on the lessons that can be drawn from the ACA's design choices and associated outcomes and how these lessons might guide health policy and reform legislation going forward. We conduct this evaluation through a close look at considerations around the ACA's coverage provisions, including the expansion of Medicaid eligibility as well as the creation of the health care exchanges. This is followed by an assessment of its reforms to the health care delivery system, including efforts to address rising health costs, such as the creation of the Innovation Center under the Centers for Medicare and Medicaid (CMS). We conclude by placing these design choices in the context of contemporary health policy and discussing future directions and implications for policymakers.

Coverage Reform

Background

Prior to enactment of the ACA, approximately 40 million nonelderly Americans—roughly 15% of the population, excluding undocumented immigrants—lacked health insurance coverage.[2] This level of uninsurance had no parallel in any other developed democracy. Underlying this figure was significant heterogeneity in the uninsured population across employment characteristics, household income, geography, and other considerations (see Chapter 1). In most cases these individuals' primary potential source for coverage was the nongroup market—a market beset by a range of access barriers in most states.[3] With average family premiums in group insurance of nearly $13,000 in 2008—or about ⅓ of the FPL for a family of 4—it is as clear now as it was then that for a substantial number of people, health insurance was simply unaffordable absent significant public subsidies.

Consistent with the first 3 principles for health reform in the president's budget—financial risk protection, affordability, and universal coverage—closing the coverage gaps for these diverse groups was an essential goal of the ACA. Also imperative was that the reform not imperil the coverage of those already insured, including through employer-sponsored insurance (ESI). The considerations motivating this "do no harm" approach to coverage expansion were manifold. First, surveys in 2008 and 2009 indicated that perhaps 70% to 80% of Americans with health insurance saw their coverage as either "good" or "excellent" and that limited public support existed for proposals that would, for example, eliminate ESI outright.[4] Second, to the extent that the ACA's coverage expansion "crowded out" existing private insurance, it would increase public expenditures without resulting in a net increase in covered Americans. Shifting enrollees from private to public insurance is challenging at any time, and it was especially challenging when Republicans were already criticizing the administration for substantially increasing government spending through the stimulus legislation. The deficit also rose at the time because of the economic contraction and its concomitant rise in outlays (e.g., via Medicaid and unemployment benefits) and shortfall in tax revenues, reaching nearly 10% of GDP in 2009—the highest level in the post–World War II era. Third, the potential labor-market adjustment costs for proposals that eliminated the health insurance industry, which Bureau of Labor Statistics data suggested employed as many as a million or more US workers,[5] were particularly concerning at a time when the civilian unemployment rate was nearly 10%. Finally, while many economists believe that ESI is inefficient, the additional dislocations caused by shifting from one system to another would be far reaching and protracted—and could extend beyond the administrative strains of transitioning 150 million beneficiaries. It is unclear, for example, how wages would respond to eliminating ESI. Although the evidence is strong that firms would shift spending on health benefits into wages in the aggregate, this shift could vary across workers.[6] At its core, though, the judgment to maintain ESI was political: the legislation would not pass without retaining it. Most of these constraints persist to this day, though some, such as the dire economic conditions, have abated, while others, such as the government deficit and debt levels, have not.

Pathways to Coverage Expansion

The central tenet of preserving coverage for those who already had it ruled out single-payer proposals that would eliminate private insurance. Broadly speaking, given the nature and fragmentation of the nonelderly uninsured population, this left 3 main pathways to expanding coverage. The first was to extend coverage through a public health insurance program. The second was to target reforms to the private individual—or nongroup—insurance market by instituting consumer protections, such as the popular ban on coverage denials for preexisting conditions, and addressing affordability challenges with public subsidies for individuals and families purchasing coverage. The third was a hybrid approach combining elements of the first 2. This was the approach adopted in 2006 by the Massachusetts health reform effort that coupled an expansion of Medicaid eligibility with regulatory changes and new subsidies for the nongroup market. In Massachusetts, Medicaid expansion and the nongroup market reforms each accounted for about an equal share of the coverage gains.[7]

Each of the first 2 pathways brought with it a distinct set of tradeoffs that look today much as they did in 2009: neither was a panacea. As a general rule, the public coverage approach, especially one founded on Medicaid, offered unique fiscal, design, and administrative advantages. For an equivalent benefit level—for example, coverage of 100% of health care costs, or 100% actuarial value—Medicaid coverage could be offered at lower per-enrollee costs. These lower federal costs primarily reflect lower provider reimbursement rates compared to commercial insurance. Relative to provider prices in commercial insurance for outpatient professional services, prices in Medicare are generally more than 30% lower, and in Medicaid prices are perhaps more than 50% or 60% lower on average (per Kaiser Family Foundation data).[8] Similar price dispersion is seen in inpatient care and other health services. Moreover, Medicaid's program design—unlike that of commercial insurance and Medicare—was and continues to be tailored to the health and care needs of the lower-income beneficiaries who dominated the then-uninsured. One example is retroactive coverage, in which Medicaid allows beneficiaries to receive coverage for medical expenses incurred up to 3 months prior to applying for enrollment—an important safeguard for financially vulnerable enrollees and one that materially alleviates enrollment burdens. Another example lay in opportunities for cross-program enrollment between Medicaid and other forms of support for low-income families—such as the Supplemental Nutrition Assistance Program (SNAP), the food stamps program—as a means of increasing take-up and simplifying administration. As of 2013 the Medicaid- and SNAP-eligible populations exhibited considerable overlap, and beneficiaries in both programs often had children covered by CHIP.[9] Furthermore, in most states Medicaid featured enhanced coverage of medical (e.g., behavioral health) and nonmedical (e.g., nonemergency transport) services that remain critical for low-income enrollees, and subsequent research has corroborated the utility of such programmatic features for this population.[10] For many of these reasons, a large number of states had already voluntarily expanded Medicaid eligibility in some form as of 2009, precedents that federal legislation could build upon and harmonize across states.

Conversely, an approach centered on reforms to the individual market preserved choice for those with pre-ACA nongroup coverage by maintaining and improving this market. It also sidestepped potential stigma associated at the time with extending Medicaid coverage; that program was then mostly focused on categorical coverage for individuals with disabilities, low-income retirees, and pregnant women, among others. Research prior to the start of Medicaid expansion in 2014 suggested that stigma may have played an important role in limiting Medicaid take-up among the Medicaid eligible.[11] Furthermore, it bypassed the "patchwork" nature of Medicaid coverage with benefits, eligibility, and program structure varying considerably across states. Above all, expansion via nongroup coverage mitigated any provider-access concerns associated with lower levels of provider reimbursement in public programs and likewise mitigated any concerns about disruption to existing beneficiaries in those programs. This reimbursement difference posed a political hurdle as well. The prospect of replacing the commercial rates paid to providers by existing nongroup insurance plans with lower rates in public insurance (Medicaid or Medicare) put providers' support for coverage expansion at risk.[12]

The hybrid approach embodied in the ACA sought to capitalize on the best of both the public and private pathways—though at the cost of complexity in administration and eligibility—and in hindsight, its diversified structure played a prudential role. The landmark June 2012 Supreme Court decision in *National Federation of Independent Business v. Sebelius* vividly illustrated the prudential point: it declared unconstitutional the requirement that states implement expanded Medicaid eligibility in order to maintain existing federal funding for Medicaid.[13] In effect, this unexpected ruling rendered Medicaid expansion optional for states. The aftermath is one we continue to deal with today: as of spring 2020, 14 states have yet to adopt expanded eligibility for their enrollees, leaving approximately 7 million individuals without Medicaid coverage.[14] In nonexpansion states the exchanges have crucially extended coverage to those in the so-called coverage gap whose incomes fall below the range eligible for exchange premium and cost-sharing subsidies but above state Medicaid eligibility thresholds.[15] Even more strikingly, had the ACA's individual-market coverage expansion instead been channeled entirely through Medicaid, perhaps 4 million additional Americans in nonexpansion states would today be uninsured.[16] There is some cause for optimism that over time the 14 nonexpansion states will expand Medicaid. Public approval for the ACA continues climbing, state referenda forcing state governments to expand Medicaid are being passed even in Republican-dominated states, and the numerous benefits of expansion continue to be borne out. Yet in retrospect the unforeseen Supreme Court judgment afforded an opportunity to design a policy trigger in the ACA that would have extended coverage through other federal programs in states declining Medicaid expansion. Because the possibility of such an option for states was seen as almost nonexistent in early 2010, the CBO would have likely "scored" this failsafe as very low or zero cost.

In turn, Medicaid in expansion states not only came with the budgetary and other advantages discussed previously but also helped ease pressures on exchange coverage. Operationally, these pressures include the complications in launching Healthcare.gov, which have been documented extensively elsewhere.[17] From a policy standpoint, too, the exchanges have long been buffeted by a series of efforts by some lawmakers to annul the ACA, including the zeroing of the individual mandate in the Tax Cuts and Jobs Act, myriad actions by the Trump administration to impair functioning of the exchanges (such as cutting enrollment advertising and outreach budgets), the defunding of risk-corridor payments in 2015 and 2016 that were intended to stabilize premiums,[18] and the Trump administration's decision to terminate cost-sharing subsidy payments for low-income enrollees. Their cumulative effect has been to suppress enrollment and raise premiums in exchange plans.[19] Some of these annulment efforts might have been deterred with technical corrections to the ACA, such as rendering risk corridors permanent (as they are in Medicare Part D) and expressly appropriating federal funds for cost-sharing reduction subsidies. Absent such corrections, Medicaid in expansion states served as a partial salve by shielding lower-income beneficiaries from these disruptions and reducing exchange premiums by 7% on average.[20]

A principal tradeoff of bifurcating coverage expansion between Medicaid and the exchanges is the burden on enrollees churning between the programs for those with income fluctuating around the exchange subsidy eligibility threshold (138% of the FPL). Again, technical corrections to the law across Medicaid and the exchanges could have stemmed the administrative aspects of this burden. One example is that the ACA could have aligned income-eligibility standards between Medicaid and the exchanges by, for instance, equalizing treatment of married couples filing separate tax returns. However, the concern that splitting coverage expansions between Medicaid and the exchanges would materially increase churn issues relative to the pre-ACA status quo does not seem to have become the problem that some feared.[21]

Additional Options for Reform

In light of the 15 million Americans who continue to lack insurance coverage and are ineligible for Medicaid or CHIP, it is helpful to reconsider 2 major dimensions along which the coverage provisions of the ACA entailed policy tradeoffs.[22] The first is with respect to increasing the subsidization of the nongroup exchanges to make coverage more affordable, either at the individual level through more generous tax credits or at the plan level through reinsurance. There is growing evidence that affordability remains a significant barrier to taking up exchange coverage, especially for consumers in households with incomes above 250% of the FPL. Roughly 15% of the uninsured population today is ineligible for premium tax credits on the exchanges, and another 25% is eligible for only partial subsidies.[23] States that provide additional subsidies to enrollees in the form of premium assistance or cost sharing have achieved higher rates of coverage.[24] Massachusetts data show that every $40 reduction in net premiums increases the enrollment rate by 20 to 24 percentage points;[25] so, too, have states that implemented permanent reinsurance programs. Evidence from Avalere suggests that these programs reduce premiums by 20% on average.[26]

The conventional binding constraint on larger subsidies is space in the federal budget for the associated cost. This "fiscal space" may have widened substantially since the ACA's drafting, notwithstanding growing deficits from the 2017 Republican tax cut. There are 2 main reasons why higher subsidies are possible: the larger-than-expected slowdown in health care spending following the implementation of the ACA's cost-reduction reforms (discussed below) and falling interest rates on federal debt. One overall measure, developed by economists Alan Auerbach and William Gale, is the fiscal gap, which compares the present value of projected federal tax revenues with that of expenditures. According to their most recent estimates, the fiscal gap since 2010 has declined by nearly 30%.[27] In parallel, the affordability challenge for many low- and middle-income families in purchasing insurance has become starker given the emergence of plans with lower co-pays and co-insurance and higher deductibles (Figure 2.1). Though the subsidy design of the ACA ensures that households earning from 138% to 400% of the FPL have premium costs capped as a share of income, the shift toward larger deductibles means that total out-of-pocket costs can be as high as double the annual premium before first-dollar coverage kicks in.

Another policy choice worth revisiting in hindsight in order to make coverage more affordable and expand choice is the addition of a

Figure 2.1 Growth of Deductibles, Copays, and Total Cost-Sharing in Commercial Insurance, 2006–2016

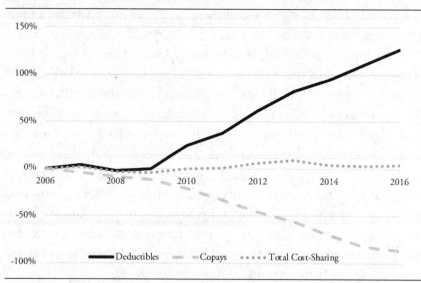

Source: Gary Claxton et al., "Increases in Cost-Sharing Payments Continue to Outpace Wage Growth," Peterson-Kaiser Health System Tracker, June 15, 2018, https://www.healthsystemtracker.org/brief/increases-in-cost-sharing-payments-have-far-outpaced-wage-growth/.

public option as an alternative to private plans, particularly in view of the roughly 20% of exchange enrollees who are currently in counties with only one participating insurer.[28] A public option could provide a modest reduction to overall premiums, particularly in regions where exchange offerings are less competitive—such as due to either a market-dominant insurance carrier, a market-dominant provider, or both. (It could also serve as a backstop for workers unsatisfied with ESI, though given that ESI is tax subsidized and predominantly employer funded, retention rates would be expected to remain high.) Holding overall benefit levels constant, the primary affordability advantages of a public option derive from 2 factors: (1) the potential to use lower Medicare payment rates for providers and (2) the potential for enhanced insurer competition on the exchanges. These factors lowering premiums would be muted by other factors, at least in some markets that feature low-cost private insurers. In such markets, low-cost plans pare premiums through care management and narrow provider networks as well as execute provider contracts priced closely to Medicare rates.[29] By contrast, in counties without low-cost carriers, the public option could have greater impact, conditional on securing provider network access at lower reimbursement rates. Interestingly, Washington state's public option proposal, signed into law by Governor Jay Inslee in February 2019, set payment rates for the public plan at 160% of Medicare, a modest discount to average commercial contracted rates today.

Delivery-System Reform

Background

Understandably, public commentary on health reform efforts in 2008 and 2009 underscored the large and persistent gaps in coverage. However, equally core to the ACA's design were reducing the cost and improving the quality of care provided by the delivery system. Some critics at the time argued that the ACA could and should have been enacted with only its coverage expansion provisions. That argument seemed both politically and substantively wrong at the time and still seems so today. Politically, it still seems implausible to us that new legislation would have been enacted with a substantial increase in spending and the budget deficit at a time when, rightly or wrongly, Congress was concerned with the fiscal implications of the stimulus legislation. Substantively, failing to incorporate delivery-system reforms would have been a missed opportunity.

In the 2000s real per-enrollee health expenditures in commercial insurance and Medicare were rising at about 4.5 and 2.0 percentage points, respectively, above the rate of real per-capita GDP growth. This high cost growth and overutilization was ultimately being passed on to American families in the form of higher premiums and cost sharing, lower wages, and worse health outcomes.[30] After all, roughly 80 cents of every dollar of health care costs were and are spent in the delivery system; this figure rises to well over 90 cents on every dollar if retail sales of prescription drugs and medical devices are included.[31] Reforming the delivery system to "bend the cost curve" was necessary for relieving financial burdens on families and promoting coverage affordability. It was also necessary for reducing the fiscal pressure on public health expenditures.[32] In 2009 and 2010 emerging research, drawn chiefly from Medicare claims data via the Dartmouth Atlas Project and other sources, revealed a target for potential savings in the delivery system: significant geographic variation of health care expenditures throughout the country with limited observable relationship to health outcomes.

During the debate over the ACA and in its aftermath, the research was attacked as unreliable; since then, however, subsequent research has underscored substantial variation in costs that cannot be explained by the health status of patients in different areas. In ESI, a significant share of this variation involves price differences; within Medicare, however, almost all of the variation involves utilization. Evidence from movers in Medicare and the military has corroborated that practice variation, not population variation, is a major driver of variation in utilization.[33] This finding suggests that value-based payment models could achieve real savings by incentivizing providers to deliver high-value care.[34] Such research has both reinforced the motivation for targeting delivery-system reform while refining policymakers' understanding of the sources of variation.

Pathways to Delivery-System Reform

The central premise of delivery-system reform in the ACA was to bring down system-wide cost growth by reducing spending variation. The most direct instrument for bringing down variation was to use Medicare payments to incentivize high-value care. This encountered 3 binding constraints. The first was the scarcity of data on evidence-based delivery-system reform programs that could be effective on a national scale in reducing spending variation. At the time of the ACA's enactment, for example, there were only 2 main implementations underway of what we now deem population-based payment models: the Massachusetts Alternative Quality Contract (AQC) and the Medicare Physician Group Practice (PGP) pilot. In addition to other models focused on episode-based payments, both programs were starting to put to action the promise of shifting providers' financial models away from fee-for-service (FFS) payments and toward value to reduce costs and promote health outcomes. Though such models carried great promise for Medicare and have subsequently demonstrated empirical success in reducing costs, at the time of the ACA's drafting they were early instantiations in limited geographies and with comparatively limited available performance data.

The second constraint was the pace at which the delivery system itself could change and the corollary desire to smooth the costs of transition away from FFS. The extent of necessary change and associated transition costs were seen as significant at the time and, if anything, appear larger in hindsight. To succeed with new payment models, clinicians and administrators have frequently needed not only a wholesale cultural reorientation but also a litany of new investments and capabilities, including care-management tools, IT and data analytics, and different mixes of facilities and services (such as home care). For instance, a 2011 report commissioned by the American Hospital Association estimated that 5 hospital accountable care organizations (ACOs) necessitate start-up capital of over $12 million on average toward clinical information systems, care coordination and quality improvement, data analytics, and other investments as well as annual operating expenses of roughly $14 million.[35] Likewise, digitizing health records—in many facets a precursor for software and analytics tools that enable value-based care—would ultimately take a period of several years following the ACA enactment to achieve wide-scale penetration in the delivery system, and as of 2009 fewer than half of US office-based physicians had adopted electronic medical records, a figure that rose to over 75% just 5 years later (per ONC [Office of the National Coordinator for Health Information Technology] data). As with coverage expansion, easing the delivery-system reform transition for providers was seen as especially imperative in the midst of the postcrisis labor-market recovery, with labor costs constituting the majority of hospital operating budgets and the likely incidence of lower utilization on inputs.

The third constraint was Medicare's limited purchasing power. In 2009 Medicare comprised approximately 20% of national health spending,[36] and 70% of that flowed through traditional Medicare. A reasonable expectation in 2009 was that the formulation of value-based payment models in Medicare would spill over into commercial contracting over time, particularly given the outsized role that Medicare fees play in determining private reimbursement rates.[37] However, absent this spillover, the vast majority of provider revenues would continue to be tied to FFS payments, even assuming full conversion of traditional Medicare reimbursements to value, thereby blunting the impact of these payments on low-value care.

The first 2 constraints drove policy design that allowed for near-term progress on key delivery-system reform goals while maintaining flexibility to innovate and tinker with new payment models that would, over time, nudge the delivery system toward value. This was accomplished most prominently through the formation of the Center for Medicare and Medicaid Innovation (CMMI), which could promulgate new value-based payment demonstrations in traditional Medicare; the Hospital Value-Based Purchasing program, which linked Medicare hospital payments to care quality; and the Independent Payment Advisory Board (IPAB), an independent body with the authority to put delivery-system reform proposals into effect in Medicare payments if high spending growth continued. The last decade has underlined the value of this flexibility via the significant and ongoing evolution in the Medicare Shared Savings Program and other ACO programs. Placing this flexibility in the hands of regulators has allowed Medicare's value-based payment programs to evolve to accommodate results on efficacy as well as assessments of burdens on providers. Although this flexibility brought with it the tradeoff that CMMI left subsequent administrations latitude in implementing value-based payment models, this latitude has not slowed model promulgation.[38] As much as 40% of spending in traditional Medicare is now flowing through alternative payment models based on shared savings.[39]

Meanwhile, the third constraint helped spur the creation of the excise tax on high-cost health plans, commonly referred to as the "Cadillac tax." In principle, the Cadillac tax could help drive adoption of value-based models in commercial insurance by gradually limiting the tax subsidy for ESI, providing an additional incentive for employers to curtail health expenditures. Despite its potential utility as a tool for delivery-system reform and its widespread support among economists, in recent years Congress has repeatedly delayed the initiation of the Cadillac tax, and in July 2019 the House of Representatives voted to repeal the provision. Nonetheless, data from the Health Care Payment Learning and Action Network and others demonstrates significant and growing take-up among commercial insurers of alternative payment models. This may testify to the clout that Medicare and, more generally,

Figure 2.2 Real Per-Enrollee Spending Growth by Payer

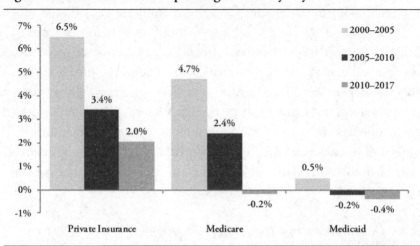

Source: CEA ACA Report, National Health Expenditure Accounts, and authors' calculations.

the federal health policy apparatus have in overcoming private-sector coordination failures and driving provider contracting. This response may also suggest that private insurers and providers are realigning care and coverage models in response to expectations set by federal policymakers regarding the long-term direction of change in the health care system, akin to the role that forward guidance as a monetary policy instrument can play in influencing long-term interest rates.

Dramatic Slowdown in Health Care Cost Growth

History may bear out the combination of many smaller steps—that together pointed to a new direction in payment models—as being a critical force behind delivery-system reform. In the years following the enactment of the ACA and through the present day, health care cost growth has slowed dramatically (Figure 2.2). Whereas from 2000 to 2005 real per-enrollee health expenditures in private insurance and Medicare were growing at nearly 7% and 5% each year respectively, since 2010 these figures have averaged 2% and -0.4%. In fact, prior to its repeal in 2018, not once since the ACA's enactment had the cost-growth threshold that triggers the initiation of IPAB been reached. Scores of studies have attempted to identify the causes of this slowdown—from the business cycle, to specific provisions in the ACA (e.g., provider productivity rate adjustments), to a slowdown in medical technology development. One recent study suggests that as much as ¼ may be attributable to advances in cardiovascular medications.[40] Still, no combination of potential explanatory factors at present can explain the magnitude of the slowdown. Though the jury is still out, there is at least anecdotal reason to believe that the delivery-system reform foundations laid down by the ACA have fundamentally altered the national conversation around health care expenditures among provider and insurer executives and in boardrooms. This "spotlight effect" may be doing more than any individual provision to advance delivery-system reform.

New Developments in the Delivery System and Additional Options for Reform

Since the ACA's enactment, research has continued to reveal new insights on the sources and drivers of spending variation in the delivery system. We now know, for instance, that as much as ¾ of the geographic variation in Medicare spending is driven by postacute care.[41] Accordingly, focusing delivery-system reform provisions in the ACA more directly on postacute spending—such as by reforming payments to skilled nursing facilities (SNFs) in Medicare, as CMS proposed in its 2018 update to the SNF prospective payment system—seems, with the benefit of hindsight, warranted. More broadly, with a delivery system primed for value and mounting evidence backing these models (e.g., with postacute care a key source of savings[42]), the time may be ripe to set mandatory targets for the share of public and private health spending that is tied to value-based payment models. This would require that providers increase the share of their revenues that flow through value-based models in order to comply with the targets, analogous to rising fuel-economy standards for automobile manufacturers. Similar targets could be put in place for linking insurer health care spending to value-based payments. In the case of ESI, this would provide a more targeted alternative to the Cadillac tax in pulling health spending toward value.

Meanwhile, Medicare Advantage (MA) is becoming a remarkably important frontier for commercial insurers that are adopting new models of care delivery and financing, including those focused on

Figure 2.3 Medicare Advantage Penetration (Trustees Report)

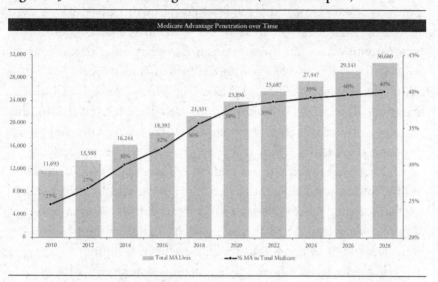

Source: 2019 Medicare Trustees report.

driving savings in postacute care. In fact, in order to finance coverage expansion, a core judgment made in the ACA was that payment rates to MA plans could be reduced to about 101% of Medicare FFS rates without threatening MA coverage. These payment reductions, totaling $150 billion over 10 years, led to projections from the CBO that MA enrollment would fall by 30%. This projection was, to put it mildly, inaccurate. Even with the payment reductions, MA enrollment since 2010 has grown by 50%, to 20 million (Figure 2.3), and private-sector analysts project that by 2024 the majority of Medicare beneficiaries will be enrolled in MA plans.[43] Fueling the growth of MA is its position at the forefront of value-oriented models. As one example, MA plans exhibit postacute care costs that are 16% lower than those of traditional Medicare.[44] MA also features prominently in the recent proliferation of vertically integrated payer-provider models. These models, spurred by the ACA's delivery-system reform provisions, among other factors, are promising chassis for aligning economic incentives, health IT, and patient experience to reduce practice variation.[45]

Another source of variation that has become more salient in recent years is care associated with medical malpractice law—so-called defensive medicine. Historically, research exploiting differences in state malpractice liability caps has concluded that medical malpractice plays a limited role in explaining the level and growth of health care costs as well as their geographic variation.[46] Recent research, nevertheless, turns attention to "customary practice" exemptions in malpractice laws, under which physicians whose treatment choices for a given malady conform to that of local physicians are protected from malpractice litigation. Researchers examining states that have relaxed this locality rule in favor of a rule that ties customary practice to national practice standards demonstrates that this change can close the gap between local and national utilization rates of procedures (e.g., cesarean deliveries) by 30% to 50%, suggesting that tort reform encouraging national safe harbors may be an overlooked lever for delivery-system reform.[47] This had been considered in the internal Obama administration debates over the ACA but was ultimately excluded from it.

Perhaps the most salient epistemological development in the economics of the delivery system since the ACA's passage hearkens back to an expression made famous by Gerard Anderson, the late Uwe Reinhardt, and colleagues from a 2003 article in *Health Affairs*: "It's the prices, stupid."[48] Recent work has reinforced this perspective. For example, research from Zack Cooper and colleagues, using claims data from Medicare and commercial insurers, has highlighted the importance of prices in the private sector. While geographic variation in Medicare expenditures is almost entirely a product of utilization variation, geographic variation in commercial insurance expenditures is at least as much a product of price variation linked to differences in local provider market structure as it is to variation in utilization.[49] Along the same lines, researchers looking at cross-country comparisons of health expenditures have found that the major cross-country differences in health spending per capita are driven largely by differences in provider pricing and administrative costs rather than differences in utilization of health care services.[50]

Both federal and state governments have long played a significant role in influencing payments to health care providers from commercial insurers; public payers are responsible for about 40% of health spending across Medicare, Medicaid, and other programs. While the ACA made payment adjustments in Medicare (to account for economy-wide productivity growth) that directly impact provider price growth, the magnitude of savings from further payment adjustments could be significant—particularly if they are made to commercial payment rates. Zack Cooper and colleagues calculate that capping commercial payments for inpatient care at 130% of Medicare rates could reduce such expenditures by around 15%, holding utilization constant.[51] These payment adjustments would need to be balanced against a careful assessment of provider-access implications. As seen in congressional activity around "surprise billing," developing proposals from the right and the left (e.g., draft legislation from Representative Jim Banks [R-IN]) regarding price caps in geographies with limited provider competition and recent price-cap regulation at the state level (e.g., Washington state public option), such tools could play a leading role in future health reform efforts.

Conclusion

The ACA was a product of tradeoffs and constraints, and its success in achieving both coverage expansion and a realignment toward value in the delivery system is remarkable. The direst predictions regarding its impacts look even more ridiculous in retrospect. Private enterprise has not stopped. Death panels have not been formed. Patients are not waiting endlessly to see their physicians. The health system has not collapsed. But even more sophisticated concerns, such as that the ACA would lead to substantial dropping of employer plans or a large reduction in MA enrollment, have not been borne out. The fundamental design choices of the ACA have stood the test of time well.

The pathway forward from here will involve many of the same tradeoffs contained in the ACA: the political viability of moving away from ESI, ways to expand coverage further, and the appropriate pace for the continued shift away from FFS payment, to name a few. Certain of these tradeoffs (e.g., fiscal constraints) may today be made on more favorable terms partly because of the ACA, creating new avenues for progress. Other avenues (e.g., postacute care) have been uncovered since 2009 due to new data and empirical findings. Both cases present exciting and thoughtful focus areas for ongoing progress on health reform, extending the lessons and legacy of the ACA.

CHAPTER 3

THE ROAD NOT TAKEN

Joseph Antos and James C. Capretta

The Affordable Care Act (ACA) was enacted in an environment of deep partisan division. The law did not completely remake American health care as some hoped and others feared. Although it adopted some of the trappings of market competition, the ACA increased federal regulatory control over the insurance market, backed up by billions of dollars in new or expanded subsidies for health coverage. Insurance became affordable for many because of those subsidies and the law's new rules protecting patients with expensive conditions. But insurance also became less affordable for others, who were not allowed to keep their less-expensive health plans.

The next reform must move decisively toward a better-functioning marketplace that reduces unnecessary spending by bringing more discipline to the way patients receive care. Although the ACA did not meet all of its objectives, the public strongly supports the law's provisions that reduce costs for people with expensive health conditions and subsidize private coverage for lower-income households. Republicans failed to reach agreement on a replacement plan for the ACA, but there may be Republican support for market-oriented reforms that are missing from the ACA.

Joseph Antos, PhD, is the Wilson H. Taylor Resident Scholar in Health Care and Retirement Policy at the American Enterprise Institute (AEI) and previously held senior positions at the Congressional Budget Office and the US Department of Health and Human Services.

James C. Capretta, MA, is a resident fellow at the American Enterprise Institute and served as an associate director for health programs in the White House Office of Management and Budget (2001–2004).

The health system needs stronger financial incentives for reducing costs and improving value, particularly in employer coverage and Medicare. Consumers can play an important role in this effort, but they need better information about their treatment options and the savings they would receive by choosing efficient and high-value care. An example of what works is reference-based pricing, which offers standard coverage if the patient chooses cost-effective providers but also requires substantially higher cost sharing if more expensive alternatives are selected. Moreover, prices for major elective procedures do not remain fixed in the face of vigorous competition. The potential loss of market share as patients shift to lower-cost providers could force competing providers to lower their prices by substantial margins.[1]

Republicans generally support reforms that give consumers better insurance options and more control over—and more responsibility for—their health care choices. Shifting to a system of automatic enrollment in place of the failed ACA mandate would promote coverage but allow consumers the freedom to drop out if they choose. Broadening the types of insurance to allow lower-cost plans is another element in promoting affordable coverage. Restructuring Medicaid subsidies to encourage states to expand eligibility while giving them greater flexibility to provide support for high-cost patients is an additional goal shared by many Republicans.

The ACA made significant changes to the insurance market but left untouched much of the waste and inefficiency that plagues the provision of care to patients. To be sustainable in the long run, we must address the underlying causes of rising health care costs. Given the size and complexity of this challenge, repeated reform efforts will be necessary.

Where the ACA Went Wrong

The Affordable Care Act created a complex mix of market mechanisms, government controls, and new federal subsidies to increase the number of Americans with health insurance. Health insurance exchanges offer a choice of health plans and incorporate new federal premium subsidies to simplify enrollment. New federal regulations require insurers to offer coverage to those with preexisting conditions, standardize the benefit package, and take measures intended to improve the operation of the individual and small-group insurance markets. While private coverage increased in those markets, the Medicaid expansion led to much larger enrollment increases.

Although the ACA made coverage affordable for more people, it failed to perform as many of its supporters had hoped. Several factors—including design failures, unanticipated reactions by insurers and consumers, and opposition from many Republican officeholders—contributed to this outcome.

Many people—approximately 2.6 million—buying their own coverage on the individual market could not keep their pre-ACA insurance.[2] The imposition of "essential benefits," guaranteed issue, and community rating forced up premiums as higher-risk people gained coverage. Older coverage was dropped in favor of plans with more expansive benefits, more expensive premiums and cost sharing, and narrower provider networks.

New premium subsidies are limited to families with incomes between 100% and 400% of the federal poverty level (FPL),[3] and cost-sharing reduction subsidies are limited to those between 100% and 250% of the FPL. Above 300% of the FPL ($37,470 for an individual, with $13,260 added for each additional family member), a family would need to pay 9.5% of its pretax income in annual premiums for a narrow network plan that might require a $5,000 annual deductible. This gives many middle-income families without access to employer-sponsored insurance no choice but to pay more than they had paid for insurance before the ACA or drop their coverage.

The individual mandate was supposed to force younger, healthier people into exchange coverage to lessen the impact of adverse selection. The financial penalty was well below the savings many healthy people could gain by not buying insurance and not paying premiums—and those savings would grow with every year of noncoverage. Other policies worked against enrolling younger people in exchange plans, including letting people under age 26 stay on their parents' coverage and age rating that shifted some of the cost of older enrollees onto premiums paid by younger ones.

The Medicaid expansion was originally intended to be universal, but instead of raising federal eligibility standards, the ACA imposed confiscatory penalties on nonexpansion states. In *National Federation of Independent Business vs. Sebelius,* the Supreme Court found that the nonexpansion penalty was unconstitutionally coercive.[4] Despite the promise of federal payments initially covering the full cost of the expansion population and tapering down to 90% of cost beginning in 2020, 14 Republican-leaning states have not expanded eligibility. That leaves no realistic insurance options for individuals who were not previously Medicaid eligible with below-poverty incomes living in nonexpansion states. Moreover, larger federal subsidies are available for Medicaid enrollees who are not poor than for those who are. This violates the principle that federal support should be the most generous for households with the least resources.

The failure to permanently appropriate payments to exchange insurers for cost-sharing reduction (CSR) subsidies has led to distorted prices in the exchange market and higher federal cost. Without a formal congressional appropriation, CSR payments are arguably unconstitutional. President Trump suspended those payments in October 2017, causing insurers to resort to "silver loading" to make up for the uncompensated cost of the subsidies.[5] Federal premium subsidies increased because they are tied to the premiums for the second-lowest-cost silver plan. Anyone not eligible for premium credits—those over 400% of the FPL—is faced with large premium increases, causing some to drop coverage.

The ACA also failed to permanently enact a reinsurance program to stabilize the exchange market. Reinsurance lowers the risk that an insurer will be left with a disproportionate number of higher-cost cases. With that risk removed, all insurers can lower their premiums with more confidence, and the overall cost drops for consumers. The ACA's reinsurance program expired after 3 years. Consequently, the average exchange enrollee pays a higher premium than would have been necessary otherwise.

Cost-containment measures in the ACA have been rescinded or delayed or had limited impact.[6] Claims that the ACA was responsible for slowing the growth of national health expenditures (NHE) ignore the fact that a slowdown began in 2002, well before the ACA was even being considered, when annual growth in NHE as a share of gross domestic product dropped from 6.4% to less in 1% in 2004 and remained low through 2017.

It is not possible to determine the net effect of the ACA on health spending growth, accounting for the increased cost of coverage, ACA savings provisions, and numerous other changes affecting the health sector and the economy. It is clear, however, that spending trends have not changed significantly over most of the past 2 decades. Between 2003 and 2010 NHE, adjusted for inflation, grew at an average annual rate of 2.7%. Between 2010 and 2017 NHE, adjusted for inflation, grew at the same rate.

There are several reasons for this. First, the Independent Payment Advisory Board (IPAB) was supposed to enforce spending reductions in Medicare if program growth exceeded a target. President Obama never nominated anyone to serve on the IPAB, which was repealed without being implemented. Second, the Cadillac tax on high-cost employer plans is opposed by unions and employers. It was to start in 2018, well after President Obama's 2 terms and the 2016 election. Anticipation of the tax might have helped slow costs if employers assumed it would not be delayed, although there is no evidence of this. But Congress did delay it—twice. It now is scheduled to go into effect in 2022, but both parties in Congress are now lining up behind another delay or perhaps full repeal. Third, accountable care organizations (ACOs)—groups of physicians, hospitals, and other providers who share savings with Medicare for delivering more efficient care—do not actively engage beneficiaries; instead, beneficiaries are assigned to an ACO based on their use of physician services and are not obligated to use ACO providers. Even the most favorable review suggests savings that are a small fraction of overall Medicare spending.[7] Furthermore, the Center for Medicare and Medicaid Innovation (CMMI) has undertaken numerous demonstration projects, many with overlapping mandates. Savings from those projects have been modest after 9 years of operation. Currently, only 2 CMMI initiatives have been expanded to nationwide implementation based on the Medicare actuary's certification that they would reduce overall program costs.[8] Finally, the ACA made substantial cuts in Medicare payment rates for providers and Medicare Advantage (MA) plans, accounting for $332 billion in savings to partly offset about $900 billion in additional spending for coverage expansions.[9]

It might be argued that the ACA fell short of reaching certain objectives in part because of opponents' concerted efforts to repeal or weaken its provisions. The Trump administration has taken several steps, including reducing funding for outreach to the uninsured, which may have reduced the ACA's ability to achieve some of its goals. But some responsibility for these failures falls on those who wrote and passed the law. The Medicaid provision trampled on state prerogatives so aggressively that it was sure to invite a constitutional challenge— and did. Many Democrats viewed the IPAB as encroaching on the legislative role of Congress. It was eventually repealed on a bipartisan basis. Further, the authors of the ACA should have known that fully implementing such wide-ranging legislation would require bipartisan cooperation. The rush to enact the ACA through 2 separate pieces of legislation on a partisan basis was sure to create continued opposition from Republicans in the states and in Congress.

An Alternative Vision

The debate over the ACA brought to the surface of American politics a long-standing divide over the proper orientation of health care policy. On one side are those who tend to promote more federal control and government regulation over insurance markets and the organizations delivering services to patients. On the other side are those who are more inclined to support consumer incentives and market mechanisms to improve the value and quality of patient care. There is overlap in the kinds of policies advanced by the 2 sides in this debate, but the underlying philosophical disagreement is deep and makes reaching broad-based consensus difficult.[10]

The ACA was not an attempt to fully remake American health care; rather, it built upon the existing complex web of public regulations, government subsidies, and private-sector organizations and incentives that have characterized the system for decades. While the ACA retained this basic structure, it tried to make improvements by substantially increasing the federal role in that system, with additional regulatory controls as well as new public subsidies for insurance enrollment.

Despite—and in some ways because of—the ACA, our health system is still badly in need of reform and revitalization. The ACA established policy objectives that set a base for future reforms: (1) give everyone access to coverage regardless of their health status, (2) provide financial assistance to help low-income families afford coverage, (3) offer families a choice of insurance rather than defaulting to a one-size-fits-all plan, and (4) bring more cost discipline to the provision of care. Although some argued for a full repeal, the Republican alternative that passed the House was aimed at achieving those same objectives.

The alternative vision of reform has several common themes. They would shift from government controls to market-based reforms and greater decentralization. Federal subsidies for insurance (including Medicare) would be converted to defined contribution payments, giving consumers stronger incentives to seek out high-value, low-cost options for their coverage and their medical care. Medicaid reforms, such as adjusting the matching rate system to promote lower costs and stable budgets, would promote more effective state management of the program's wide array of acute-care and long-term-care services. Health Savings Accounts (HSAs) would become an integral part of coverage to enhance and strengthen the consumer role in the market. Meaningful price and quality transparency would improve decision making on the part of providers and consumers.[11]

This approach to reform is challenging technically and politically. Consumers would be required to take more financial responsibility for the choices they make, which is an unpopular position. Republican opponents of centralized control often embrace a more market-oriented approach to reform more in theory than in practice.

This conflict between philosophical objectives and technical and political feasibility was evident in the 2017 debates over repeal-and-replace legislation. Although House Republicans were able to pass a repeal-and-replace bill that year, that legislation fell well short of what would be considered a well-designed, market-driven plan. For starters, House Republicans dropped a provision to place an upper limit on the tax preference for employer-provided health care. This is key to bringing more cost discipline to the system, and dropping it substantially weakened the GOP case that the party's bill had more effective cost controls than the ACA. Further, the bill did little to reform Medicare, which is the most important source of financing for most providers and, thus, is instrumental in financing inefficiency in care delivery. A market-driven health system would require major reform of Medicare—a challenge for politicians regardless of political party.

Republican Roads Not Taken

Republican opposition resulted in numerous proposals to repeal, defund, or delay provisions of the ACA. The Republican victory in the 2016 election led to a concerted attempt to repeal and replace the ACA—one that eventually failed.

The House narrowly approved the American Health Care Act (AHCA) on May 4, 2017, following intense debate among Republicans over the scope of the bill. The conservative House Freedom Caucus argued that the AHCA did not go far enough in repealing major sections of the ACA, including insurance rules such as the "essential health benefits" requirement.[12] Concern that anything short of full repeal would be "Obamacare Lite" has been an underlying political theme of the ongoing Republican unease over the ACA.

However, a slim Republican majority in the Senate meant that a repeal bill could only pass under reconciliation rules to avoid a filibuster. Senate rules generally prohibit provisions that are extraneous to achieving the budgetary goals established in the budget resolution. Changes to the ACA's insurance rules were likely to be dropped for that reason and were not included in the proposed bill.

Nevertheless, the AHCA contained significant changes that addressed many Republican policy concerns about the ACA.[13] They included:

- Repealing the new taxes and tax increases imposed by the ACA. CBO estimated that the AHCA tax changes would have reduced federal revenue by $992 billion between 2017 and 2026.[14]
- Reducing the enhanced matching rate for the Medicaid expansion and conversion of the federal Medicaid payments

to per-capita allotments, with a state option to receive a block grant. These provisions addressed concerns that the Medicaid expansion undercuts the private insurance market, unfairly treats states that did not expand Medicaid, and allows states to artificially increase federal payments that do not necessarily result in better health care for low-income families. CBO estimated that federal Medicaid spending would fall by $834 billion and reduce enrollment by 14 million in 2026.[15] That raised concerns among Democrats and Republicans about the impact these policies would have on access to care for low-income families and on state budgets.[16]

- Repealing the mandate penalties. Repealing the penalties would not eliminate the requirement to have insurance but would limit the government's ability to enforce the mandate.
- Converting the ACA's premium credits (which vary according to the enrollee's income and the cost of the second-lowest-cost silver plan) to flat credits that increase with the enrollee's age.
- Allowing states to modify ACA insurance regulations, including raising the default limit on age rating and replacing the federal "essential health benefits" with their own requirements.
- Promoting continuous insurance coverage. States could allow insurers to impose a premium surcharge on customers who have a lapse in coverage or allow insurers to set premiums based on health status for customers with a lapse in coverage.
- Providing $138 billion to states to fund high-risk pools or other assistance to high-risk individuals.

The Senate considered several proposals to repeal and replace the ACA, including the Better Care Reconciliation Act (BCRA), all of which failed to pass. A repeal-and-delay bill, giving Congress 2 years to enact a replacement strategy, was brought to a vote as it became apparent that Senate Republicans had not reached agreement about what, if anything, should be substituted for the ACA.[17] That bill also was defeated.[18]

The BCRA and the subsequent Graham-Cassidy plan retained many of the major provisions of the AHCA.[19] Unlike the AHCA and the BCRA, the Graham-Cassidy bill would end premium tax credits, cost-sharing reduction payments, and enhanced Medicaid expansion funding.[20] They would be replaced by block grants to the states to promote enrollment in insurance, stabilize markets, reduce cost sharing, and provide coverage to the Medicaid expansion population. The goal of the proposal was to move authority and funding from the federal government to the states. Although it gained support from some Republicans, there were questions about whether the states could implement their own subsidy programs within 2 years.[21] Moreover, there was concern that the level of funding would fall below the level promised by the ACA, which could lead to a significant loss of coverage.

Congressional Republicans worked hard to reach an agreement on a replacement for the ACA that would shift control over health care from the federal government to the states and to consumers. Policy differences were not resolved, and no legislation was enacted. Despite years of criticizing the ACA, Republicans entered 2017 without a consensus on what the replacement should be or even whether there should be a replacement. Moreover, they were unable to agree on how to protect people with preexisting conditions and provide support for low-income families while reinforcing private markets and reducing tax burdens. These are the main goals that a realistic Republican plan must fit within if it is to be successful.

A Way Forward

The ACA changed the rules of the insurance market to ensure greater access to health coverage for millions of people who previously were left out. It did not fundamentally change the public-private nature of our health system, a point of contention within the Democratic Party. That would have been a step too far. The public supports actions that would make coverage less expensive without sacrificing access to medical advances, but they are unwilling to jettison the health insurance they have now for a new government-run program.[22]

A more practical approach to reform would emphasize transparency and consumer choice by injecting stronger market principles into current arrangements without exposing consumers to undue financial risk. The following discussion summarizes specific policies that could be adopted to reduce the number of uninsured, bring greater cost discipline through market principles, return power and control to individuals and the states, and improve the long-term fiscal outlook.

Insurance Market Reforms

A number of policies should be adopted to increase insurance enrollment and promote efficient coverage. Although the ACA extended coverage to many who could not otherwise obtain insurance because of preexisting conditions or cost, others who previously purchased coverage on the individual market have been squeezed out of the market because of increased costs. The Trump administration has taken steps to provide new coverage options outside the constraints of the ACA's rules, including short-term duration plans. Those options should be preserved, but more needs to be done to make lower-cost coverage available to consumers who buy insurance outside of the employer setting.

A new, permanent reinsurance program would reduce premiums across the entire individual insurance market. This could be structured as a state-implemented effort spurred on by an initial injection of federal funds. States would have some flexibility in structuring reinsurance or other mechanisms to reduce the financial burden on plans experiencing a disproportionately large number of high-cost cases. With adequate funding, reinsurance (or high-risk pools) removes the highest-cost outliers from the premium calculation, making premiums consistent with the lower health risks that most people have. Lower premiums would also reduce federal premium subsidies, offsetting some of the initial federal cost of establishing these programs.

The ACA's insurance rules and the difficulty of attracting younger purchasers leaves the non-group market vulnerable to adverse selection. Healthy consumers can opt out of coverage and enroll in later open-enrollment periods without penalty. Congress should counter this tendency by making it as easy and painless as possible for consumers to remain covered through the use of automatic enrollment techniques.

Many people who remain uninsured are eligible for subsidized coverage but either do not know of their eligibility or have failed to take advantage of it. Maryland is the first state to use income tax filing information to automatically enroll those who are eligible for Medicaid but do not have health coverage.[23] The federal government could facilitate state-led automatic enrollment efforts by making federal data necessary to determine eligibility readily available to the states and by providing seed money to offset the initial administrative expenses that states would incur. Residents who are eligible for premium assistance could be enrolled directly into plans and then given the option to opt out if they prefer.

For job-based coverage, Congress should either retain and implement the ACA's Cadillac tax or replace it with an upper limit on the exclusion from income and payroll taxes of premiums paid for employer-sponsored health insurance. By setting a maximum premium beyond which employer-paid coverage will trigger tax consequences, employers and employees would be encouraged to favor lower-cost options. The current policy of unlimited tax subsidies for job-based coverage dilutes the incentive for cost-control and leads to coverage that is more expensive than would otherwise be the case.[24]

The growth of higher-deductible plans has made more consumers sensitive to the cost of care. However, it is difficult for them to compare prices because pricing is opaque and medical care is complex. In addition, consumers with generous coverage and modest cost-sharing requirements do not have a strong financial incentive to comparison shop. Physicians could guide their patients to lower-cost services or providers, but they typically lack both the incentive and information specific to the patient's insurance to make that possible.

The federal government should adopt policies to help consumers and their physicians determine the most cost-effective course of treatment and which providers offer the best value. For instance, pricing prior to use should be available for all medical procedures and services that allow for consumer discretion and choice. This does not mean every person needing a medical service will shop around, just as not everyone who buys consumer goods shops for the best price. If even a fraction of consumers become active price shoppers, however, the market will function better for all patients. Better price information, combined with objective information on provider performance, would enable physicians to more effectively advise their patients and would help shift utilization to higher-value care.[25]

Medicare Reforms

Medicare is pivotal to an effective reform of US health care because of its size and dominant regulatory role. Beneficiaries should be given clear coverage choices, and the government's financial support should be restructured to encourage enrollment in lower-cost coverage. Policies should be adopted to modernize the program, promote more effective competition, and encourage value-creating innovations in health care delivery. They include:

- Combining Part A and Part B into a single program subject to a single premium and simplified cost-sharing requirements—that is, a single deductible rather than multiple deductibles and uniform coinsurance for all covered services.[26] These changes would help beneficiaries select between traditional Medicare and competing MA plans.
- Giving beneficiaries selecting traditional Medicare the option to enroll in an ACO rather than being assigned through attribution.
- Improving the Medicare plan finder system to include information on plan options, drug coverage, and supplemental benefits (including Medigap policies) to provide beneficiaries a clearer understanding of the costs and benefits of their coverage options.
- Realigning Part D incentives by placing greater financial risk for high-cost beneficiaries on Part D plans and drug manufacturers as well as protecting beneficiaries by imposing a cap on out-of-pocket spending.
- Establishing price competition between traditional Medicare and MA plans through direct bidding in local markets.

Medicaid Reforms

The Supreme Court ruling that the ACA's penalty on states for opposing Medicaid expansion was unconstitutional opened the door to large disparities in coverage across the nation. In states that declined the ACA's now-optional Medicaid expansion, 2.5 million poor uninsured adults fall into the coverage gap and have no reasonable options for health insurance.[27] Their incomes are below the FPL but are not low enough to qualify for Medicaid in their states. They do not have access to premium credits in the ACA exchanges, which are available only to households with incomes starting at 100% of the FPL.

There should be a compromise on Medicaid that closes this coverage gap and makes other reforms that would allow states greater freedom to efficiently and fairly manage the program without federal interference. As part of this compromise, Republicans should accept that Medicaid is the nation's safety net health insurance program, and everyone below the FPL should be eligible to enroll. Medicaid should be restructured to provide strong financial incentives for every state to provide coverage at least to that income level.

At the same time, the ACA has devoted more federal resources (on a per-capita basis) to the expansion population than to lower-income enrollees. That should be corrected by moving from the current federal matching grant system to per-person federal subsidies to the states based on eligibility categories. Those amounts would grow as needed to ensure fair access to care. States that agree to this change in federal payments could be given greater flexibility to run their own programs. Currently, states are required to get federal permission for many different types of reforms. With per-capita payments, states should be able to freely implement reforms, such as changes that emphasize more consumer responsibility and choice, so long as they do not reduce benefits or eliminate eligibility categories established in federal law.

Conclusion

The ACA largely accomplished its major objective of expanding access to health insurance coverage. Political debate over what should come next has heated up among Democrats seeking their party's presidential nomination for the 2020 election. Spurred by continuing concern over the rising cost of care and a complex insurance system, some Democratic candidates and outside activists are calling for a single-payer system (or a public option that inevitably pushes out private coverage). Those are political slogans with some appeal among voters, but they would involve such expense and disruption that their broader appeal and practicality is questionable.

Republicans seem less eager to take on the risks of another major health reform. They were unable to agree on a specific replacement for the ACA in 2017, and the possibility that the courts might invalidate the entire law has not led to the development of an alternative that could be embraced widely. In general, conservatives support a consumer-driven approach to expanding health insurance coverage that promotes greater efficiency and continued medical innovation. That may be where any broad agreement ends.

We take a pragmatic view of the issue. Many ACA rules that changed the way the insurance market operates have been in effect since 2010. The exchange system, premium subsidies, and other ACA provisions have been in place since 2014. Insurers, provider organizations, and states have made significant investments to comply with the ACA. It is unrealistic to imagine upending those structural changes, but it is realistic to consider policies that specifically address real, long-standing problems of cost, quality, and access to appropriate care.

Part II

THE POLICY AND POLITICS OF IMPLEMENTATION

CHAPTER 4

PRESENT AT THE CREATION
Launching the ACA—2010 to 2014

Kathleen Sebelius and Nancy-Ann DeParle[1]

In the classic version of American democracy, once the US Congress passes and the president signs a bill, the fight is over and the new act becomes the law of the land. That is not the story of the Patient Protection and Affordable Care Act (ACA).

After a bruising legislative battle, President Barack Obama signed the ACA into law on March 23, 2010. Just 7 minutes after the president put down his pen, 14 state attorneys general filed the first in a seemingly endless series of lawsuits challenging the law's constitutionality.[2] In the months and years that followed, the law's opponents shut down the entire federal government in a failed attempt to block implementation, routinely denied ordinary and usual funding to carry out the law, blocked commonsense technical corrections to fix glitches, spread pernicious misinformation to undermine confidence in the law, and voted more than 70 times to repeal or significantly change the law.

The challenge of implementing the ACA's first phase began in March 2010 and ended in April 2014. Implementation would have been daunting—and mistakes would have been made—even under perfect conditions. The ACA is a massive, comprehensive, and complex piece

Kathleen Sebelius, MPA, is CEO of Sebelius Resources LLC and served as the 21st secretary of the US Department of Health and Human Services (2009–2014).

Nancy-Ann DeParle, JD, is a partner and cofounder of Consonance Capital Partners and served as counselor to the president and director of the White House Office of Health Reform (2009–2011) and assistant to the president and deputy chief of staff for policy (2011–2013).

of legislation, encompassing not only the new coverage for uninsured Americans that we focus on in this chapter but also hundreds of other provisions, ranging from delivery-system reforms to promote higher quality and more efficient care for Medicare beneficiaries, to a requirement that insurers spend a specified percentage of premium dollars on medical costs rather than salaries and administrative costs, to requirements that restaurants and other food establishments include calorie counts on menus to promote healthier eating. Some provisions were effective upon enactment, some later in 2010, many others in January 2014. A remaining few do not become effective until 2020.

None of it was easy. Indeed, given all the obstacles we faced, it is fair to say that nothing about the implementation of the ACA remotely resembled anything taught in a civics classroom about what happens when a bill becomes a law.

How We Started

While the ACA's initial implementation phase would not be completed until the first open enrollment period ended in spring 2014, the work to craft a nationwide framework to allow consumers to shop for health insurance as well as to create the opportunities for states to expand Medicaid for lower-income adults (at 100% federal expense initially and slightly lower cost sharing in later years) began in 2010. Insurance is regulated at the state level, with responsibility over markets carried out by insurance commissioners in each of the 50 states and the District of Columbia. The ACA did not change that regulatory framework—notwithstanding frequent false claims that it represented a federal takeover of health care—but it probably would have been easier had the claims been true.

We had the responsibility to lead the implementation effort, and our goal was to write regulations that would encourage state control within a federal framework, recognizing that states were likely the best experts on their own health insurance marketplaces. It seemed logical—especially to us, as former state officials—that states would welcome the opportunity to run their own health insurance marketplaces with federal financial assistance rather than deferring to the federal government to operate the marketplaces. But we were wrong; politics won over precedent.

The March 2010 lawsuit brought by a group of Republican state attorneys general was just the first sign that logic might not prevail. It was clear that those states and some others would refuse to participate in setting up their own state-based marketplaces or expanding Medicaid eligibility. Soon legislatures in some 30 states were considering legislation blocking elements of the health care bill, further complicating the job at the federal level. It was against this backdrop of resistance from both federal- and state-level opponents that implementation commenced.

Three federal departments—Health and Human Services (HHS), Treasury, and Labor—were charged with jointly implementing the law. While rulemaking is never easy, it became even more challenging with 3 agencies at the table, dealing with a brand-new area of federal authority: creating a framework for the private insurance marketplaces where consumers would buy health insurance, providing tax credits and subsidies to help eligible consumers pay premiums and cost sharing, and acting as the default regulator for states that did not participate.

At HHS we quickly established an Office of Consumer Information and Insurance Oversight[3] as the focal point of implementation and hired experts with state-level regulatory experience. We were also working furiously to meet a timeline set in the law, requiring that benefits be available to consumers on January 1, 2014—45 months after the bill was signed.

But there was no timetable for judicial clarity about constitutionality and no way to determine state participation until deadlines were set and either met or ignored. This made our already very complicated implementation task even more challenging. We had originally assumed that only a small number of states—maybe a dozen, based on the states that had filed the lawsuit on the day the ACA was enacted—would not move forward to operate their own exchanges, as states had clamored to retain control over their exchanges throughout the ACA's drafting process. But the litigation meant that we had to prepare for every contingency—from a scenario where the federal government would run every exchange, with constant resistance from a handful of states, to a scenario in which every state would eventually decide to operate its own insurance marketplace. The traditional conservative approach to government—which strongly argues for states' rights—was turned on its head as the more conservative states deferred to (or dared) the federal government to implement the health law and refused to take control.

Early Benefits for Seniors and Families

Within weeks after the ACA's passage we launched a number of benefits that Congress had designed to take effect right away so that people would see immediate positive effects from the ACA: for seniors, closing Medicare's so-called donut hole gap in prescription drug coverage, and for families, requiring health plans to cover adult children of their enrollees until age 26. By September 2010 there was a "first, do no harm" effort to stabilize employer retiree markets with reinsurance. Then we established a federal high-risk pool, the Preexisting Condition Insurance Plan, to provide bridge coverage for those who were denied insurance, had serious health conditions, and needed help to pay medical bills until the new marketplaces were up and running in 2014.

These efforts—because they required "notice and comment" rulemaking and cost-benefit analyses pursuant to the federal Administrative Procedure Act—were very labor intensive. We published dozens of major regulations during the summer of 2010, including a set that together encompassed a Patient's Bill of Rights that banned lifetime caps on health insurance, prohibited companies from rescinding health insurance plans for people who got sick, prohibited medical underwriting for children under the age of 19, and improved consumer appeals processes. Many of these benefits and protections applied to those who had employer-based insurance lacking these critical protections. For about 75 million Americans the ACA ensured that health insurance plans added full payment for cancer screenings, immunizations, and women's health benefits that were classified with an A or B rating by the US Preventive Services Task Force. We hoped that these tangible early benefits for consumers would counter the negative charges about what the ACA would "take away" from consumers, lower the uninsured rates among young adults, and provide some stability for retirees and those with desperate health needs.

"If You Like Your Health Plan, You Can Keep Your Plan"

Bridging the gap between the health insurance available to consumers when the law passed in 2010 and when the new, improved health plan offerings would be available in January 2014 was a major challenge. There were no perfect solutions. On the one hand, we wanted people to have access to the improved coverage and benefits of the ACA-compliant plans right away, but we also wanted to ensure that the limited number of people who liked and wanted to keep their pre-ACA plans had viable, affordable options. Thus, we decided to allow "grandfathering" of those noncompliant plans to continue. This meant that some very low-benefit plans—so-called skinny plans—were allowed to continue selling and renewing coverage until 2014, even though they did not meet minimum consumer protection and benefit requirements. But insurers had to continue the benefits at the existing 2010 levels and could not drastically increase premiums to continue to qualify for the grandfathering protections that lasted until 2014.

The law's impact on the remaining skinny plans proved to be among the most contentious issues in implementation. As plans had to meet new coverage requirements and could no longer cherry pick enrollees based on health status, their premiums increased or, in some cases, the plans were discontinued. The ACA's opponents seized on this as evidence that President Obama was breaking his pledge that "if you like your health plan, you can keep your plan."[4] In December 2013, a month before the new marketplace coverage took effect, one Republican congressman declared on national television that 80 to 100 million people were receiving cancellation notices.[5] Predictably, such sensationalized warnings received widespread media attention. In crafting a common-sense response to the inevitable complications of transitioning to a new system, we tried to defuse what the law's opponents thought was their most lethal attack to topple the new law at the time. Unfortunately, the political attacks about "taking away health coverage" continued, and the grandfathering policy added instability to the fragile new markets by removing individuals who chose to retain their old plans because their good health status afforded them low rates.

In reality, there were fewer than 3 million cancellation notices, half of which were to consumers eligible for newly subsidized and often better insurance. But there were still over a million people—of the more than 200 million in the individual or employer insurance market—who previously had health insurance that they deemed satisfactory and would now be offered plans that were more comprehensive but also more expensive.

To help families with incomes above 400% of the federal poverty level who were not eligible for cost-sharing subsidies, in December 2013 HHS made clear that the law's hardship exemption, for low-income individuals who still could not afford health insurance, could also allow "unsubsidized individuals" to avoid the mandate to purchase insurance if they certified that the policy was not affordable. A team of consumer specialists at HHS worked with affected consumers to help them find the best options available, and in virtually all cases they were successful.

As these early coverage options and financial protections were being rolled out, the battle to strike down or repeal the ACA raged on at the state and federal levels. And the airwaves were full of dire predictions about what would happen when the ACA was fully implemented. Those claims were not limited to the phony estimate that 100 million people would lose their health plans; there were also claims about exploding deficits, devastating job losses, death panels, unaffordable premium spikes, and death spirals for health plans. Every one of those claims was proven false.

Plans for Expanded Coverage

The ACA provided 2 new options for health insurance for Americans. The lowest-income workers were eligible for expanded Medicaid, and higher-income individuals above 100% of the federal poverty level had the option to buy a private plan with a sliding scale of federal subsidies and protection against preexisting condition discrimination. Both required a federal framework and implementation rules.

Medicaid was already the largest transfer of federal funds to states. To encourage rapid expansion of Medicaid to cover low-income uninsured people, the ACA offered states an incredibly generous deal: the federal government would cover 100% of the cost of the newly insured population for 4 years, to be gradually reduced to a 90% federal share over a decade. States could expand Medicaid immediately, and some, like California, hit the ground running. Other states were fighting us or were not sure what they wanted to implement and sought concessions and waivers to cover less than the population intended by the law. Following the Supreme Court decision making the expansion optional,[6] we had to engage in tedious and often tendentious state-by-state negotiations. Miraculously, by January 1, 2014, 23 states, including 6 headed by Republican governors, expanded Medicaid.

As we worked to expand Medicaid, efforts were underway to set up the marketplace systems. But there was still no certainty about when the litigation—hovering over us as an existential threat to the ACA—would be concluded or whether states would participate or resist. Thus, everything was done on a dual track.

In October 2010, on the eve of the midterm elections, Senate Majority Leader Mitch McConnell (R-KY) declared that the "single most important thing we [Republicans] want to achieve is for President Obama to be a one-term President."[7] The 2010 elections delivered new recruits to the effort to resist, repeal, and replace the ACA. Republicans picked up 63 seats in the House, achieving a decisive majority, and won 7 additional seats in the Senate, where Democrats retained control. And 6 additional Republican governors took office in 2011. Thus, far from a more conciliatory congressional and state landscape, we faced reenergized forces working against us, resisting cooperation at the state level and blocking or defunding implementation in Congress.

Show Me the Money

The funding issues were quite dire. When the ACA was drafted, Congress and the administration assumed, as had been the case with every other previous piece of major legislation, that Congress would appropriate implementation funding in the ordinary course. There-fore, the law included only $1 billion for implementation, assuming that the president would request—and Congress would appropriate—additional funding as needed. The Congressional Budget Office (CBO) estimated that fully implementing the law would cost $10 billion. The president's budget requested funding every year, but it was consistently blocked. And over time Congress inserted language to block the secre-tary's options at HHS to transfer appropriated money to use for imple-mentation, severely limiting the opportunities to educate consumers and promote the new benefits to those who were uninsured.

To put this in context, the ACA was considerably more complex than the Medicare Modernization Act, which essentially only added a prescription drug benefit for seniors. That law was passed in November 2003 and became effective on January 1, 2006—and Congress appro-priated more than $3 billion for implementation, 3 times what it was willing to spend on implementing the ACA.

Further compounding this inadequate administrative funding, additional funds that insurers had relied on to enter and stay in the new marketplaces were cut in 2014. Senator Marco Rubio (R-FL) led the successful effort to eliminate the statutorily guaranteed "risk cor-ridor" funds, which he called insurance bailouts, designed to com-pensate companies that attracted a higher share of high-cost enrollees. The insurers sued HHS for failing to make more than $12 billion in payments; this litigation has been ongoing and is now pending in the Supreme Court.[8] House Republicans challenged other payments to insurers, known as cost-sharing reduction payments, as not properly authorized by the ACA. Ultimately, that litigation was settled,[9] but not before uncertainty over the future of the payments caused significant market instability.

"Hot Button" Issues

Although there were hundreds of "hot button" issues during imple-mentation, 2 features of the law received particular focus: essential health benefits and contraceptive coverage.

Essential Health Benefits

In an effort to avoid one of the legislative pitfalls of the Clinton health reform effort, Congress chose not to specify the benefits to be covered in the law. Because insurance was regulated and controlled at the state level, the benefit packages and mandated coverage varied widely among states. Congress chose not to preempt these state decisions but instead set a floor for the essential health benefits that an insurance policy had to include. The HHS secretary was directed to define these essential health benefits—10 categories of health services and treatment to be included in a benchmark plan in every state. These services, such as maternity care and mental health treatment, were often missing from individual insurance plans. Many consumers believed that they had comprehensive health insurance, only to learn after an accident or diagnosis that their policy did not cover the ambulance ride or the necessary treatment or the birth of their child, leaving them with thousands of dollars in medical bills and dire choices about treatment.

HHS, in turn, asked the Institute of Medicine (since renamed the National Academy of Medicine), an independent expert panel of health care providers, to advise the secretary about how to implement this section of the law. Not surprisingly, there were many ideas. Some of the most vocal disease advocates wanted HHS to impose various treatment mandates nationwide. Others, including some employer groups, argued for national uniform standards for each category, recommending that HHS prescribe very specific limits on insurers' discretion.

While the Institute made recommendations on process and cost targets, it did not recommend how the HHS secretary should arrive at a benchmark plan or give advice on specific definitions within the 10 categories of essential health benefits. We concluded that attempting to impose national mandates and national standards on 51 different state marketplaces would be almost impossible and could cause increased resistance to the ACA in general. And because insurance was regulated and priced at the state level and that had not been changed by the passage of the ACA, we had little authority to regulate prices that would be proposed with any national directive.

Therefore, our decision, which we hoped the states would welcome, was to conform these new policies to those already marketed and popular in each state. This provided each state with 10 different plan choices to use for its benchmark plan for essential health benefits: the most popular small group plans, state employee plans, federal employee plans in the state, and the largest commercial HMO plan.

We also needed to decide how to handle additional insurance benefits, like autism screening, mandated in some states but not in every market. Again, our effort was to strike a balance and a glide path to the improved plans. Although our new rules did not nationalize various mandates—much to the dismay of various advocacy groups that hoped this would eliminate their state-by-state battles—we resisted insurance industry efforts to eliminate all state mandates and allowed states to include their specific insurance mandates, with federal funding for the first 2 years. And if a state chose as its benchmark a popular plan that did not include all the essential benefits outlined, the state had to add those categories of coverage to all plans in the individual and small group markets by January 1, 2014.

Almost no decision pleased everyone: every decision was mischaracterized as "vast overreach" by opponents of the federal law and as "consumer neglect" by advocates who had hoped for more sweeping and uniform federal rules.

Contraception Coverage

Another controversial decision involved no-cost access to contraception. HHS was directed by Congress to develop a list of preventive services for women that would be included in individual and employer insurance plans without co-pays or deductibles. The ACA required this benefit to be available by August 2012.[10]

HHS again turned to the independent Institute of Medicine for expert recommendations, which included a series of benefits—including well-woman visits, domestic violence screening, and contraception—that should qualify as preventive care, along with cancer screenings and immunizations graded as an A or B by the US Preventive Services Task Force. In July 2010 HHS quickly issued an interim final rule including all the Institute's recommendations on preventive services. We requested public comments and promised guidance by August 2011, with the goal of a 2012 final rule to provide clarity for women about their new benefits and financial responsibilities.

We struggled to find a policy that would balance the religious liberty of employers with the health needs of their female employees and dependents. Our initial proposal used the most common religious exemption, one enacted in several states mandating contraception coverage, which had withstood federal court challenges. The policy was designed to accommodate the special concern of religious organizations about providing contraceptive coverage and was written narrowly, knowing that about 99% of American women have used contraception at some point in their lives,[11] and more than half of women of child-bearing age struggle to afford their prescribed birth control.[12]

The interim rule and final rule generated a huge outcry from opponents and proponents alike. Republicans and conservative media accused the president of trampling on religious freedom and ignoring church leaders' requests to exempt employees of all religious schools, universities, and hospitals, which could have blocked these benefits for millions of women who were students, workers, or spouses or dependents of workers in those institutions. Women's health advocates and proponents of affordable contraception, who saw contraception as a health benefit but also as an essential element in the effort to reduce abortions and reduce teen and unwanted pregnancies, celebrated the new coverage but expressed concern about any religious exemptions.[13]

The ACA has made an estimated 50 million women eligible for no-cost contraception coverage,[14] and teen pregnancies and abortions have been reduced.[15] But the debate about religious exemptions from the requirement to provide contraception continues. Employers have filed numerous cases, including ones that reached the US Supreme Court, notably the Hobby Lobby case, decided in 2014,[16] and the Little Sisters of the Poor case, resolved in 2016,[17] which resulted in broader exemptions for employers claiming religious objections to the mandate for contraception coverage for employees.

The Supreme Court Weighs In

The US Supreme Court granted *certiorari* in 2011 in the case of *National Federation of Independent Business v. Sebelius*,[18] an 11th Circuit ruling on a Florida case declaring the ACA to be unconstitutional.

The case was argued in late March 2012, just 2 years after the ACA became law—and after 2 years of feverish work and many changes already made in order to reform insurance markets, strengthen the health care delivery system, expand Medicare benefits, and provide coverage to millions of Americans.

We knew we needed to maintain our momentum toward implementation, so we projected confidence that the Court would uphold the law and continued work full steam ahead. But although our case was strong, no one knew how the Supreme Court would rule, and we all anticipated it would be a close decision. And at the state level, opponents could argue that any move toward implementation or cooperation with us undercut their argument on constitutionality. Thus, the looming Supreme Court decision gave further resolve to states who chose to sue or resist putting an implementation framework in place.

At the federal level, that meant we needed to plan for all possible contingencies, recognizing that a negative decision would impact millions of patients, providers, and insurers. During the months leading up to the decision, we faced increasing questions from states about whether they should move forward with developing state-based marketplaces or stop and wait for the Supreme Court decision. Should they continue to press for legislation expanding their Medicaid programs? And insurance companies that were preparing to sell policies and make changes in existing plans were uncertain about whether to commit resources to the new marketplaces. The already heated political rhetoric in DC became louder and more partisan, with daily releases from members of Congress, governors, and state attorneys general announcing that the law was clearly unconstitutional, confusing consumers and worrying providers and plans.

In all the scenarios discussed as possible outcomes, no one ever suggested the decision that was rendered on June 28, 2012. As predicted, it was a closely divided court, with Chief Justice John Roberts writing for the majority in a 5–4 decision. While the vast majority of the law was found to be constitutional, the court also found that Congress could not "coerce states" to expand Medicaid by threatening to revoke existing Medicaid funding if they failed to create a new program for the expanded Medicaid population. Although the news was very good for the new marketplaces and the whole array of other health benefits, suddenly

Medicaid expansion, which had been seen as the most efficient and economical way to provide health coverage for millions of low-income workers and families, was at risk because the Court's remedy was to make it optional. And because the ACA was structured as a seamless continuum of access, with Medicaid expansion as the foundation in every state for the lowest-income uninsured, workers in states that refused to expand Medicaid were suddenly "too poor" for subsidies.

Furthermore, while the Court essentially "blessed" the tax penalty and gave a green light to setting up an individual marketplace with some uniform rules in every state in the country, the proximity of the reelection campaign gave opponents continued fuel for opposition. The Republican nominee, former Massachusetts governor Mitt Romney, vowed to eliminate the ACA if elected, which had a chilling impact on insurers in "hostile" states and gave political leaders little incentive to cooperate with the federal government.

The Court decision created chaos for the national Medicaid expansion efforts. Suddenly we had to deal with an optional expansion and negotiate with individual states. Even with the most generous federal/state cost-sharing formulas ever offered to states, the political calculations of governors and legislators became the only determining factors about whether constituents in a state would have access to the benefits of the ACA.

We did a lot of hands-on, state-by-state work with Republican and Democratic governors, making it clear that if state lawmakers had strategies to insure the qualified population and improve the Medicaid plan, we were eager to work with them through the Section 1115 waiver process. States like Arkansas and Indiana had state-specific ideas that we concluded were broadly consistent with the law and approved with continued oversight. Other states asked for 100% federal funding to provide benefits to individuals up to only 100% of federal poverty levels instead of the threshold of 138% set by the ACA, which we rejected. And some states wanted to expel people from their health plans if they did not follow certain rules; again, we rejected those proposals.

We tried to draw a bright line, giving flexibility to states that wanted some plan variation but intended to insure the entire eligible population with federal funding. And we rejected requests for limiting the number of eligible individuals or adding nonhealth requirements, like work, to qualify for federally funded health benefits. Again, our decisions left many on both sides unhappy. Many states knew that the financial bargain was too appealing to turn down and moved to expand Medicaid. But 9 years after the law passed, 14 states—including Florida and Texas, with large numbers of uninsured Americans—still have not expanded Medicaid.

A Reelection Reset?

We hoped that the Supreme Court decision would mark a turning point in the politics, that it would bring Republicans to the table to help us make the law work for the American people. But by the time the decision was issued, the 2012 election campaign was already underway. So the debate about the ACA continued throughout the campaign, even though it was Romney who had, in 2006, signed a Massachusetts bill into law that had been the model for the ACA. The debate over the ACA raged on even after the resounding reelection of President Barack Obama and a Democratic Senate.

Republicans in the House and Senate immediately renewed efforts to defund and repeal the law. In spite of frequent and contentious debates in the 2012 presidential election about health care—and the strong election results for President Obama, who won 26 states and DC, won the popular vote by 5 million, and captured 332 electoral votes—the battle continued as if the voters had not been consulted.

The Healthcare.gov Rollout

As Obama took his second oath of office, 2013 was a sprint to put all the pieces of the puzzle in place so that open enrollment could begin on October 1, 2013. Our team wanted consumers to have 3 full months to shop and enroll in plans before benefits began in January 2014. Open enrollment would then continue for the first 3 months of 2014, giving first-time shoppers and procrastinators ample time to learn about insurance and choose a plan that was a good fit for them and their family. The enrollment system was designed to be mostly online, gathering information from a consumer at the beginning of the process and verifying an address, income level, and citizenship status to qualify for the proper tax subsidy. Then consumers could choose from a set of qualified insurance plans in their state that were priced according to their individual subsidy.

The process of developing the first-of-a-kind national website to sell health insurance while simultaneously qualifying individual customers for tax credits based on citizenship status, employment data, and family size, with unique benefits and prices in every state in the country, was supervised by the Centers for Medicaid and Medicare Services (CMS), with close oversight from HHS leadership and our White House partners. CMS hired several preapproved government contractors to build the various parts of the online shopping experience, including the qualification and verification process; the hub that connected to government data from several agencies, including the Internal Revenue Service and the Department of Homeland Security; the shopping experience customized for each state marketplace; and the pricing with individualized subsidies calculated by family, with the insurance product priced for the home state. Even state marketplaces needed to connect to the federal hub for the data held by federal agencies. And unfortunately, the arcane government contracting system prevented the newest generation of technology companies from bidding to do this work.

We had outside reviews from experts at prominent consulting firms to give us insight into potential problems and provided Congress and the president frequent updates about whether the system would be ready on October 1, 2013, as promised. The site was tested, but we could not do "beta testing"—actually allowing some consumers to enroll—before the launch. About a week before the launch all the key contractors appeared at a congressional hearing and were asked, one at a time, whether the system was ready, and all said yes—both to Congress and to CMS and the HHS/White House team.

We knew that there were likely to be issues and glitches when the system first opened for business. Even though the site had been built to handle volume significantly larger than the Medicare.gov website, the government's most popular website, no one really knew how big the demand would be. And because we had very limited funds for outreach and promotion—nothing remotely like the resources a private company would spend when launching a new product—we hoped that a lower traffic volume before insurance benefits were available on January 1 would give some time for the system's bugs to be discovered and worked out.

As intense work was being done to finalize the web offerings and shopper experience, the congressional opposition grew louder and more frantic. In August 2013 several senators launched a Defund Obamacare Town Hall Tour, and 80 House Republicans wrote to Speaker John Boehner (R-OH) to "continue efforts to repeal Obamacare in its entirety" and defund it in the meantime.[19] Facing an October 1 deadline to pass a budget or run out of money, the Republican House sent several short-term funding bills to the Senate that included proposals to defund or delay the ACA. The Democratic Senate responded with its own short-term proposals, stripped of language that would delay the October 1 launch of the Healthcare.gov marketplaces.

On September 30, after more failed attempts to reach a compromise, the president warned that a government shutdown would delay vital services to millions of Americans and hurt the economy. But he also assured Americans that the health insurance marketplaces would open on October 1 and said, "The Affordable Care Act is moving forward."[20] When the House and Senate failed to reach an agreement before midnight on October 1, 2013, the federal government shut down for the first time in 17 years, furloughing approximately 800,000 federal employees, including 40,000 from HHS.

The government was closed, but the Healthcare.gov website, which had been touted as an experience as easy for consumers as booking a plane ticket online, was open for business on October 1, 2013. Within a few hours we knew there were serious issues. By October 3 we knew that in the first 2 days, more than 7 million people had visited Healthcare.gov, more than 7 times the number of visitors to the Southwest Airlines website in a month.

What initially appeared to be difficulties caused by the high volume of potential customers was determined within a few days to be major glitches in the entire process, leading to some rapid decisions. We knew that one of the significant flaws was that while the individual components of the system might adequately function, when they were joined as an online process of verification, shopping, and enrollment, there were huge glitches. Although there is no shortage of ideas on what could have been done better, the constraints of the cumbersome government procurement system, the decision that buying component parts was likely less expensive and less risky than an end-to-end new build, and the failure to have a project integrator whose only job was to make the website function end-to-end were critical mistakes.

The information technology leader at the White House who had worked closely with HHS from the beginning called on behalf of the president for reinforcements from the tech community. The president brought in an experienced manager to be the website czar, and we worked together to choose and hire an outside consultant to drive the project to fix the website. We placed calls to the CEOs of all the major contractors involved, requesting their personal involvement and commitment to deploying their best employees to help fix the problems.

Once a thorough review determined that the site could be upgraded and relaunched by December 1, we went to work assuring advocates, consumers, insurers, and others that they would be able to have health insurance when benefits were available on January 1.

After 16 days and billions of dollars of losses to the economy, the federal government re-opened in mid-October. One of us (Sebelius) testified before the House Energy and Commerce Committee on October 30, apologizing for the deeply flawed launch of Healthcare.gov and pledging to fix the website before any consumer missed the opportunity to receive benefits on January 1. (It is ironic that the legislators who acted to shutter the government because they wanted to delay the ACA were outraged that the website was not performing well.)

An accomplished team of private-sector software engineers responded to the president's call for help and came to work at CMS. They joined the existing contractors and government employees who had built the system to identify and fix problems that blocked customers from completing their purchases. During October and November the president and the HHS secretary traveled the country, visiting with advocates, insurers, and health partners and assuring allies that the problems would be fixed. As promised, on December 1, 8 weeks after the badly flawed initial rollout and one month before insurance plans or Medicaid benefits would be available to consumers, a much-improved website was relaunched. One million customers enrolled by Christmas in state and federal marketplace plans, and millions of other previously uninsured low-income Americans were able to enroll in state Medicaid programs.

Given the extreme dysfunction and negative publicity in the early days of open enrollment during the government shutdown, we extended open enrollment from mid-March to mid-April 2014. By April 19 HHS announced that 8 million people had enrolled in health insurance marketplace plans, exceeding CBO projections of a first-year enrollment of 7 million consumers. And millions more newly and previously eligible Medicaid beneficiaries enrolled in state Medicaid plans.

Between the time the bill was signed and the first open enrollment period ended almost 4 years later, millions of Americans gained health insurance coverage through private marketplace plans or Medicaid programs. Consumers enjoyed new benefits and, for the first time, true health security with their existing plans. Seniors received additional Medicare benefits and cost savings on prescription drugs. And in spite of ferocious opposition from congressional Republicans and unceasing litigation, the ACA survived to protect Americans with preexisting health conditions, support women who had paid discriminatory prices for plans that did not include essential women's health services, and help millions of Americans who could not afford insurance and risked financial ruin with every illness or accident.

Lessons Learned

If we had it to do over again, what would we do differently? Without a Congress willing to roll up its sleeves and help, we did not have the luxury of contemplating this question. But with the benefit of hindsight, there are many things we would change. For example, in retrospect, a national marketplace might have been easier to implement than 20-plus state marketplaces. But the major lessons we learned were ones we already knew from high school civics.

First, bipartisanship helps. There is no question that the ACA would have been stronger—and implementation would have been easier— had some Republicans voted for it. Certainly, President Obama did everything he could to garner Republican support, as evidenced by the hundreds of provisions championed by Republicans that ended up in the bill. And there were years of bipartisan efforts by health policy experts and congressional leaders leading up to the 2008 election, resulting in a broad consensus around the framework that ultimately became the ACA: an individual mandate, tax credits and subsidies, Medicaid expansion, private plans offered through online marketplaces, insurance reforms, a strengthened delivery system, and a bill that is fully paid for and does not increase the deficit. The ACA embodied all of these ideas—some would say Republican ideas—and yet Republicans in Congress chose not to support it. We wish Republicans had supported the bill and know that it would have made implementation smoother and better. But in the end, it was their choice. They chose not to support the ACA not because of its policies but because of their politics.

Second, trying to implement a major piece of legislation without adequate resources is a train wreck waiting to happen. Again, we knew this but depended on the settled expectations of hundreds of years of history pursuant to which Congress has appropriated adequate funding to implement laws it has enacted, whether it likes them or not. In this regard the ACA experience is a cautionary tale; officials charged with implementing future legislation would be wise to ensure that the funding is mandatory, not discretionary and subject to the whims of the annual appropriations process.

During the Obama administration, health care inflation hit its lowest growth rate in 50 years, and when Obama left office the number of uninsured Americans had reached an all-time low. Patient safety efforts were beginning to show signs of success, with fewer hospital infections and preventable readmissions.[21] The goals of the ACA for expanded affordable health insurance, better care for patients, and lower health costs were being realized. And most Americans now believe that those who need health insurance the most should never be denied coverage because of a preexisting condition. That is a final civics lesson: the ACA is not perfect—no major law is—but it was worth fighting for.

CHAPTER 5

IMPLEMENTING THE INSURANCE EXCHANGES
A View from the Trenches

Joel Ario

The team assigned to implement the health insurance exchanges was full of optimism in 2010. The exchanges were the centerpiece of the Affordable Care Act (ACA)'s individual market reforms: the place where an estimated 20 to 25 million people would go to purchase health insurance. The exchanges would offer comprehensive and affordable coverage to those who fell through the cracks of our balkanized health insurance system, extending health security to many of those not eligible for employer coverage, Medicare, or Medicaid. The exchanges would work in tandem with Medicaid expansion to bring the uninsured population under 5%.

While the ACA fell short of these ambitious goals, the incremental progress achieved through it remains a major step forward in America's painstakingly slow march toward universal coverage. Medicaid is now a more-popular-than-ever safety net for 75 million people; further, there are 10 million exchange enrollees. Although these numbers fall short of the Obama administration's goal, they nonetheless represent a vastly larger, more stable risk pool for those who could have been denied coverage or charged more due to preexisting conditions prior to the ACA. The Medicaid and exchange markets have begun to show signs

Joel Ario, MDiv, JD, is a managing director at Manatt Health and served as the first director of the US Department of Health and Human Services' Office of Health Insurance Exchanges (2010–2011) and as insurance commissioner in Pennsylvania (2007–2010) and Oregon (2000–2007).

of converging, but the exchanges remain a separate and unique market segment primarily for subsidized enrollees up to 400% of the federal poverty line.

Much went right in implementation; much went wrong. Both experiences highlight lessons learned for what might come next.

Three Goals

In the fall of 2010 the exchange team faced 3 challenges:[1] (1) supporting states in setting up state-based exchanges in as many states as possible; (2) collaborating with insurers ready to implement guaranteed issue and other ACA reforms; and (3) creating a federal exchange to identify synergies that might aid state exchanges and act as a back-up exchange for states that defaulted to the federal government.

State Exchanges

Conventional wisdom holds that the ACA's implementation was destined to be partisan because it passed on a party-line vote. This view is belied by the fact that 5 months later, in August 2010, 49 of the 50 states applied for $1 million planning grants to establish state exchanges. This was not surprising at the time because the law's preference for state exchanges was a compromise in which the state-oriented Senate bill prevailed over the House preference for a federal exchange.

The one hold-out was Minnesota's Republican governor Tim Pawlenty, who refused to apply for the planning grant despite pressure from Democratic legislators.[2] Foreshadowing the partisanship that was to come, Pawlenty argued that Republicans should not cooperate with the Obama administration and subsequently used his early opposition as a talking point in his campaign for the 2012 Republican nomination for president. Despite this, Minnesota became one of the first states to move forward on a state exchange when a Democrat, Mark Dayton, was elected governor of Minnesota in November 2010.

The rise of ACA-related partisanship became an acute problem when the Republicans flipped 11 states from Democratic to Republican governors in 2010, including the bellwether states of Florida, Pennsylvania, Ohio, Michigan, and Wisconsin. In every one of those states, the new Republican governor, as part of a broader trend in which the Republicans saw political advantage in opposing the ACA, reversed course and decided not to establish a state exchange. Ultimately, only 3 states with Republican governors (Idaho, Nevada, and New Mexico) established state exchanges. All 5 states that flipped from Republican to Democratic governors in 2010 (California, Connecticut, Hawaii, Minnesota, and Vermont) moved forward with state exchanges, as did 8 other states with Democratic governors as well as the District of Columbia. In sum, the 2010 midterm elections were the real game changer in sharpening the partisan lines that have been a feature of ACA implementation ever since.

As a former governor, Secretary Kathleen Sebelius directed the exchange team to work with the states, but the reaction to ACA implementation was strikingly similar across all the red states. By the 2010 election the Office of Health Insurance Exchanges (OHIE) had forged relationships with the career staff in state agencies in virtually every state. These agencies generally continued to strategize with the exchange team on maintaining momentum for state-based exchanges, regardless of whether a state had flipped Republican in 2010. But this mostly happened under the radar, and the political headwinds were fierce enough that Sebelius regularly received rhetorical letters from Republican governors demanding unworkable concessions to state proposals not in compliance with the ACA.

In addition to the fraught political environment, in Denver in the spring of 2011 at a sobering meeting with states, it became clear that even some of our leading exchange states were having trouble meeting their technology milestones for setting up a state exchange. This was compounded by the fact that none of the early innovator states developed a successful prototype (see the Federal Exchange section below). By May the exchange team presented a deck to the White House team predicting 40 or more federal exchange states if states faced a bifurcated choice between a full state exchange or default to the federal exchange. While the challenges were primarily political in most states, even states that were strongly supportive of the ACA were concerned about the technical challenges and welcomed federal support.

In the face of these difficulties, the exchange team developed a spectrum of state partnership options to get the states on board with implementation. Ultimately these options did salvage a lot of goodwill between state and federal officials, allowing the exchange team to build some very creative working relationships,[3] but the creation of state exchanges remained a problem. Some at HHS pushed for shared authority in these partnership exchanges; however, this proved unworkable. The lawyers involved insisted that a clear hierarchy was not optional for a functional working relationship—that "someone has to be in charge"—and the career staff at Centers for Medicare and Medicaid Services (CMS) would not compromise on bottom-line federal control at the operational level for any form of partnership.

The skirmishing went on until late 2012, when, in the end, 34 states defaulted to the federally facilitated exchange (FFE), commonly known today as Healthcare.gov.[4] Interestingly, the decisions made then did not change until the 2017 and 2018 elections brought a wave of new Democratic governors. In between, 5 of the 16 state-based exchanges (SBEs) were forced by technology failures to fall back into relying on the federal technology platform as well. Three of these SBEs (Nevada, New Mexico, and Oregon) carved out a new category, called SBEs on the federal platform (SBE-FP). This nomenclature reflected the fact that they wanted to preserve their state governance of nontechnical functions. Kentucky was the only state with a successful technology platform to voluntarily dismantle it for political reasons when a Republican governor, Matt Bevin, was elected in 2016.

As of August 2019 the exchange landscape consists of 12 state-based exchanges (11 states and DC), 5 state-based exchanges on the federal platform, and 34 FFE states. However, this is changing. Nevada, New Mexico, and Oregon are at various stages of returning to their own state technology platforms.

In addition, Pennsylvania and New Jersey enacted statutes to become SBEs for 2020.[5] They filed blueprints on August 1, 2019, to become SBE-FPs in 2020 and then to move to full SBEs in 2021. Their motivation is twofold: (1) exchange technology has decreased in price to the point where states can assess exchange user fees themselves, and save money on technology costs by becoming SBEs, and (2) the federal technology platform constrains state policy flexibility to pursue all but the most anodyne "state innovation waivers" under Section 1332 of the ACA. In addition, some of these states are concerned about changes the Trump administration has made to Healthcare.gov, including severe cuts in consumer outreach budgets as well as the promotion of short-term plans and other health benefit options that undermine exchange risk pools.[6]

ACA implementation would likely have been much smoother had 40 or more states established their own exchanges. The federal government could then have focused on fewer states and counted on more cooperation from states in charge of their own exchanges. Moreover, it would have been harder for red states to remain opposed to the ACA in general if they had ownership over their own state exchanges and had to answer to their constituents for how well those exchanges functioned. For example, Idaho is a deep-red state that has an SBE. It uses the state Medicaid agency to determine eligibility for both Medicaid and exchange tax credits and has one of the largest per-capita exchange enrollments of any state. Nevertheless, Idaho is not totally immune to ACA-related partisanship; the state is still fighting over Medicaid expansion and flirting with innovation waivers that could end up undermining the exchange risk pool. But the conversation is different in Idaho compared to FFE states, which can attack the ACA with virtual impunity.

Was there anything more that could have been done to overcome the polarization that followed the Republican gains in the 2010 election? It is doubtful. Once the political advantages of opposing the ACA became clear to Republicans, that strategy was impossible to resist. In general, the exchange team remained as nimble and deferential to the states as possible unless their actions violated the ACA protections for people with preexisting conditions, which some states wanted to do to reduce premiums for healthy people. Although there were discussions of taking a more forceful hand with recalcitrant states, the Obama administration generally avoided legal confrontations with states that were arguably not "substantially complying" with the ACA, despite their inaction rising to the legal standard for federal action. This overall attitude of deference, however, would come to impact various technological problems with the exchanges in 2013, as elaborated below.

Insurer Collaboration

Successful implementation of the ACA required robust insurance participation, as individuals looking to enroll in the exchanges had to find health plans worth buying. This need for insurer participation made it imperative that the exchange team fully engage with insurers and patiently work through many differences on regulatory issues with them. Fortunately, the team could afford to be selective: there were more than 1,000 health insurers in 2010. The vast majority of these companies relied on a business model that depended on finding the healthiest individuals and denying coverage to those who most needed it. Prior to the ACA all but a handful of states had allowed medical underwriting and rating to deny coverage to people with preexisting conditions or charge them more based on their health status. Because the ACA prohibited that kind of discrimination, insurers were required to change their business model or exit the individual market, as many did. There were, however, 3 groups willing to work with the exchange team to eliminate underwriting and achieve large and balanced risk pools that did not discriminate based on health status.

The first of these 3 groups was the 39 (now 36)[7] Blue Cross Blue Shield insurers (Blues) and their national association. The Blues started in the 1930s and 1940s as local insurers sponsored by hospitals (Blue Cross) or physicians (Blue Shield) and had become a leading national association with more than 100 million members across all 50 states. The Blues came to the ACA with a history of insuring a broad cross-section of healthy and unhealthy individuals; it is perhaps unsurprising that they became the mainstay in most state exchanges. Gaining their support was critical because the Blues were the dominant insurer in virtually every state's individual market, often holding market shares in excess of 50% in the smaller states. The Blues continue to be the largest insurers in most states, and where the local Blue insurer did not participate in the exchange, such as in Iowa and Mississippi, the exchange market suffered from a lack of competition. In the doldrums of 2016 and 2017, when some national insurers pulled off the exchanges, it looked as though there might be so-called bare counties with no insurer participation. In most of those cases it was a Blue insurer who agreed to be the single remaining insurer.

State insurance markets are typically strengthened when deep-pocketed, for-profit national insurers compete with the local Blue insurer and other competitors. The exchange team worked closely with the top 5 national health insurers (Aetna, Anthem, Cigna, Humana, and United) on issues like network adequacy and essential health benefits, where they generally wanted a delicate balance between a level playing field across states and as much flexibility as possible. Although these 5 companies were cautious participants in year one (2014), they all were major participants in 2015, with United expanding its footprint to more than 30 states and Aetna, Anthem, and Humana to more than a dozen states. As it turned out, however, the national insurers were not the best fit for the exchanges because they lacked the deep connections to local providers that made it easier to craft affordable products with narrow networks. Without the same allegiance to local markets and state regulators as the Blues, the national insurers tended to leave exchange markets rather than reform their business models.

In 2016 and 2017 the Blue insurers responded to affordability issues by moving toward narrow network or HMO-type products. The national insurers, meanwhile, mostly turned their attention to other markets. Anthem was a special case because it was both a Blue and a for-profit insurer, as it was composed of 14 state Blues who had converted to for-profit status. As the only for-profit Blue insurer, Anthem did threaten to pull back from less-competitive rural areas. However, Anthem also continued to reflect its roots in the nonprofit Blue world by responding to public pressure and often reversed course when federal and state regulators pressed the company not to pull out of counties that would have no insurer at all if Anthem left.

Ironically, all 5 national insurers have become huge players in the more heavily regulated Medicare Advantage (MA) and Medicaid managed care organizations (MCOs) markets, both of which have been growing more rapidly than the exchange market. All 3 of these programs share a common model in which government defines the health product and various rules of the road but contracts with insurers to deliver the product to enrollees. The government allows varying levels of innovation and, in the case of value-based purchasing and other delivery-system reforms, actively encourages or even requires innovation. While the exchanges initially attracted the most attention as a place for innovation, the national insurers quickly moved away from them when they attracted smaller enrollment than expected, resulting in greater price fluctuations and ultimately a good deal of political uncertainty after the 2016 election.

It is unclear why insurers, who generally espouse market-oriented approaches, have shifted away from the exchanges (the most market-oriented of the 3 programs) while embracing the more heavily regulated Medicare and Medicaid managed care programs.[8] Part of the answer is simply volume: there are more than 20 million enrollees in MA and more than 50 million enrollees in Medicaid MCOs, compared to 10 million in the exchanges. But a more important lesson may be that insurers do not have a problem with regulation if it leads to a more stable and predictable program, especially on price, than the still-evolving exchange market.

Beyond the Blues and national insurers, which collectively cover more than ⅔ of the health market, regional provider-sponsored plans are an important force in many local markets. The best of these are the Kaiser-like plans (e.g., UPMC, Geisinger, Intermountain) that are integrated provider-insurer systems, typically with narrow networks that are more tightly managed than traditional PPO networks. Locally based plans, with strong ties to local providers, have been important exchange players in their states and in recent years have been supplemented by Centene and other Medicaid MCOs expanding their business models to compete on the exchanges as well as for Medicaid contracts. A common strategy for both provider-sponsored plans and Medicaid-based plans has been to offer narrow or "selective" networks to keep prices down for their exchange products.

As yet it is unclear whether the national insurers will begin to use their Medicaid MCO subsidiaries instead of their commercial chassis to compete in the exchanges. If so, this could further an evolving convergence between exchange and Medicaid markets around issues like network formation and provider reimbursement. Such a convergence also would exacerbate an increasing disparity between public programs and employer-based coverage, where broad networks that generally include the most expensive providers keep prices higher.[9]

The Federal Exchange

The exchange team planned for the development of a federal exchange to be done concurrently with state-based exchanges, both because it would help illuminate the challenges faced by states and because it was always likely that at least some states would default to the federal exchange. It did not turn out that way.

Policy, not technology, was the central focus of the group, as demonstrated by the fact that I—a technophobe with 15 years of state regulatory experience—led the team. It has been reported that there were conversations going on among senior officials about a technology czar, and it seems obvious in retrospect that the federal exchange should have been a higher priority for the exchange team. But it had been made clear from the start that the job of the exchange team at HHS was to bring the states along. There was little or no dissent from the view that investing major resources in the federal exchange, especially given the severe limits on our resources overall, would provoke a major political backlash from ACA opponents and make working with red states that much more difficult.

The exchange team did make efforts on the technology side. The team created a $250 million program for states to develop technology prototypes in the fall of 2010, but the program did not succeed, at least in part because several early innovators, including Wisconsin and Oklahoma, pulled out when new Republican governors were elected in 2010. In addition, the exchange team worked with web-based companies who had experience with selling individual insurance over the web. These companies maintained extensive networks of business relationships designed to help them reach potential customers, such as individuals leaving employer-based coverage. The result was a program now called enhanced direct enrollment (EDE) that authorizes "web brokers" who meet rigorous privacy and security standards to enroll people in ACA-compliant coverage through their own websites rather than redirecting them to Healthcare.gov, which does not offer the ideal user experience for all prospective enrollees. EDE partners now account for almost 20% of FFE enrollment.

While SBEs have yet to embrace EDE partners, there is growing recognition that the best way to reach a broad and diverse group of potential enrollees is to have a broad and diverse set of partners. That includes diversity in web-based partners as well as diversity in community partners. Alternative websites can also be invaluable during service outages. An early version of EDE was included in the first wave of 2012 regulations, and had it been made a top priority, the problems with Healthcare.gov in 2013 might not have been headline news; instead, President Obama could have gone on television in November of 2013 and said, "Healthcare.gov is down, but here are 6 other websites run by government-certified companies that can offer you the same website experience, down to how plans are sorted and presented."

This does not, of course, excuse the failure to develop a world-class federal exchange for the October 2013 launch of the exchanges. Although it may have been correct that too much attention to the federal exchange would have provoked a political backlash, it was clear that the federal exchange would be necessary in at least some states. Moreover, we know in hindsight that the website woes of October and November 2013 were turned around quickly by a crack team of technology experts. Casting a broader net earlier might have been a winning strategy, even if it would have been more politically challenging than confining our initial procurement to a preapproved list of technology vendors.

Common Issues

Two major issues permeated the exchange team's work: regulating in a highly complex environment and deciding, on a case by case basis, when state flexibility made sense and when national uniformity was needed. To that end, it is interesting to note that HHS described its July 2012 rules on market practices and qualified health plan (QHP) certification as maximizing state flexibility and its August 2012 rules on eligibility and enrollment as a simple and seamless approach.

"Keep it simple" was a recurring theme as OHIE struggled to write the administrative rules that were its primary day-to-day responsibility, but CMS was staffed by many health policy experts who saw the ACA regulations as an opportunity to embed their best ideas into federal law. A pattern emerged in which first drafts were overly complex and would gradually be pared back, especially following meetings with the White House team. Brevity commanded a level of respect at the White House that was difficult to achieve on the ground at CMS, where there was less appreciation for the cost-benefit tradeoffs of regulation.

The resistance of the states also presented an inherent policy dilemma: How far should the exchange team go to engage the states in developing their own SBEs, as opposed to seeing their unexpected resistance as an opportunity for the federal government to exert more national control over health care? Three key policy decisions concerning essential health benefits, network adequacy, and exchange eligibility illustrate the ongoing debates about these countervailing considerations.

Essential Health Benefits

Defining essential health benefits (EHBs) was an early test case. From a policy perspective, the ideal solution to defining what benefits should be required in ACA benefit plans would have been to assemble the country's leading medical experts and let them put together the package. However, this approach had helped derail the Clinton health plan in the 1990s, when defining the benefit package became a metaphor for too much complexity. Because the secretary and others in HHS (including me) had been state insurance regulators, we knew that states had deep experience with resolving debates about benefit mandates. We also knew that defining benefit mandates was an inherently political exercise in which political power too often trumped good medicine. Perhaps the Obama administration could have overcome the political challenges in a pristine federal process, which is what the ACA seemed to envision, but that did not seem likely, and we had many other priorities. In light of these issues, the administration resolved to largely delegate the EHB issue to the states, with regulatory guardrails designed to achieve more or less similar results across states. The key guardrail was that state EHBs had to be based on benchmark plans, such as the best-selling plans in each state. The states embraced the EHB regulations, and many engaged in elaborate processes to compare their benchmark choices and find the best option.

Network Adequacy

Defining network adequacy was another challenge. Again, the exchange team's collective state experience was helpful as the team labored to steer a middle course between lax guidelines that would result in substandard plans and prescriptive standards that would drive up premiums. The key flash point was whether to stick with the broad qualitative standard found in the statute[10] or to add a set of quantitative standards such as time and distance requirements to measure the proximity of providers, wait times for appointments, and so on.

The team largely stuck with qualitative standards with some exceptions, such as a requirement to develop a roster of "essential community providers," a statutory term that referred to providers in low-income communities who might not be included in standard commercial networks. Three arguments prevailed: (1) the National Association of Insurance Commissioners (NAIC) was actively engaged in updating its network adequacy model, and states pushed for deference to the qualitative approach that was the centerpiece of the NAIC model; (2) Kaiser and other integrated systems typically had quite narrow networks, and these plans often scored well on MA quality ratings; and (3) the team knew that the ability to form selective networks would give insurers critical leverage in keeping premiums as low as possible. Interestingly, CMS has vacillated on this issue over time, moving toward quantitative standards at the end of the Obama administration and then moving to even greater state deference than the original regulations during the Trump administration. Finding the right balance is a constant challenge based on the number and distribution of providers across widely divergent urban and rural markets.

Eligibility and Enrollment

Eligibility and enrollment (E&E) was another hotly debated regulatory challenge and, in retrospect, may have been a missed opportunity to implement a single, national eligibility system outside the exchanges, with hand-offs to the exchanges for helping consumers choose and enroll in a plan. The statute allowed this approach, stating, "The Secretary shall establish a system . . . under which residents of each State may apply for enrollment in, receive a determination of eligibility for participation in, and continue participation in, applicable State health subsidy programs."[11] The team did not, however, give it a great deal of consideration due to another statutory mandate requiring a seamless coverage continuum between Medicaid and the exchanges. Because Medicaid eligibility was a state function, the exchange team believed eligibility for tax credits should be handled at the state level as well. As a consequence, every state exchange was required to work with the state Medicaid agency to build its own eligibility and enrollment technology platform, even though income eligibility for tax credits was required to be exactly the same in every state (except for the variations in who was eligible for Medicaid because those eligible for Medicaid are not eligible for tax credits).

Many of the state exchanges did achieve a high level of Medicaid-exchange integration, though even minor tweaks to the eligibility rules for tax credits continue to complicate exchange operations. Ironically, due to a combination of political and technical reasons, the FFE did not achieve the same level of integration, so that in FFE states an individual coming through Healthcare.gov who appears to be Medicaid eligible is handed off to the state Medicaid agency. There also are cases, of course, in which an individual coming through the state Medicaid program appears to be eligible for a tax credit and is handed off to the exchange. These hand-offs inevitably result in some people falling through the cracks and suggest the potential value of a uniform national approach to eligibility with hand-offs to the exchanges or Medicaid for enrollment.

Exchange operations would be simpler and cheaper if the exchange's job was limited to helping individuals with precertified eligibility review plan options in their local area to enroll in a plan. A national eligibility service would ensure consistency across states, and because it would have to incorporate the income-related Medicaid eligibility rules for every state to ensure appropriate placements between the exchange and Medicaid, it would streamline Medicaid eligibility as well, with the caveat that there are other Medicaid eligibility categories and there will always be a small number of complicated cases that cannot be handled online. Not every state will prefer streamlined enrollment into Medicaid because—unlike the exchange tax credits, which are federally funded—Medicaid involves a mix of state and federal funding. However, the ACA calls for a seamless, "no wrong door" approach to eligibility, and the simplest and most direct way to achieve this would be a national eligibility service run by a world-class, customer-service-oriented technology company under strict federal oversight.

Taking Stock and Looking Ahead

Although the exchanges have stabilized over the last 2 years, they continue to suffer from low enrollment and high prices. There are many exchange issues that remain fluid and many lessons learned for future reform efforts.

Federal and State Exchanges

After 5 years of relative stability in the lineup of SBEs and FFE states, many of the 34 FFE states are reconsidering their options now that the price of technology has come down. This price drop has made it possible for states to charge insurers the same user fees as those insurers currently pay HHS and generate savings to increase consumer subsidies or otherwise bolster state markets. New Jersey and Pennsylvania are the test cases for 2020, and if they succeed, there could be a wave of states pursuing the same path for 2021. Cost savings are always attractive, but an even more important decision driver could be the policy flexibility that SBE states enjoy. The ACA will always be a complex mix of federal and state prerogatives; hence, there is no way for any state to insulate itself from the consequences of the 2020 election. Nonetheless, both red and blue states that look carefully will find reasons for trying to control their own destiny rather than speculating on what might happen in 2021. As a former state insurance commissioner in 2 states, I am an unabashed advocate for SBEs as a useful instrument of state policymaking. Indeed, SBEs give states a deeper investment in their individual insurance markets and the flexibility to be innovative in ways that Healthcare.gov simply cannot accommodate without a fundamental overhaul.

Role of Insurers in Government Health Care Programs

There are many lessons to be learned from the exchanges about the role of insurers in public programs. First, national insurers can be enthusiastic participants in public programs, even ones with a heavier regulatory overlay than the exchanges. In fact, insurers have proven remarkably flexible in accepting high levels of regulatory direction over how they deliver their products in exchange for stable pricing in Medicare and

Medicaid. This fact points to the next stage of reform as one in which the government (federal and state) sets the rules of the road, including whatever level of price regulation is deemed necessary, and then allows insurers to compete under those rules to enhance innovation.

Medicare for All has been a topic of particular focus since the 2018 election and is likely to continue to be a center-stage subject of debate through the next presidential race. But the fact that 75% of Medicaid beneficiaries and more than 30% of Medicare beneficiaries are served by insurers rather than directly by the government makes something like Medicare Advantage for All or Medicare for All that gives private insurers a role more likely than a Medicare for All program fully operated by the government. Limits on loss ratios and compliance with market rules can and should be part of holding insurers accountable, but these concerns do not negate the value that insurers are bringing to Medicare and Medicaid today as they operate within strict, government-set parameters that also offer insurers strong incentives to negotiate the details of innovative, value-based purchasing arrangements with providers.

State Flexibility

The ACA enhanced the role of the federal government in critical ways, but the law did not eliminate the challenge of finding the right balance between asserting federal power with prescriptive rules and empowering states with flexible rules or even broader deference. Although I generally would like to see that balance struck in favor of state deference, I remain a strong advocate for the core consumer protections in the ACA, including detailed rules about rating and risk pools and a federal insurance-purchase mandate. Absent these rules, insurers will find ways to siphon off the healthiest enrollees and give them better prices at the expense of those who need or want comprehensive coverage. Conversely, states should not be put in a straightjacket on issues such as network adequacy that call for nuanced judgment based on differences in local markets. The exchanges will continue to be a volatile testing ground for how best to balance federal and state prerogatives. If the job is done well, the states will be laboratories of democracy—able to innovate and test new ideas until enough consensus is reached to enact new federal reforms that further advance our quest for universal coverage at affordable prices.

Conclusion

The questions the exchange team confronted over the course of ACA implementation may yield different answers in the next wave of reform, but hopefully those answers will build on what the team learned about empowering states and regulating insurers in ways that serve the goals of reform—however those goals are defined.

CHAPTER 6

THE ACA, REPEAL, AND THE POLITICS OF BACKLASH

Jonathan Cohn

President Barack Obama called the 2010 midterm elections a "shel-lacking."[1] He was right. Democrats had lost 64 seats in the House of Representatives, relinquishing control of the chamber's majority just 4 years after they had seized it. And although the results reflected a variety of factors, including frustration with a still-sluggish economy, they also had a lot to do with anger over the Affordable Care Act (ACA).[2]

Republicans had spent the campaign attacking "Obamacare" as a boondoggle that would make private insurance more expensive, undermine Medicare for seniors, and generally wreck everything that was good about the US health care system. With the ACA still several years away from full implementation, and the messy, year-long effort to pass the law still a fresh memory, voters seemed inclined to agree. Public opinion tilted toward disapproval of the law by anywhere from a few percentage points to more than 10, depending on the survey. Republican voters were especially angry.[3] A subsequent study by a group of prominent political scientists concluded that the health care law had cost the Democrats about 25 seats, enough to give Republicans control of the chamber. The effects were subtle and a bit convoluted: As a *New York Times* polling analyst put it, "In a tough national environment in 2010, Democrats who voted against the ACA found it easier to distinguish themselves from the national party."[4] Whatever the mechanism, the result was clear: Democrats had passed the ACA, and now they were paying a political price for it.[5]

Jonathan Cohn is senior national correspondent at *HuffPost* and the author of *Sick*.

Eight years later, in the 2018 midterm elections, it was time for another shellacking. But this time it was the Republicans losing seats—42, to be precise. Although that was fewer than the number of seats Democrats had lost in 2010, the difference was largely a by-product of gerrymandering and where Democratic voters happen to live.[6] In the national popular vote—that is, among the total number of US voters casting ballots in House elections—the Democratic margin over Republicans was nearly 9 points, which was actually higher than the GOP's advantage from 2010. That was more than enough to put Democrats back in charge of the chamber, thereby depriving Republicans of their ability to repeal the ACA via legislation for the next 2 years.[7]

And that seemed appropriate, because health care had played a critical role in the 2018 election, just as it had in 2010. The GOP repeal effort had famously come up short in July 2017, when 3 Republican senators broke ranks with the majority. That left Republicans with just 49 votes to advance a bill out of that chamber. Along the way, the effort to pass repeal legislation, which actually continued for a few months after that, had stirred up intense opposition. The biggest outcry had come from liberal activists aligned with the Democrats who, like their conservative counterparts in 2010, had staged rallies and confronted individual lawmakers at district events. But public opinion had clearly shifted too. For the first time, polls showed, more people consistently approved of the ACA than disapproved of it.[8]

The campaign, in turn, had played out as a near-perfect reversal of 2010. Voters said repeatedly that health care was their most important issue, and Democrats simply could not stop talking about it.[9] More than half of their campaign ads focused on health care, according to tracking by the Wesleyan Media Project, and it was a dominant theme of their speeches as well.[10] Republicans reacted either by trying to dodge the subject, as many Democrats in 2010 had, or simply lying about their records—insisting that their repeal votes did not mean they were trying to take away the law's popular features, like protections for people with preexisting conditions. Media fact checkers called them on the deception, and the voters simply did not buy it.[11]

The 2018 results and the popular sentiment behind them did not represent a total vindication of the ACA. Far from it. The number of

Americans expressing disapproval of the law may have ceased to be a plurality, but they still represented a substantial portion of the country—more than 40% in most surveys. Feelings about the law had a distinctly partisan tinge: Republican voters still did not like it; Democrats did. But the ambivalence also reflected ongoing frustration with the ACA's performance. Even with the law fully in place, millions were still struggling to pay for health care, sometimes because they remained uninsured and sometimes because the insurance they had cost too much or covered too little. Heading into the 2020 elections, health care remains a top issue according to the polls, in part because so many people are eager for more help in some form or fashion and want Washington to act.

And yet the shift in public opinion, however tentative, is meaningful all the same. It is a reminder of why passing any major social reforms in the United States—but especially health care reforms—is difficult. It is a sign of growing polarization in American politics. And it is a signal that, for all of its well-documented flaws, the ACA has provided the public with something that it truly values and does not want to give up.

The Democrats Succeed—at a Cost

The US political system thwarts change, and that is very much by design. The framers of the Constitution, wary of reckless majorities giving in to political passions, insisted that passing laws require assent of both the president and Congress—and, even then, from 2 separate, differently constituted houses, one of which had members serving staggered 6-year terms.

But change for the last few decades has been decidedly more difficult for Democrats than for Republicans because the clustering of their supporters in cities and suburbs, especially along the coasts, tilts representation in the House and, more so, the Senate toward relatively conservative parts of the country.[12] Another reason change is especially difficult for Democrats trying to enact progressive (or, as it used to be called, liberal) legislation is that such initiatives frequently run up against powerful wealthy interests in the business community that have leverage over Congress through advertising, direct lobbying, and campaign contributions.[13]

Throw in the filibuster, which in the 1990s evolved from an occasional outburst of legislative obstruction to a de facto shield against simple majority rule, and the daunting scale of obstacles standing in the way of progressive reforms finally come into view. In principle, senators representing less than one-fifth of the country's population have the power to block a bill.[14] Or, to put it another way, a Democrat looking to enact an ambitious, sweeping piece of progressive legislation—say, an overhaul of the US health care system—could in theory have to win over senators representing more than 80% of the American public.

That kind of threshold is virtually impossible to meet, given the deep investment so many powerful interests have in the status quo. It is not just the insurance and drug industries that profit from the existing system and resist major changes; it is also the hospitals and doctors and other care providers, whose bills together account for the majority of health care spending, and to some extent groups like unions, who despite their progressive ideological leanings are wary of anything that threatens existing arrangements they have negotiated in collective bargaining. The aversion to change—any change—extends to the public as well, which despite its frustrations with the problems of American health care also gets skittish about alternatives. It is all part of a phenomenon that political scientists call "path dependence," and it helps explain why transforming health care might be the single hardest thing for progressive Democrats to attempt.[15]

This political environment was very much on Obama's and the Democrats' minds as they embarked upon their reform effort in 2009. They were determined to act because Obama had promised it as a candidate and because the cause of universal health care—of making sure it is a right, not a privilege, so that nobody struggles to get the care they need—had been such a core part of the Democratic Party's identity going all the way back to the 1940s. But they also tailored their plans in a way they hoped would overcome—or at least get around—all of those familiar obstacles.

In particular, they adopted a scheme heavily reliant on private insurance partly because at least some Republicans and conservatives had supported versions of it in the past. Democratic leaders courted individual GOP lawmakers, especially members of the all-important Senate Finance Committee, chaired by Montana's Max Baucus. They pledged to keep the proposal budget neutral, partly out of principle but partly out of political necessity, as more conservative Democrats (like Kent Conrad, the North Dakota senator and chairman of the Budget Committee) insisted upon it. In yet another nod to the Republicans and conservative Democrats, they gave states power over implementation. They negotiated directly with health care's special interests, eventually announcing deals with almost every sector. And they decided to leave the predominant form of insurance for working-age Americans, employer-sponsored coverage, largely as it was.[16]

Each one of these decisions entailed tradeoffs, and those tradeoffs help explain the skepticism and hostility that the ACA has generated for most of its legislative life. The extended negotiations with Republicans, which eventually netted one GOP vote in committee (from Maine senator Olympia Snowe) but nothing on the final floor vote, turned the proposal into a punching bag for opponents—never more clearly than in August 2009, while negotiations in Finance had bogged down and Tea Party protesters first descended upon Democratic lawmakers back in their districts. That anger only grew as the process dragged on, in no small part because concessions they had made to get their 60 Senate votes, like dropping a public insurance option, had disheartened their supporters. It also did not help that, in order to secure the final vote, Democratic leaders agreed to deals like extra money for hospitals in Nebraska, home of a key senator.

The Republicans Fight—and Nearly Win

When Obama signed the ACA legislation in March 2010, many hoped the debate would enter a new phase—one in which the intense feelings about the law might die down so that officials could get to work on implementing the law and, if need be, lawmakers could adjust it along the way.

Those hopes did not last long. Republicans introduced bills to repeal the ACA immediately after it became law and turned the cause into one of their defining goals, as central to their party identity as the cause of universal coverage was to the Democrats. Between 2010 and 2016 House Republicans passed repeal bills more than 50 times.[17] Although the votes felt largely symbolic, given that the GOP did not control the Senate until 2015 and did not control the White House until 2017, those votes were part of a much broader campaign to undermine the law.

The most consequential element of that campaign was, arguably, the actions by GOP state officials who refused to expand their Medicaid programs as the law's architects had hoped. They could do so because of leeway the Supreme Court had given them in the first of 2 major challenges to the law.[18] The terms of the expansion, with the federal government picking up nearly all of the cost, were still highly favorable to states—so much so that plenty of Republican governors, despite their open opposition to the ACA, grabbed the money because of what it could mean for their uninsured residents and the health care providers that served them. But in states like Florida, Georgia, and Texas, what seemed to many like obvious self-interest gave way to partisan interest—and literally millions of low-income people remained uninsured as a result.[19]

The GOP officials in these places made no secret of their feelings about Obamacare, trashing the program at every opportunity and joining lawsuits against it (including one working its way up through the courts as this goes to press[20]). In taking these steps, state-level Republicans were taking their cues from Washington, where congressional leaders had long since embraced the call by Senate Majority Leader Mitch McConnell (R-KY) to oppose Obama at all costs and spent the years after the ACA's enactment seeking ways to sabotage its implementation.[21]

Sometimes this intense, relentless opposition to the ACA produced nothing more than spectacle, as when GOP leaders provoked a government shutdown in 2013, demanding that Democrats agree to repeal the law. (They did not, and the GOP had to back down.) But sometimes the opposition had real-world effects. A case in point was Republican attacks on the ACA's so-called risk corridor program, which was designed to insulate insurers from excessive losses. Conservatives attacked it as an insurer bailout, even as a similar program had long existed in Medicare Part D without controversy, and in late 2015 Marco Rubio, the Florida GOP senator, secured a provision inside a year-end spending agreement to eliminate the program's funding. In the coming years, with payouts from the program a pittance of what the government had promised, insurers had to jack up prices, and some smaller carriers had to shut down altogether.[22]

Those problems did not help the ACA's public image, although, to be clear, frustration with the law also had a lot to do with its design and function. The botched rollout of the Healthcare.gov website, which was basically nonfunctional after its launch, turned into a public relations disaster for the Obama administration. The public took notice. In early and mid-2014 opposition in the Henry J. Kaiser Family Foundation tracking poll hit and exceeded 50%, its worst result ever.[23]

The public's reaction was not simply about the website problems, though. The actual insurance options available through the ACA left a substantial number of Americans unhappy and more than a few irate. Insurers were canceling old plans (despite Obama's promise that people could keep their plans if they liked them) and charging higher premiums for the new ones because now they had to offer more benefits and cover people with preexisting conditions. Both of those things cost money. The ACA's subsidies offset the increases for many but not all of the people buying them. In the years that followed, especially in states where GOP officials were at best disinterested and at worst hostile to the law's implementation, insurers had to raise premiums substantially or abandon markets altogether, fueling more resentment of the law. Worries about "bare counties" with no insurers left became an annual ritual, and a few places came close, although no county ever lost insurers completely.

Subsequent research found that the number of people who actually lost plans because of the ACA was relatively small. One reliable estimate put the figure at 2.6 million—a substantial number of people in absolute terms but just a tiny portion of the population.[24] Many of them ultimately found cheaper plans, while even those spending more were usually getting coverage with benefits and protections for people with preexisting conditions that their old plans had lacked. But especially in an era of such intense party polarization, a vast swath of Americans, whom the ACA had not affected in visible ways, simply took their cues from partisan leaders. Intensity was predominantly on the Republican side, which was united in its desire for total repeal and, by 2015 and 2016, had come to see the law as symbolic of everything they hated about Obama and his administration. Democrats dissented but always with qualifiers because, after all, they too saw the flaws and wanted something better.[25]

Nor was it just what the politicians were saying. Republicans had a loyal partner in right-wing media, especially Fox News, which pumped out negative coverage of the law while barely acknowledging its accomplishments, if it acknowledged them at all. On the left, the more partisan outlets were already looking ahead to how to improve upon the ACA or replace it with the kind of single-payer system progressives had wanted all along. As for the mainstream news media, which conservatives dismissed as a tool of liberals, it covered the ACA story the way it covers all issues: it focused on the conflicts and shortcomings.[26]

What effect all of this media coverage and partisanship had on perceptions of the ACA is impossible to say with any certainty. But it probably did not increase the law's standing with the public, and it most likely diminished it.

Repeal (Mostly) Fails and the Law (Mostly) Survives

That set the stage for 2016 and the Republican wins, especially President Donald Trump's victory, that seemed to make repeal a near inevitability. It had been the GOP's signature crusade for nearly a decade, after all, and it was among the promises that Trump, as a candidate, had made most vocally and relentlessly.[27]

Republicans came awfully close to succeeding. With just a little more deliberation (to address the frustration that Arizona senator John McCain expressed over the rushed process) or just a few more adjustments on the policy side (to address the qualms that Maine senator Susan Collins and Alaska senator Lisa Murkowski had about the impact on their constituents), it is possible that GOP leaders could have pried loose the one vote they needed to get a bill out of the Senate and into a conference committee negotiation with the House, which had passed a bill back in May.

But long before that late-night debate when McCain gave his memorable thumbs-down gesture on the Senate floor, the GOP repeal effort was in big trouble because of promises its leaders had made and had no way to keep.

Going all the way back to the very first repeal votes and really all the way back to the initial ACA debate in 2009 and 2010, Republicans said they had a superior alternative—a health care plan that would provide better coverage to as many or more people for less money. The most audacious promises came directly from Trump, who as a candidate and then a newly elected president vowed that "we're going to have insurance for everybody," that "everybody's going to be taken care of much better than they're taken care of now."[28] Once he took office, his lieutenants echoed and amplified these promises, like when House Speaker Paul Ryan (R-WI) vowed that Republicans would make sure "no one is worse off."[29]

Republicans also boasted that repeal would reduce federal spending—and on that count, they were telling the truth. Reducing government's reach into health care was the whole point of the repeal project. They wanted less federal spending, fewer regulations, and lower taxes. Their plans reflected these imperatives, and an honest defense of them would have emphasized how they advanced longtime conservative and GOP goals, like allowing businesses and overall markets to operate with less interference from the government while minimizing taxes, especially taxes on the wealthy. In the conservative worldview all of these are good for the economy and society more broadly.

But Republicans could not escape the tradeoffs of policy any more than Democrats could 10 years before. The tradeoff of scaling back regulation, spending, and taxes is that government cannot do as much to help people get health care. It is simple math, really. Insurance is so expensive that the only way to put it within reach of everybody, at least in the short term, is to have the government spend a lot of money in the form of subsidies or direct provisions of coverage. Any system that relies on private insurance, even in part, will require a lot of regulation because otherwise insurers will avoid covering expensive services and the people who are likely to need them. Scale back regulation and spending, and many more people will end up struggling to pay their health care bills.[30]

As the CBO eventually confirmed, that math held for every reform proposal that Republicans considered, including the one that eventually passed the House and the variants that came up for votes on the Senate floor.[31] This did not sit well with the public. Since the ACA's enactment, millions had gotten coverage through the Medicaid expansion, whose funding Republicans were going to eliminate, or with the help of federal subsidies for private coverage, which Republicans proposed to redirect and shrink. Others had come to count upon guarantees of coverage for people with preexisting conditions, which Republicans had proposed to undermine, albeit in roundabout ways.

The numbers who stood to lose coverage reached into the tens of millions, dwarfing those who had faced plan cancellations when the ACA's regulations were implemented. (Conservatives complained that CBO overestimated the coverage loss and CBO itself later reduced its estimates, but even under more favorable assumptions, the coverage loss would have been massive.) The number of Americans who benefited one way or another from preexisting condition protections was even larger than the number who had gained coverage, in the sense that most people either had a serious condition or knew somebody who did. Repeal now sounded a lot less appealing.[32]

Even at the nadirs of the ACA's popularity, after enactment and then again during the Healthcare.gov fiasco, polls showed that most of the law's elements were extremely popular, even with Republicans[33]— just as the Medicaid expansion, long thought to be politically vulnerable because its constituency was poor, traditionally powerless people, turned out to have deep reservoirs of support in some of the most politically conservative parts of the country. One reason for this was the nation's opioid epidemic, which had been hammering places like Ohio and West Virginia. In those states expanded Medicaid programs had become a primary funder of treatment programs.[34]

Repeal's last gasp in 2017, which happened not when McCain said no but in September, when GOP leaders backed off plans to vote on a new bill from Senators Bill Cassidy (R-LA) and Lindsay Graham (R-SC), did not end the party's interest in eliminating the ACA. Two years later, even after the 2018 midterms, Trump insisted he had not given up—and bragged that he had already taken several steps to weaken it.

The boast, such that it was, was legitimate. The administration had canceled funding for outreach, stopped paying a key set of subsidies for insurers, and rewritten regulations about the kind of insurance that private insurers could sell.[35] It had also changed the rules about how states could design their Medicaid programs, making it possible for states to add work requirements. Congress got in on the action too, passing a tax bill reducing to zero the ACA's individual mandate penalty for people who did not carry insurance. Trump, who had supported the provision, signed it.[36]

The effects of these moves were not always what the administration and its allies had intended. The removal of those subsidies to insurers, for example, actually made insurance cheaper for many poorer people because of the way the ACA linked tax credits to the price of coverage.[37] And the changes to Medicaid ran into some skeptical federal judges who halted, at least temporarily, their implementation. But the cumulative effect was to reduce the ACA's reach, especially into the middle class. By 2019 the number of Americans without insurance had started to rise for the first time since the law's enactment. Many experts believed Trump administration policies were a significant factor in that shift.[38]

Still, the program on its tenth anniversary seems to be stable in terms of policy and politics—or at least as stable as government programs can be. It remains under assault in the legislatures and in the courts partly because so many people continue to struggle with health care and partly because Republicans remain so committed to its demise. But the efforts at repeal had reinforced what the polls had said all along: Americans wanted to build on the ACA rather than wreck it, to keep moving toward universal coverage rather than away from it. The debates over Obamacare would never stop, just like the debates over health care policy would never stop. But they would never look quite the same either.

CHAPTER 7

THE ACA AND THE REPUBLICAN ALTERNATIVE

Eric Cantor

The Background

To understand the Republican perspective on the ACA, you need to rewind to the health care debate during the 2008 campaign and the process that led to the enactment of the 2009 American Recovery and Reinvestment Act (a.k.a. the stimulus).

The 2008 Campaign

It is not well remembered now, but in 2008 Senator John McCain, the Republican nominee for president, unveiled his own ambitious health care reform proposal.[1] Senator McCain proposed to provide every family without access to or who declined employer-provided health insurance a $5,000 tax credit for the purchase of health insurance. For those with preexisting conditions, the McCain proposal included funding for states to develop high-risk pools and other mechanisms to ensure access to coverage. McCain paid for his proposal by limiting the exclusion from taxation of employer-provided health insurance.

Senator McCain's approach was consistent with longstanding conservative views on health care reform. It would expand insurance coverage through an individual tax credit and break what was viewed as the accidental connection between health insurance and employment (a

Eric Cantor, JD, is the vice chairman and a managing director at Moelis & Company and served as a US congressman from Virginia (2001–2014), including 4 years as House majority leader (2010–2014).

result of employer-provided health insurance not being subject to federal wage controls during World War II and the IRS determining that such insurance would be exempt from taxation). Putting consumers in charge of buying their own insurance would also make them more cost conscious, which would ultimately lower health care costs. The McCain approach drew praise from conservative think tanks, including the Heritage Foundation and the CATO Institute.[2]

Senator Obama, however, was relentless in his attacks. In speeches and ads he called the McCain plan "radical," said that McCain would tax health care for the first time ever, and that 20 million Americans would lose their employer-provided health insurance, neglecting to mention that the same study indicated that 21 million would buy insurance in the private market. Although the senator and his allies could have focused on net coverage, it was clear that the politically winning argument was what voters might lose.[3]

That argument was so powerful that Senator Obama promised that under his plan, if you liked your health care plan, you could keep it. As he said during one of the debates, "Number one, let me just repeat, if you've got a health care plan that you like, you can keep it. . . . All I'm going to do is help you to lower the premiums on it. You'll still have choice of doctor."[4]

Many Republicans concluded that although McCain may have had the right policy, the politics were simply unwinnable. Indeed, a 2008 exit poll found, "One-in-three voters said they are very worried about being able to afford the health care services they need, and these voters backed Obama by a 65%-to-32% margin."[5]

In the decade since 2008 the GOP has never once seriously considered limiting the exclusion for health insurance. This is perhaps the biggest contributing factor to the GOP being unable to develop a comprehensive alternative to the ACA: without the revenue from limiting the exclusion, it was difficult to fund insurance for low-income individuals lacking employer-provided insurance.

But Republicans were probably right about the politics. In 2019, the Democrat-controlled House of Representatives passed a bill 419–6 to permanently repeal the ACA's tax on high-cost employer-provided health insurance plans (the so-called Cadillac tax), which was a modest, back-door version of eliminating the tax exclusion.[6]

The Stimulus

The first legislative priority for President Obama was an economic stimulus package. The nation had entered what would be the worst economic downturn since the Great Depression, and taking steps to stabilize the economy was at the top of the to-do list for Republicans and Democrats alike.

President-elect Obama set the tone for how he envisioned proceeding on the stimulus when he visited the Capitol 2 weeks before the inauguration to hold a meeting with the bipartisan congressional leadership.[7] The president-elect made clear that he wanted a bipartisan bill and that he wanted not just to hear Republican ideas but also to include them.

House Republicans took the president-elect's offer seriously. We began to develop a set of proposals that we thought Democrats could support. A couple of days after the inauguration I presented the president with a 5-point plan. The president remarked, "Nothing on here looks outlandish or crazy to me."[8] Although we certainly had our differences, it was clear that there was an opening for a bipartisan stimulus package.

At the same meeting, however, the president also curtly cut off a discussion he disagreed with, declaring, "Elections have consequences, and I won." This was a sentiment that Democratic leaders—with their majorities in the House and Senate—seemed to embrace. So which path would we go down—bipartisan negotiations or to the victor go the spoils?

Within a week we had our answer: the initial draft of the stimulus bill passed the House without the support of a single Republican, and within 3 weeks the final version passed the same way. What had happened?

The Democratic majority in Congress, well on their way to drafting the bill, were not very interested in pausing to negotiate over including Republican ideas. In addition, some of the president's advisers thought they would win some GOP support without having to engage Republican leaders or even rank-and-file members. After all, the president was popular and supporting the economy was something that had to be done.

Unrecognized at the time was how the stimulus negotiations—or lack thereof—would set the tone for negotiations on legislation for the next 2 years, including the ACA: Republicans were convinced that Democrats were not really interested in our ideas, and Democrats were convinced that Republicans would never help them pass anything.

The Leadup: January to August 2009

The development of what would become the ACA followed a script familiar to the stimulus, just over a longer period: bipartisan public entreaties, partisan legislative development.

Having pledged as a candidate to televise the negotiations over health care, President Obama launched his reform effort with a televised "White House Forum on Health Reform."[9] Attendees included representatives of various health care sectors, interest groups, think tanks, and Republican and Democratic members of Congress.

Real negotiations do not take place in front of cameras, and Republicans viewed the forum for what it was: a media stunt.

Only slightly better were the White House's efforts in the spring of 2009 to court a handful of moderate and vulnerable rank-and-file House Republicans with private meetings such as the one in May with White House Chief of Staff Rahm Emanuel and nearly a dozen Republicans.[10] Often leaked to the press, such meetings seemed more about feigning an interest in bipartisanship than an effort to really negotiate a bipartisan deal.

More promising were the negotiations of the Senate's so-called Gang of Six, 3 Republicans and 3 Democrats led by Senate Finance chairman Max Baucus (D-MT).[11] If there was going to be a bipartisan deal, it would likely emerge from such a gang.

Yet the fundamentals of arithmetic and political pressure hamstrung productive negotiations: Democrats did not need Republican votes in the House or even in the Senate, given the 60 seats Democrats held. Liberals in the House and in the Senate were pushing for a more progressive approach than Republicans would ever support. Indeed, in June of 2009 House Democrats unveiled a draft proposal with no Republican input, and various elements—including a public option— that would never lead to a bipartisan agreement.[12] Not to be outdone, in July of 2009 the Senate Health, Education, Labor, and Pensions

Committee, chaired by the ailing Senator Ted Kennedy (D-MA), approved its version of health care reform with a "strong public option."[13]

If there were any push for moderation and a more bipartisan approach, it would need to come from the administration. But from my conversations with them, including with Nancy-Ann DeParle, who was heading up health care for the White House, it was clear that the administration was going to stick with the approach being developed by congressional Democrats. When I would note that nothing even close to the current proposals could pass with Republican support, the response was essentially: "So be it."

Rather than serving as a starting point for potential future negotiations, these partisan proposals solidified Republican opposition and deepened the differences between the parties. And as the opposition within the Republican base grew, it made it even more difficult to find common ground. Members went home for the August recess to raucous town halls where the pending health care bill was roundly pilloried.[14] By the time Republicans returned to the Capitol, any hope of a truly bipartisan deal was dashed, and even the Gang of Six threw in the towel.

Partisanship Rules: September to December 2009

In an effort to reclaim momentum, President Obama addressed a joint session of Congress in September. Yet the speech was almost immediately remembered for the outburst by Representative Joe Wilson (R-SC), who shouted "You lie!" when the president said his proposal would not cover undocumented immigrants.[15] Leaving aside the obvious, terrible breach in decorum, the moment accurately captures the gulf between the parties on health care. There would be no bipartisan deal.

On November 7 the House passed its bill 220–215, with 39 Democrats joining all but one Republican in opposition.[16] In a dramatic Christmas Eve vote, the Senate passed its version of the health care bill 60–39, with no Republican support.

Some Democrats were hopeful that Senator Olympia Snowe, a moderate Republican from Maine, might support the bill. She had supported an earlier version in the Senate Finance Committee. But

Senator Snowe shared the concerns of other Republicans about the impact of the new taxes on employment and the vast new government bureaucracy that was being created. Before the Christmas Eve vote she expressed her "extreme disappointment" in the way the bill had evolved, noting that "there was zero opportunity to amend the bill or modify it, and Democrats had no incentive to reach across the aisle."[17]

Like the stimulus, at the end of the day the political pressure on Democrats to go it alone without compromise was stronger than the desire for a truly bipartisan deal.

The Massachusetts Bombshell

On January 19, 2010, the unbelievable happened: Massachusetts voters elected a Republican, Scott Brown, to fill the remainder of the late Senator Kennedy's term. Brown ran on a pledge to be the 41st senator against Obamacare.

With Brown in the Senate, it appeared that the Democrats would need to start over if they wanted to pass a health care bill. I even suggested, somewhat in jest, that the place to start was the House Republican alternative.[18] Although I knew Democrats would never simply accept our plan, my point was clear: it would take more than tinkering around the edges of the Democrat bill to produce a truly bipartisan reform.

Déjà Vu

On February 25, 2010, President Obama convened a 7-hour bipartisan summit at Blair House to discuss the pending health care bill. Unlike the White House summit a year earlier, this meeting included the committee and legislative leaders from both parties. But crucially, just like the 2009 meeting, it was to be televised. We knew it was a show, an attempt to feign bipartisanship for the cameras without any real negotiation. The House Republican leadership convened our members who would be participating in the summit and developed our game plan:

we would make the case for starting over by exposing what we saw as the flaws in a 2,400-page, trillion-dollar takeover of the American health care system.

I even brought a copy of the bill to the summit, prompting the president to scold me for bringing a prop.[19] It was a prop, but the truth is that the president had invited us Republicans as props to sit before the cameras. We saw the meeting as a precursor to the Democrats' go-it-alone strategy—a possibility that was reported simultaneously with the summit.[20] And indeed, the president concluded the summit with a veiled threat that Democrats were prepared to go it alone and test who was right with the voters that November. Needless to say, we did not mind taking our case to the voters.

Enactment

Less than a month later House Democrats passed the bill that had passed the Senate on Christmas Eve by a vote of 219–212, without a single Republican vote. At the same time, the House and Senate passed amendments to the bill using a process known as reconciliation that only requires 51 votes in the Senate. It was a bold exercise of raw, political, majoritarian power.

Tensions were high as Congress passed the bill with protests, vandalism, and even threats of violence.[21] These passions would not simply fade away. The Democrats now owned Obamacare, a moniker even the president began to embrace, and Republicans had become defined in large measure by our opposition.

As the president had suggested, we would let the voters decide.

The Voters Have Their Say

Election Day 2010 was a tidal wave for Republicans. We won 63 seats, capturing control of the House of Representatives. In the Senate, Republicans picked up 6 seats, with Democrats only preserving their majority as a result of the makeup of the seats up for election that year.

The view of voters when it came to the health care law could not have been clearer. Exit polls showed 81% of Republicans and 53% of independents wanted it repealed.[22]

For the Tea Party, which had started as a rebellion against government spending, repeal became the top priority. Republicans might not be able to reverse the stimulus—the money had been spent—but they could repeal Obamacare.

Divided Government

Our new House Republican majority was keen to keep our promise of repeal. On the first day of the new Congress I introduced H.R. 2, the Repealing the Job-Killing Health Care Law Act. The title reflected not just the ongoing concern about the economy but also the fact that the nonpartisan CBO had estimated that the ACA would reduce the amount of labor in the economy.

After 7 hours of debate the House passed the bill 245–189. With 3 Democrats voting for repeal, repeal had more bipartisan support than the law's passage. But with Democrats in charge of the Senate and Obama still in the White House, it was only a symbolic victory; indeed, the Senate never took up H.R. 2.

Over the course of 2011 and 2012 numerous opportunities arose to repeal or defund various individual pieces of the law. We viewed such efforts as not only consistent with our electoral mandate but also as potential opportunities for incremental success. Indeed, over a half dozen provisions of Obamacare were repealed as a result of our efforts. But politically speaking, the effort began to backfire. As the press ran headlines like "House Obamacare Repeal: Thirty-Third Time's the Charm?,"[23] our mandate began to be portrayed as an obsession.

Of course, the only way to actually repeal Obamacare would be to elect a Republican president and a Republican Senate.

Heading into the 2012 election, we were optimistic. While no one was measuring the drapes, our staff had begun preparing for the possibility of a unified Republican government come January 2013. One of the first orders of business would have been to set up a reconciliation bill: the same procedural tool that had gotten Obamacare across the finish line would be used to quickly repeal it. Because the exchanges would not open until 2014, we could enact repeal and then focus on a Republican version of health care reform.

But the planning was for naught. President Obama was reelected and Democrats slightly expanded their Senate majority. Republicans still controlled the House. Republican voters still wanted repeal, but there was no path to legislative victory.

As the 113th Congress got underway, Republicans and Democrats returned to normal fights over spending and regulations. We continued our oversight of Obamacare and had occasional votes on the most unpopular aspects of the law, like the individual mandate.

As October 2013 approached, it was clear that the Obamacare exchanges would come online.

The Futile Fight

Spurred by outside groups, Senator Ted Cruz (R-TX) and his allies in the House led an effort that resulted in a 16-day government shutdown in October 2013. The strategy, if you can call it that, was that the Republican majority in the House could force a defunding of Obamacare by refusing to pass a bill to keep the government open unless it contained a defunding provision. The obvious problems were that the Democrat-controlled Senate would never pass such a defunding (they stripped out the provision), and even if they were to pass it, President Obama would never sign it.

It was a doomed desperation play from the beginning. So why did Republican congressional leaders go along? Simple: for Republican base voters, it had quickly become a test of whether you were willing to truly fight to stop Obamacare before it took full effect. Few Republicans wanted to go home and explain why what we all wanted to happen could not happen. Ironically, the government shutdown distracted public attention from what, by all accounts, was a disastrous rollout of the ACA enrollment website.

The shutdown, along with the media assessment of the numerous repeal votes, gave the Democrats an opening: they could portray Republicans as simultaneously obsessed with relitigating the past and being ineffective. In his 2014 State of the Union Address Obama put it this way:

> Now, I do not expect to convince my Republican friends on the merits of this law.
>
> [Laughter. Chuckles. Laughter.]
>
> But I know that the American people are not interested in refighting old battles. So again, if you have specific plans to cut costs, cover more people, increase choice, tell America what you'd do differently. Let's see if the numbers add up.
>
> [Applause.]
>
> But let's not have another 40-something votes to repeal a law that's already helping millions of Americans like Amanda.
>
> [Cheers. Applause.]
>
> The first 40 were plenty. We all owe it to the American people to say what we're for, not just what we're against.[24]

What We Are For

It became almost cliché to say the GOP did not have an alternative to Obamacare. In truth, House Republicans offered an alternative in 2009 when Obamacare was being considered in the House. Mindful of what Senator McCain had just gone through with his plan, we avoided touching the employer exclusion and instead took a more limited approach. Rather than guaranteeing universal coverage, like the Democratic plan, we focused on lowering costs.

Our plan would have protected consumers by preventing insurers from imposing annual or lifetime spending caps or unjustly canceling policies. It empowered individuals by allowing them to use Health Savings Accounts (HSAs) to pay insurance premiums. A new Universal Access Program expanded high-risk pools and reinsurance programs to protect those with preexisting conditions. Medical liability reforms and expanding association health plans helped lower costs. The nonpartisan CBO estimated that our plan would lower premiums in the small-group market by an estimated 7% to 10% and in the individual market by an estimated 5% to 8%.[25]

But by 2014 this alternative was long forgotten in the public debate. I was tired of the attacks that the GOP had no plan and was convinced that a comprehensive alternative was our last and only hope to push back on Obamacare. Two days after Obama's State of the Union Address, I announced that House Republicans would vote on an alternative to Obamacare that year.[26]

Two major hurdles stood in the way.

First, after Obamacare's enactment, the test for an alternative was a comparison of coverage numbers. (Never mind that the growing concern of the American people was affordability, and premiums were rising.) Republicans would never agree to an individual mandate, and it would be impossible to maintain Obamacare's coverage numbers without one.

Second, expanding coverage for those without employer-provided insurance and ensuring access for those with preexisting conditions (without an individual mandate) costs a significant amount of money. And as the Democrats discovered, there are no easy pay-fors. The obvious place to go was some limitation on the employer exclusion. Even though it was 6 years after then-candidate Obama's very successful attacks on the McCain plan for taking away employer-provided health care and so much had changed in the debate since then, no one viewed this as a viable approach.

Many Republicans viewed rolling out a plan with pay-fors as simply inviting new rounds of attacks. Why do it if you cannot make law? And with Obama in the White House, there was no way to make law.

I left Congress in the summer of 2014. The House never did consider a comprehensive replacement bill.

Now It Is for Real, but the Debate Has Changed

The 2016 election was not fought on the issue of health care, but it managed to produce the unified Republican government we were hoping for in 2012.

And Republicans dusted off the plan from 2012 to use reconciliation for a quick strike. But it was not meant to be. The divisions among Republicans of how much or how little of Obamacare to repeal proved to be insurmountable. (Full repeal was no longer an option even for the most strident Obamacare opponents.)

Ironically, even though 28 million Americans remained uninsured in 2016,[27] the great cause that drove the enactment of the ACA—universal coverage—was supplanted by a bigger concern for most voters in 2018: cost.[28] The country had moved on from the debates that surrounded the ACA.

The Democrats Attack the ACA

As America heads toward its 6th election since the enactment of the ACA, it is remarkable to note that today the attacks on the law are more likely to come from the left than from the right.[29] Some of the leading contenders for the Democratic presidential nomination have embraced Medicare for All as a replacement for the ACA.[30] Even the most moderate candidates lament that the ACA failed to include a public option.[31]

Conclusion

Looking back on the past 10 years and how health care reform continues to bedevil our country and dominate our politics, it is hard not to wish that we had found a way to come together as Democrats and Republicans and enact true and durable reforms—reforms that would have both expanded coverage and truly bent the cost curve for all Americans.

There are many reasons that did not happen. For Democrats, the ability to "go it alone" in unified government meant that maximizing policy preferences was more important than bipartisan compromise. (This affliction is not unique to the Democratic Party. The same was true of Republicans when they had unified control of government and were passing tax reform.)

For Republicans, the initial public backlash against Obamacare and the political opportunity it created was simply too strong to ignore. Taking advantage of it helped us secure the majority in the 2010 elections. (Again, not an affliction unique to the Republican Party: today the electoral benefits of opposing President Trump at virtually every turn are more appealing to Democrats than compromise.)

Where do we go from here? If I could make one recommendation, it would be for both parties to pull back and take a different tack. Rather than relitigating the ACA or pursuing a universal government plan, both parties would benefit from focusing on how we bend the cost curve. Reforming the payment system to focus on outcomes and quality rather than the rate paid for individual procedures performed or services provided is a crucial first step. Policy experts in both parties have done good work on how we can begin to reform the system. The benefits would accrue not just to government programs like Medicare and Medicaid but also to the millions of Americans who have private insurance through their employer.

Admittedly, quality-based payment reforms, incentives for disease prevention, and chronic disease management do not fit well into political stump speeches or 30-second ads. But after a decade of partisan battles, maybe that is just the prescription our country needs.

Part III

LAW AND GOVERNANCE

Constitution's "original meaning." It was, in many aspects, a challenge to the legitimacy of much of the domestic policy progress made since the New Deal.

The judicial battle over the ACA has unfolded in 3 phases. The first was litigation over the law's constitutionality, which began the day the ACA was enacted and culminated in the Supreme Court's 2012 decision in *National Federation of Independent Business v. Sebelius (NFIB)* upholding the law.[1] The second phase, which began almost as soon as the first ended, involved litigation over whether the statutory terms of the law contained a flaw that had the effect of precluding tax subsidies to make the purchase of insurance affordable in many states—a technical issue but one that would have decimated the ACA in much of the country had the Supreme Court ruled against the government. The ACA survived that challenge too, as the Supreme Court held in *King v. Burwell* that subsidies were available in all states.[2] The third phase is unfolding now. The legal issues at each phase have been different, but at bottom it has been just one fight. It is the fight over the legitimacy of using the power of the federal government to provide affordable health care for all Americans.[3]

Round 1:
National Federation of Independent Business v. Sebelius

The Challenges

President Obama signed the Affordable Care Act into law on March 23, 2010. An onslaught of litigation soon ensued, focusing on 2 challenges that had been developed by jurisprudential conservatives working in academia, policy positions, and law firms: that the ACA's individual mandate—the requirement that people maintain health insurance or pay a tax penalty—exceeded Congress's power to regulate interstate commerce because it did not regulate existing commerce but instead "regulated inactivity" (or forced citizens to engage in commerce) and that the law's Medicaid expansion violated the 10th Amendment's "anticoercion" principle (a principle that had never before been invoked to invalidate a federal law) by forcing states to accept the expansion because they would suffer an unsustainable blow of losing all existing Medicaid funding if they did not.

The Individual Mandate. In one sense, it was no surprise that the attack focused on the individual mandate. The requirement that people purchase health insurance or pay a tax penalty was deeply unpopular. As a legal matter, it could be characterized as a step beyond what had previously been understood to be the furthest extension of the commerce power. As most law students learn, the outer bound of Congress's power to regulate interstate commerce had long been thought to be the Supreme Court's 1941 decision in *Wickard v. Filburn*, which upheld a law that restricted the amount of wheat that farmers could grow.[4] Congress enacted that New Deal measure to combat the collapse of agricultural commodity prices; it sought to stabilize prices in the wheat market by limiting supply. A farmer who claimed he grew wheat solely for his own consumption challenged the law. He argued that applying the law to him exceeded Congress's power to regulate interstate commerce because his wheat never became part of commerce. Rejecting that challenge, the Court upheld the law on the theory that comparable conduct by many farmers could reduce aggregate demand and undermine the law's aim of stabilizing wheat prices.

The ACA's insurance mandate was like the law at issue in *Wickard* in that it sought to stabilize an interstate market—the individual insurance market—that Congress has the power to regulate under the Commerce Clause. However, it imposed a purchase requirement, not a prohibition. It could, therefore, be characterized as compelling commerce—that is, forcing people to participate in a market they otherwise would avoid, which is a step beyond *Wickard*. Even worse, the challengers claimed, the power to compel commerce was a power without limit. Theoretically, if Congress could require every American household to purchase insurance in order to stabilize that market, it could also compel Americans to purchase automobiles in order to prevent the collapse of the domestic auto industry. Congress could even compel the purchase of broccoli (what Justice Ginsburg would later dub the "broccoli horrible") to prevent the collapse of broccoli prices.

In another sense, however, this line of attack was surprising. The individual mandate had been a cornerstone of conservative health care reform proposals for decades because it relied on private markets to provide coverage and enforced a norm of personal responsibility. This approach had been consciously designed as a market-based alternative to the health care reform proposals made by Democrats during the Clinton administration. And it was and remains a market-oriented alternative to what has come to be called Medicare for All. To add insult to injury, the ACA's insurance market reforms—including the mandate—were modeled on reforms that Massachusetts had enacted some years earlier under the leadership of then governor Mitt Romney, who would campaign for the presidency in 2012 on a pledge to repeal the ACA.

Medicaid Expansion. The Medicaid expansion was a classic example of Congress's "spending power" under Article I of the Constitution. Congress provides funding to carry out a social program—here, health care for the poor—to any state that agrees to provide some percentage of the funding for the program and to abide by legal requirements (defining eligibility and other matters) as a condition of receiving the funds. The ACA's Medicaid expansion substantially increased the availability of Medicaid coverage in the states—making any citizen with an income below 133% of the federal poverty level eligible[5]—with the federal government paying almost all the cost. The ACA gave states an either-or choice: they could agree to the Medicaid program in its expanded form, or they could choose to opt out of Medicaid altogether and relinquish the funding they were already receiving to support pre-ACA Medicaid programs.

The challengers argued that this was no choice at all because no state could endure the cut-off of existing Medicaid funding. States depended on that funding to pay for medical care for the poor and disabled as well as nursing home care for the elderly. Ending that funding, these states argued, amounted to coercion in violation of state sovereignty guaranteed by the 10th Amendment. Although the Supreme Court had previously suggested that coercive federal spending programs might be unconstitutional, the Court had never invalidated a federal program on those grounds. The challengers sought to make this case the first.

The Defense

Commerce Clause. The most natural way to defend the mandate was as an exercise of Congress's power to regulate interstate commerce. Even the challengers agreed that the overall structure of market reforms the ACA put in place to prevent discrimination against people with preexisting conditions was the kind of national economic regulation Congress had the authority to enact; the mandate was simply a means that made these otherwise uncontroversial market reforms work. If these problems the ACA addressed were within the authority of Congress's commerce power, then Congress should certainly have the power to fashion an appropriate regulatory response. That was doubly true because Article I of the Constitution authorizes Congress not merely to regulate interstate commerce but also to adopt any measures that are "necessary and proper for carrying into execution" its enumerated powers, including the commerce power. Congress could reasonably conclude that the individual mandate was necessary and proper to carrying out the ACA's insurance market reforms.

By the time I took over as solicitor general, the argument that the mandate was an unprecedented attempt to "regulate inactivity" or "compel commerce" had gained considerable traction in litigation in the federal courts and in the broader public discourse. Several district court judges (the trial-level courts in the federal system) had embraced it, and one federal court of appeals, the 11th Circuit, would soon do so. The scholars and litigators who had developed the argument were relentless in promoting it. One blog, the *Volokh Conspiracy*, became the locus for their efforts.[6] Day after day, week after week, they published blog posts explaining their theory, responding to their critics, and urging the courts to follow their lead. Professor Jack Balkin of Yale University has described this as the transformation of a legal argument from an "off the wall" to an "on the wall" position—from extreme to mainstream. Of the many lessons to emerge from the experience of defending the ACA, one of the most important was a recognition of the enormous influence that new means of communication—the blogosphere and, increasingly, Twitter—had come to wield on high-stakes litigation before the Supreme Court.

At the Department of Justice (DOJ) we knew it would be imprudent, given the prevailing climate, to underestimate the appeal of the "regulating inactivity" argument. We would acknowledge the limits the Supreme Court had previously identified and point out that the ACA's mandate transgressed none of them. It regulated the operation of interstate insurance and health care markets, and it did not intrude on spheres traditionally reserved to the states like education or domestic relations. Beyond that, we tried to situate the ACA's insurance market reforms, including the mandate, as an *interstate* problem and not merely a national one. We accepted that the Commerce Clause authorized federal regulation only to deal with problems that were truly interstate in character, either because they involved economic activities that themselves crossed state lines, regulated activities in one state with spillover effects in another (such as water pollution), or dealt with "collective action" that would hinder a state's ability to handle problems on its own.

Even with these limitations, I remained concerned. It was not difficult to posit situations involving collective action problems or spillover effects that would justify a purchase mandate under our approach but would seem quite extreme. Could Congress really require that every American family purchase a car from an American automobile company every 3 years in order to preserve the domestic auto industry? Against the backdrop of the then-recent GM bankruptcy, that question had a lot of bite. Staving off the demise of the auto industry was a problem of great national consequence that individual states could not address on their own. But would 5 justices ever agree with a theory that supported such a result?

So we went narrower still. A brilliant conservative jurist on the US Court of Appeals for the 6th Circuit, Jeff Sutton, showed us what such a narrower justification might look like. In an opinion upholding the ACA—a courageous ruling for a man whom many considered a strong candidate for an eventual Supreme Court appointment—Judge Sutton explained that the mandate was nothing more than a before-the-fact regulation of commerce that was certain to occur eventually. It seemed clear that Congress could constitutionally enact a law saying that only people with health insurance could obtain medical care. Such a law directly regulates commerce—the transaction for medical care itself. It does not require anyone to purchase insurance. Viewed from that perspective, the main difference between a law requiring that health care be available only to people with health insurance and a law requiring people to purchase health insurance in advance of needing health care was just a difference in timing that ought to be within the authority of Congress to decide as a matter of policy.

This was the place where I decided we should make our stand. We would argue that the mandate was consistent with every limit the Court had previously articulated. But we would rest on the proposition that the ACA's mandate was simply anticipatory regulation of commerce that was certain to occur.

Tax Power. Even narrowed in these ways, the Commerce Clause defense continued to be a cause for worry. We needed a fallback argument that would allow the Court to uphold the mandate on an alternative ground if we could not persuade 5 justices to uphold the law as a regulation of interstate commerce. This was the now-famous "tax power" argument.

One of the enumerated powers given Congress in Article I of the Constitution is the power to tax. Historically, Congress had used that power to achieve regulatory objectives as well as to raise revenue. Consider the mortgage deduction: it uses a tax break to create a financial incentive for home purchases. The ACA's mandate was similar. It created an incentive: you either maintained insurance or you paid a tax. To be sure, the ACA described the payment as a penalty, not a tax. But it lent itself to being characterized as a tax measure. The relevant ACA provisions were amendments to the Internal Revenue Code. You reported whether you had the required insurance on your Form 1040, and those without it paid an amount to the IRS based on a percentage of their income on April 15 along with whatever other tax they might owe. And the only consequence of failing to maintain insurance was payment of the tax. If you did not maintain the required coverage but paid the tax, you were not a lawbreaker.

The tax power argument had real advantages. It offered the Supreme Court the option of upholding the mandate on a narrow ground that did not imply limitless congressional power to command individual behavior. It also reinforced that the ACA was an innovative, market-based response to a social problem.

As the argument took shape, it was increasingly clear to me that the issue would come down to a fight over nomenclature. That was favorable terrain for us. Although the statute used the word "penalty," the fact remained that Congress could have done exactly what it did by simply using the word "tax" instead. The Supreme Court had made clear for a very long time that Congress does not need to identify what source of authority it relies on to enact a law, including a tax law. The question is one of substance, not form: Does the Constitution give Congress the authority to do what it did? Supreme Court precedent also made clear that a law can be a valid exercise of the tax power even if the law aims to regulate behavior as well as generate revenue. Most importantly, framing the argument in this way allowed us to anchor our position in a core principle of constitutional adjudication. As the Supreme Court has recognized since the early part of the 19th century, courts have a duty to interpret Congress's enactments in a manner that avoids a constitutional objection if the law can be fairly construed to do so. This avoidance principle reflects respect for the judgments of the democratically accountable branches of government. If a statute can reasonably be read to operate in a manner that is within Congress's constitutional authority, then a court has a duty to read it that way to vindicate the will of the people expressed through their elected representatives.

The Medicaid Expansion. As obsessively as we focused on defending the mandate, in retrospect it is clear that we underestimated the challenge to the Medicaid expansion. We thought the defense was straightforward: the expansion did not force states to do anything. They had the same option they always had: participate in the federal Medicaid program and receive substantial federal funding in exchange for a commitment to supply state funding and abide by federal regulations governing the program. From the outset the Medicaid statute reserved to Congress the authority to change the program in ways that would expand it and increase the states' financial obligations under it. Thus, states were on notice. To the extent that a state might risk losing billions of federal dollars, that risk was a result of voluntary decisions the state had made over the years to take advantage of options under Medicaid to provide additional services to its residents. And to the extent that a state no longer wanted to participate, that was not "coercion." A state always remained free to opt out of the federal program and provide health care to its poor citizens on its own. Given the strength of these points, we thought it unlikely that this would be the first case in which the Supreme Court would find that Congress had exercised its spending power in violation of the 10th Amendment.

Oral Argument

The Supreme Court held oral argument over the course of 3 days—March 26 to 28, 2012. In the modern era, devoting what amounts to an entire week of the Court's argument calendar to one case was extremely unusual.

I argued on each of the 3 days. The first day, which focused on a threshold question of jurisdiction, was uneventful. The second day, which focused on the constitutionality of the mandate, was anything but. I argued first and got off to a terrible start. I had a problem with my throat, could not get my words out, and lost focus. I lost control of the argument and was quickly hit with a barrage of hostile questions. It took what felt like an eternity for me to climb out of that hole, regain my footing, and begin to make our case. I thought that I managed to get our commerce power points out eventually, and I fought for the opportunity during the latter part of the argument to make sure the justices understood that the tax power argument was an important part of our defense. But when I sat down, I knew we were in a bad place. And my opposing counsel, Paul Clement and Michael Carvin, were quite effective during their turns at the lectern. When I got back up for a brief rebuttal, I mustered all the focus I could to summarize the strongest version of our case. When I finished, I thought we had gotten the arguments across. But impressions were formed based on those first few minutes of my opening argument, and the reviews were rough. A consensus quickly hardened among commentators and the public: the ACA was toast, and it was my fault.

By the time the third day rolled around, I was running on fumes. My argument that day focused on the Medicaid expansion. But toward the end I thought it was important to step back and put this fight into a broader context. Here is what I said:

> There is an important connection, a profound connection, between [this] problem and liberty. And I do think it's important that we not lose sight of that. That in this population of Medicaid-eligible people who will receive health care that they cannot now afford . . . there will be millions of people with chronic conditions like diabetes and heart disease, and as a result of the health care that they will get, they will be unshackled from the disabilities that those diseases put on them and have the opportunity to enjoy the blessings of liberty.
>
> And the same thing will be true . . . for a husband whose wife is diagnosed with breast cancer and who won't face the prospect of being forced into bankruptcy to try to get care for his wife and face the risk of having to raise his children alone. And I could multiply example after example after example.
>
> In a very fundamental way, this Medicaid expansion, as well as the provisions we discussed yesterday, secure the blessings of liberty. And I think that that is important, as the Court is considering these issues, that that be kept in mind.

Here is what Paul Clement, characteristically eloquent and effective, said in response:

> I would respectfully suggest that it's a very funny conception of liberty that forces somebody to purchase an insurance policy whether they want it or not.
>
> And it's a very strange conception of federalism that says that we can simply give the states an offer that they can't refuse, and through the spending power, which is premised on the notion that Congress can do more—because it's voluntary, we can force the states to do whatever we tell them to. That is a direct threat to our federalism.

I thought then and still think that this exchange captured the fight over the legitimacy of the ACA about as well as it could be captured.

The Supreme Court's Decision

The Court announced its decision on June 28, 2012. As solicitors general customarily do, I sat in the courtroom to hear the announcement. I do not know that I have ever experienced anything quite as emotionally intense as that announcement.

After the Court worked its way through several other cases, the chief justice stated that he would announce the Court's decision in *NFIB*. He began by explaining that a 5-justice majority had concluded that the ACA's mandate exceeded Congress's commerce power. "Under the Government's logic," he said, "that authorizes Congress to use its commerce power to compel citizens to act as the Government would have them act. *That is not the country the Framers of our Constitution envisioned.*" My heart sank. My defense of President Obama's signature achievement had failed, and the promise of health and security for so many Americans was probably gone.

Then came the word "but." Something about the chief's tone of voice told me that we had prevailed on the tax power argument. And we did, for the reason we thought had the most force. Even though the ACA used the word "penalty" rather than "tax," it could reasonably be read as an exercise of the tax power. Because the ACA could be read that way, the Court's duty to respect the will of the majority required that the ACA be read that way. My heart soared.

The chief then addressed the Medicaid expansion. This time he spoke for 7 justices in ruling that the expansion violated the 10th Amendment. The threat of losing existing Medicaid funding was a coercive "gun to the head" that went beyond what Congress could constitutionally do. Again, my heart sank. But there was another "but." The ACA could be—and therefore should be—read to give states a choice to either opt into the expansion or to reject the expansion but remain in the existing program. That was, I remember thinking at the time, as good as an affirmance. What states would turn down the opportunity to vastly expand health care for their poor citizens with the federal government picking up most of the tab?

We left the Supreme Court on June 28 confident that the future of the ACA was secure. The law had survived a brush with death and would be implemented as planned. Then came the infamous leak. The press reported that the chief justice had originally voted to strike down the mandate and reversed himself shortly before the decision issued. What actually happened may never be known. If the chief justice did change his mind, it would hardly have been the first time a justice altered the outcome of a case by deciding to change course. Whatever happened, it showed exceptional courage for the chief justice to rule as he did, knowing the furor that would ensue. But the leak would continue to hang over the ACA, casting a shadow on its legitimacy.

Round 2: *King v. Burwell*

Shortly after the Supreme Court's decision in *NFIB*, 2 new lawsuits were filed attacking the ACA. These suits did not challenge Congress's authority directly. But the threat they posed to the law's insurance market reforms—the protections for people with preexisting conditions in particular—was, like the cases that had just concluded, existential. That these attacks came so swiftly after the *NFIB* decision was not surprising, especially given the leak. Many on the right refused to accept *NFIB* as legitimate and treated the opinion of the chief justice with scorn.

This time, the challengers sought to turn the language of the ACA back on itself—to destroy the statute from within. Their argument rested on a technical matter of statutory interpretation, but its consequences for the ACA would have been devastating had the Supreme Court accepted it. To understand the argument, recall the overall structure and operation of the ACA's insurance market reforms. Those reforms depended on 3 main supports: (1) the tax penalty, which was designed to get individuals to purchase insurance; (2) new online, state-specific marketplaces, called "exchanges," to oversee the sale of insurance; and (3) subsidies, to be distributed through the new exchanges, to make the new insurance affordable. Individual states were to operate the exchanges if they chose; the federal government would operate a state exchange in the event a state chose not to do so. It was obvious that Congress intended that these online marketplaces would function more or less identically in every state, whether the state itself or the federal government was operating the marketplace. But the particular statutory language Congress used to authorize subsidies to make insurance affordable stated that the subsidies would be available to persons who purchase insurance "on an Exchange established by the State" under the applicable statutory provisions.

Read in isolation from the overall context, design, and purposes of the law, this phrase could be read to make subsidies available only in states that set up and ran their own ACA exchanges, not in states where the federal government operated the exchange because the state government had opted out. More than half the states had decided to opt out—many to express continuing ideological opposition to the ACA. Eliminating federal subsidies in all of those states would have made insurance unaffordable for millions of Americans. It would likely have triggered the "death spirals"—the collapse of the insurance markets—that the ACA's reforms were designed to prevent because many customers would have decided not to buy the new insurance, preferring instead to pay the penalty (and in some cases becoming exempt from the penalty, which did not apply if insurance is more than 8% of income). Only the sickest (and thus, most expensive) customers would remain. It would have turned the country into a patchwork—affordable insurance in a functioning market in some states, unaffordable insurance in crippled markets in others.

You might ask how anyone could think Congress would have wanted to create such a system, one with a built-in self-destruction mechanism. The challengers claimed, first, that this was intentional—that Congress created this powerful incentive for states to take up the responsibility of running their own exchanges: unless a state established an exchange, its insurance market would be crippled and many of its citizens would be denied affordable health insurance available under the ACA to similarly situated people in other states—essentially a Don Corleone approach to governance. Ultimately, however, they claimed that it did not matter whether Congress actually intended this result. All that mattered were the words Congress used in the statute. If Congress had done something stupid, Congress could amend the law to correct the stupidity. But a court could not. That would be rewriting the law—making law, not interpreting it.

Our experience litigating *NFIB* taught us to treat these challenges with the utmost seriousness. There was something else we learned from

NFIB, and it led us to handle this second wave of challenges differently from the first. In *NFIB* the challengers controlled the public narrative and had all the momentum. I was determined not to allow that to happen again—we were not going to let this challenge move from "off the wall" to "on the wall." As the government's lawyer, I could do little directly. I could not blog or give interviews or deliver speeches. That is not the way the solicitor general's office does business. But others could. And they did. An army of scholars and policy experts unleashed a focused, determined effort to ensure that their views would be heard in the public dialogue. That effort had 3 goals: (1) ensure that no one would take seriously the challengers' contention that Congress actually planned for the ACA to operate in the self-annihilating way they described; (2) ensure that our argument—that the "exchange established by the state" language had to be read in light of the structure and purposes of the ACA—was perceived as a conventional, mainstream legal analysis and that the challengers, in contrast, were misusing the courts to achieve a political result rather than a legal one; and (3) ensure that the public understood how many millions of people would lose their health insurance and how much disruption would be visited on insurance markets if the challengers prevailed.

The 2 challenges worked their way through the courts quickly. On the same day in July 2014 one federal court of appeals (the 4th Circuit) rejected the challengers' case, but another (the DC Circuit) accepted it—guaranteeing that the Supreme Court would need to have the last word.

After the briefing was complete, the Supreme Court heard oral argument on March 2, 2015. The argument could not have been more different from *NFIB*. As we had hoped, the challengers faced tough sledding in trying to persuade the Court that Congress was so focused on creating an incentive for states to create their own exchanges that it was willing to threaten the kind of chaos that would follow from denying subsidies to citizens of states that refused. Dealing with the text of the statute itself—"exchange established by the state"—proved more challenging. Justice Scalia led the charge. If Congress made a mistake, he asserted, it was up to Congress to fix it. Congress legislates, not the Court, and we were asking for legislation, not interpretation. We wanted the Court to change the meaning of the text to make it work. It culminated with this exchange when Justice Scalia asked me how often the Court refuses to rewrite a statutory mistake and Congress does not then step in to fix it:

> JUSTICE SCALIA: What about—what about Congress? You really think Congress is just going to sit there while all of these disastrous consequences ensue.
>
> . . . Congress adjusts, enacts a statute that—that takes care of the problem. It happens all the time. Why is that not going to happen here?
>
> GENERAL VERRILLI: Well, this Congress, Your Honor?
>
> [Laughter.]

Attempting humor during a Supreme Court argument is risky business. Attempting it in an exchange with Justice Antonin Scalia, a man whose brilliance and wit I could never have hoped to match, was borderline suicidal. But I knew I would get this question, likely from Justice Scalia. I wanted to crystallize what everyone knew to be true: if the Court ruled for the challengers, there was no way that a Republican House of Representatives under the control of Speaker Paul Ryan (R-WI) would step in to revive the ACA. I thought it imperative that the challengers—and any justices inclined to side with them—be on the hook for the disastrous consequences that would follow from a ruling against us. Fortunately, I survived the encounter unscathed.

The Supreme Court ruled on June 25, 2015. The ruling was everything we could have hoped for—and then some. The chief justice wrote the opinion for a comfortable 6–3 majority. It was a complete vindication. The opinion could not have been more clear that the Court was prepared to accept the ACA as the legitimate product of the democratically accountable branches of government. Whether the law would continue to be implemented as originally designed or be amended or repealed was a judgment for the people to make through their elected representatives. We anticipated that the Court's opinion would, finally, put an end to the legal battle over the ACA's legitimacy. We were wrong again.

Round 3: *Texas v. United States*

To state the obvious, the election of President Trump and a Republican Congress in November 2016 changed everything. With Republicans in control of the Senate and the House as well as the presidency, they had the power to repeal the ACA. Remarkably, the repeal failed, with Senator McCain's dramatic thumbs-down vote sinking the effort.

A few months later Congress did make one significant change to the ACA. It effectively repealed the individual mandate by setting at zero the tax penalty for declining to maintain insurance. I say "effectively" because Congress technically left the mandate in place. It just eliminated any adverse consequence for failing to have insurance. From Senate Leader Mitch McConnell (R-KY) to Speaker of the House Ryan on down, Republican leaders all described this step as a repeal of the mandate. Reasons of Senate procedure dictated that it be accomplished by zeroing out the tax rather than repealing the mandate outright. Revenue measures (like changes in tax rates) can be passed through reconciliation by simple majority, avoiding the need to clear the 60-vote filibuster threshold (which would have been required to repeal the mandate itself). But in effect, the mandate was gone.

This technicality created an opening, and several Republican-controlled states pounced. Congress's tax power could no longer justify the ACA, they argued, because it no longer imposed any tax. Without a tax power justification for the mandate, it is no longer constitutional. And the mandate was, at least formally, still in place. If the mandate was unconstitutional, they contended, the rest of the ACA had to fall with it because Congress would not have intended for any other part of the ACA to remain operative if the mandate were struck down. Never mind that actions of the 2017 Congress made clear that the opposite was true. After having declined to repeal the ACA in toto, Congress, in the words of its own Republican leadership, effectively repealed the mandate while leaving the rest of the law in place. It was blindingly obvious what Congress would have wanted if the mandate were formally struck down and not merely neutered by zeroing out the tax.

Remarkably, a federal district judge agreed with the challengers and struck down the entire ACA.[7] As this book went to press, the US Court of Appeals for the 5th Circuit had issued a decision reviewing the opinion and sending it back to the district court for further consideration.[8] So the battle continues.

Conclusion

What to make of this decade-long battle in the courts? First, the Republican establishment and conservative intellectuals remain tenacious in their refusal to recognize the ACA as a legitimate exercise of government power. In many ways that is as true today as it was in 2010. Second, the ACA has managed to survive as sustained an assault in the courts as has ever been brought against an act of Congress. Third, if anything explains the ACA's resilience, I think it is that over time a majority of this country has come to accept the connection between a guarantee of access to health care when they need it and their ability to enjoy the blessings of liberty.

CHAPTER 9

THE ACA AND THE COURTS
Two Perspectives, Part Two

Paul Clement

The litigation concerning the Affordable Care Act (ACA) has been outsized in every respect. The original constitutional challenge to the statute generated unprecedented amounts of Supreme Court argument time and press attention. And follow-up cases involving a single provision of the statute put approximately $12 billion at issue. Nothing about the ACA has been small, including its impact on the Supreme Court.

National Federation of Independent Business: The Constitutional Challenge

The constitutional challenge to the Affordable Care Act in general and the individual mandate in particular began long before my own involvement in this litigation. Florida and 12 other states filed the first lawsuit in the Northern District of Florida immediately after the bill was signed. A number of other actions followed suit (literally), including the challenge filed by Virginia on the same day in the Eastern District of Virginia.

Although these numerous constitutional challenges were filed immediately after the ACA's passage, the legislative debates over the Act had focused on policy, not constitutional concerns. Even when it came

Paul Clement, JD, is a partner at Kirkland & Ellis LLP and served as the 43rd solicitor general of the United States (2004–2008).

to the individual mandate, the principal objections were made in terms of the requirement being imprudent, not unconstitutional.[1] Although this is not unusual—Congress has failed to "issue spot" when it comes to other constitutional issues[2]—it does stand in sharp contrast to other major constitutional challenges in recent memory, such as those mounted against the 2002 campaign finance law, the Bipartisan Campaign Reform Act (BCRA). In BCRA, the congressional debates were constitutional debates, with much of the opposition to the Act framed in First Amendment terms that were echoed in First Amendment challenges after passage. Not so in the case of the ACA, where constitutional objections were raised only in passing and at the tail end of the legislative debates.[3]

Perhaps because the legislative debates did not condition the public to think about constitutional questions of congressional power, the early reactions to the lawsuits were largely dismissive (e.g., Charles Fried, former US solicitor general, promised to eat a hat made of kangaroo skin if the ACA were struck down[4]). I recall being on a National Public Radio show in 2010 along with another former US solicitor general, Walter Dellinger, on which the host asked us about the then-nascent lawsuits and their prospects if they ended up before the Supreme Court.

Dellinger was more familiar with the lawsuits and expressed a view that was common at the time, essentially dismissing the suits as unfounded.[5] My answer was more tentative. I had not been directly involved in the litigation and, thus, had not studied the law or the challengers' legal theories closely. I did, however, sound one cautionary note about the conventional wisdom that the challenges should not be taken seriously. Based on my own experience in the solicitor general's office defending the constitutionality of federal statutes challenged as being beyond Congress's Commerce Clause power in cases like *Gonzales v. Raich* (which concerned regulation of homegrown cannabis)[6] and *Rapanos v. United States* (which concerned federal power to regulate wetlands),[7] I thought that the challenge for the government would be articulating a limiting principle.

When the federal government can explain why Congress has the power to enact the challenged statute but not some more extreme version, the federal government generally wins because there is a near consensus that Congress's Commerce Clause power is broad. But when the federal government cannot articulate a limiting principle, it often loses because there is a near consensus that Congress's Commerce Clause power is not unlimited. After all, the framers went to a lot of trouble in articulating the specific powers granted to the new federal Congress,[8] and all that effort would be pointless if the Commerce Clause in fact gave Congress essentially plenary power. In my view, the federal government had not yet persuasively articulated a limiting principle explaining why Congress could force individuals to buy health care but not every other article of commerce.

The public attitude toward the lawsuits began to shift when 2 federal judges in short order accepted the challengers' arguments. First, Judge Henry E. Hudson in Virginia struck down the individual mandate as unconstitutional.[9] Judge Roger Vinson in Florida reached the same conclusion but additionally found the mandate not severable from the rest of the law—that is, that the rest of the law could not stand without it—and so he declared the entire ACA void.[10] It is a lot harder to be dismissive of challenges to the constitutionality of an act of Congress when 2 federal courts have not only just taken the arguments seriously but also embraced them in significant part.

Those actions, however, were not the only litigation involving the ACA, and decisions upholding the constitutionality of the new health care law followed from courts in the District of Columbia and another court in Virginia.[11] Commentators quickly noted a readily discernable pattern in the decisions with "district judges appointed by Democratic presidents upholding the law and Republican appointees striking it down."[12]

As the cases transitioned to the courts of appeals, 2 things happened: (1) the pattern of decisions became more nuanced and (2) I became involved in the litigation. As to the latter point, after the Florida decision striking down the individual mandate as unconstitutional, the number of states joining that particular challenge grew to 26, creating the remarkable spectacle of over half the states in the Union challenging a federal law in a single lawsuit. At the same time, the states became sufficiently optimistic about the prospects of eventual Supreme Court review that they decided to retain specialized appellate counsel for the 11th Circuit appeal and the Supreme Court proceedings to follow.

Once I was retained, my team set out to refine the arguments on the constitutionality of the individual mandate on which we already had prevailed and also try to rethink our arguments on the constitutionality of the ACA's Medicaid expansion, which had not persuaded Judge Vinson, notwithstanding his decision to invalidate the mandate.

As noted, the pattern of decisions that emerged from the courts of appeals became more nuanced. In the 11th Circuit case, which was heard by a 3-judge panel, 2 judges—one appointed by President George H. W. Bush and one by President Bill Clinton—voted to find the individual mandate unconstitutional. The court went on to reject the challenge to the Medicaid expansion and to find most—but not all—of the rest of the ACA "severable" from the unconstitutional mandate. In particular, the 11th Circuit found that the provisions guaranteeing availability of coverage and prohibiting the exclusion of preexisting conditions as well as the myriad provisions unrelated to private insurance could function without the individual mandate. The court wrote, "We are not persuaded that it is *evident* (as opposed to possible or reasonable) that Congress would not have enacted the 2 reforms in the absence of the individual mandate. . . . We therefore sever the individual mandate from the remaining sections of the Act."[13]

In other circuits, prominent judges appointed by Republican presidents, like Laurence Silberman of the DC Circuit and Jeffrey Sutton of the 6th Circuit, authored opinions upholding the Act as constitutional. Those decisions usefully undermined the narrative that judges were voting along "party lines" and also created something that every Supreme Court advocate prizes—a split in the circuits.[14]

The Supreme Court granted review on the ACA's constitutionality, which was no great surprise. But the way the Court granted review was a surprise and underscored the outsized importance of the case. The Court granted not only the government's petition concerning the individual mandate but also a separate petition filed by the states on the Medicaid expansion questions, even though there was no circuit split on that question, as well as the petitions raising the severability issues. The Court also made clear that it was interested in considering a jurisdictional question involving another law, the Anti-Injunction Act (AIA), that governs the timing of litigation concerning taxes, an issue that could have delayed an ultimate Supreme Court resolution by years.

The Court further underscored the importance of the case by appointing 2 different amici—lawyers specially appointed to argue positions not squarely addressed by the parties—and scheduling 4 separate oral arguments over 3 days, much more time than the one-hour argument the Court usually schedules even in high-profile cases involving challenges to important federal statutes. The prospect of having 4 separate arguments spanning 3 days was unprecedented in the modern era. Certainly, no one could doubt that the Supreme Court was taking the challenges to the ACA seriously.

The press and public interest in the cases when they reached the Court was, like everything about the cases, outsized. I thought my experience with other high-profile, closely watched cases would prepare me well to handle a case where the press was covering every filing. But I had never seen anything like the press interest in the ACA cases. Generally, Supreme Court reporters have to fight with their editors to get a few extra inches to cover an important Supreme Court case. But Supreme Court reporters were basically given a blank check when it came to the ACA. And it was not just Supreme Court reporters who were writing about the cases; given the centrality of the ACA to the delivery of health care in America, reporters with a health care beat were covering the cases intensely. And because the cases would determine the fate of President Obama's signature legislative achievement in an election year, political reporters covered the case extensively as well. It was a veritable perfect storm of press interest that resulted in more extensive coverage of the cases than anything I have seen before or since.

When it came time for the oral argument in late March, the first issue up and the exclusive focus of the first day was the critical but technical question of whether the AIA deprived the federal courts of jurisdiction to hear the case. This created a conundrum for the press. The public was ready to hear about the justices' views about the ACA, not the finer points of federal-court jurisdiction, but if the Court seized on the AIA issue, it would render all the other issues in the case beside the point, so it could not be ignored. Fortunately, although the Court had a lively 90 minutes of argument on the AIA, it did not appear on the verge of holding the case premature, and the stage was set for the main event: the second day of arguments, focused on the constitutionality of the individual mandate.

Although there were always other issues in the litigation, the heart of the challenge to the ACA was to the constitutionality of the individual mandate. And in most of the discussion about the constitutionality of the individual mandate, the question was framed in terms of Congress's power under the Commerce Clause—the power to regulate commerce between the states. The question at the absolute epicenter of the Supreme Court case was, thus, whether Congress could force individuals to purchase health insurance (or pay a penalty) as part of a congressional effort to regulate commerce in the health care industry.

But the Commerce Clause issue did not stand alone. The government had 2 alternative arguments to justify the individual mandate. The government invoked the Necessary and Proper Clause, which is the very last of the enumerated powers granted to Congress in Article I, section 8 of the Constitution. The clause empowers Congress "to make all laws which shall be necessary and proper for carrying into execution the foregoing powers." The government also contended that the individual mandate could be justified as a valid exercise of Congress's taxing power. These alternative arguments created an asymmetry in the argument over the individual mandate. The government had 3 different theories to justify the mandate and only needed to prevail on one. The challengers, by contrast, had to run the proverbial table and show that none of the 3 powers justified the individual mandate.

The much-anticipated oral argument on the mandate focused, as expected, on the Commerce Clause. And the argument appeared to go well for the challengers. Most court watchers believed that Justice Anthony Kennedy held the critical vote concerning the fate of the individual mandate, as he did in so many issues that came before the Roberts Court during Justice Kennedy's tenure. Justice Kennedy's questions at the oral argument suggested that he had real doubts about the mandate's constitutionality. In part because of those questions and in part because so many people had been relatively dismissive of the constitutional arguments, the immediate commentary suggested that a majority of the Court was skeptical of the mandate's constitutionality.

Jeffrey Toobin of CNN famously described the argument as a "train wreck for the Obama administration,"[15] while others concluded that the individual mandate was "on life support."[16] One thing was certain: after the second day of oral arguments, no one was dismissing the constitutional challenge to the ACA as a mere "political stunt" that was not to be taken seriously.

The third day of oral arguments was a doubleheader. In the morning session the Court considered the question of severability, or how much of the ACA would be invalidated if the individual mandate were to be held unconstitutional. By definition, this issue would not even arise if the Court upheld the constitutionality of the individual mandate. As a result, the Court's treatment of this issue provided a barometer of the Court's thinking about the mandate. If the justices were reasonably sure there were 5 votes to uphold the mandate, one might expect the argument on severability to have the feel of an exhibition game. In reality, not only did the arguments feel every bit as intense as the previous day's arguments, but it also appeared that a number of justices, including Justice Kennedy, were taking very seriously the possibility that the unconstitutionality of the mandate could cause the entire ACA to be struck down.

Finally, in the afternoon session the Court considered the constitutionality of the Medicaid expansion. The Supreme Court had previously held that Congress has the ability to use its spending powers to incentivize the states to take actions that would be beyond the power of the federal government to do itself or to command states to undertake. To take a classic example approved by the Supreme Court: although Congress could not, consistent with the 21st Amendment, simply enact a nationwide drinking age of 21, the Court approved Congress's decision to condition a portion of federal highway funding on the states' willingness to increase their drinking ages to 21.[17] Although the Court in that case and others suggested that certain uses of the spending power could be impermissibly coercive, the Court had not—at least since the New Deal—actually found that Congress had gone too far in an exercise of the spending power. Undeterred, the states argued that Congress had crossed a constitutional line in conditioning the availability of all Medicaid funds—those that predated the ACA as well as those made newly available to help finance the proposed Medicaid expansion—on the states' willingness to expand Medicaid to cover millions of previously ineligible individuals.

Whether because the Supreme Court had never struck down an exercise of the spending power as too coercive or because neither Judge Vinson nor the 11th Circuit majority embraced the argument, expectations were relatively modest about this last segment of the extraordinary 3-day argument section. Nonetheless, the Court's more conservative justices expressed considerable skepticism about the Medicaid expansion. And the combined effect of the Court's seeming willingness to entertain the possibility of striking down the entirety of the ACA in the morning and apparent receptiveness to the Medicaid expansion challenge in the afternoon left the pundits reeling. Toobin suggested that if day 2 of the arguments was a "train wreck" for the government, then day 3 was "a plane wreck."[18]

Efforts by politicians and commentators to influence the Court's decision-making process began almost as soon as the arguments finished. For example, Senator Patrick Leahy (D-VT) claimed on the Senate floor that "if the Supreme Court overturns the Affordable Care Act now, it will be devastating to kids, families, and senior citizens."[19] Most prominently, President Obama suggested that striking down the law would be an "unprecedented, extraordinary step" and "judicial activism."[20] Although these efforts to influence the course of the Supreme Court's decision making on a case *sub judice* were extraordinary at the time, so was virtually every aspect of the ACA litigation.

As the Supreme Court's term drew to a close, the Court's decision in the health care cases was eagerly awaited. On the term's final opinion on the final day, the Chief Justice announced that he had the Court's opinion in the health care cases. The confusion was almost immediate. Perhaps because the Chief Justice had expressed considerable skepticism about the ACA at oral argument or because the Chief Justice began his opinion announcement by concluding that the individual mandate exceeded Congress's power under the Commerce Clause, a number of major news outlets reported that the Court had struck down the individual mandate as unconstitutional. That was not the case; instead, the Chief Justice concluded that although Congress lacked the power to impose the mandate under the Commerce or Necessary and Proper

Clauses, the mandate was nonetheless a valid exercise of Congress's taxing power. At the same time, a majority of the Court concluded that the Medicaid expansion was an invalid exercise of Congress's spending power. In fact, on that issue, no fewer than 7 justices concluded that Congress had crossed a constitutional line.

What had happened? Had commentators and Court watchers simply misread the oral arguments? Part of the problem was that there was precious little oral argument about the taxing power. Although the taxing power had come up a bit during the first day's jurisdictional arguments, the Court sustained its jurisdiction and viewed the mandate as not a tax for purposes of the AIA. And in the principal arguments over the mandate's constitutionality, the taxing power had made no more than a cameo appearance. Moreover, although it might have been possible to count 5 votes against the Medicaid expansion on the last afternoon of the argument, there was little indication that Justices Stephen Breyer and Elena Kagan (both nominated by Democratic presidents) were about to join a 7-justice majority to strike down the expansion and create a new limit on Congress's spending power.

At least one reporter has concluded that the explanation for the surprising result rests in machinations that occurred after an initial vote of the justices to strike down the mandate.[21] Whatever the cause, there is no denying that the Court's decision left the vast majority of the ACA intact while providing the states with a new option to retain their pre-ACA Medicaid funds even while declining the funds provided for the expansion. There is also no denying that the Court's decision was not its last word on the constitutionality of the ACA or the legality of its implementation.

Other Major Challenges

Shortly before the House took its final vote on the ACA, Speaker Nancy Pelosi (D-CA) admitted that few members had had the opportunity to read the 2,400-page bill and that they would "have to pass the bill" to "find out what is in it."[22] A law that long, that substantial, and that rushed is destined to raise dozens of legal questions about its meaning, implementation, and legality. And given the political dynamics that produced the ACA, those legal questions were unusually likely to result in contested litigation. The challenges to the ACA fall into 2 broad categories: those that pose an existential threat to the law and those that challenge the implementation of specific provisions.

The litigation that produced the landmark decision about the individual mandate and the Medicaid expansion clearly fell into the first category. The second round of litigation posing at least a potential existential threat to the ACA culminated in the Court's 2015 decision in *King v. Burwell*.[23] This case, more than any other, may have been a direct result of the haste with which the ACA went through Congress. In providing for tax subsidies for low-income individuals who purchase health insurance on the exchanges, the ACA specified that such subsidies were available for policies purchased on "an Exchange established by the State."[24] Elsewhere the ACA makes clear that if a state does not voluntarily set up an exchange, the federal government will establish and operate an exchange in that state. The question in *King* was whether such a federal exchange constituted "an Exchange established by the State" for purposes of the tax subsidies. The problem at the heart of the case was that such a federal exchange was plainly established by the federal government and not "by the State" but that denying tax subsidies for low-income individuals in states where the exchange was federally established just as plainly made no sense. What is more, knocking out subsidies in the 34 states with federal exchanges threatened the viability of the ACA in those states. In the end, 6 justices—the majority in *NFIB* plus Justice Kennedy—rejected a plain-text interpretation of the statute that would have undermined the statute's operation.

The third round of existential-threat litigation is the ongoing litigation initiated by Texas and 19 other states in the wake of Congress's repeal, as part of its 2017 tax reform law, of the tax penalty accompanying the individual mandate. The theory of this lawsuit is straightforward and follows directly from the Chief Justice's opinion in *NFIB*. The Chief Justice there rejected the government's efforts to justify the individual mandate as a valid exercise of Congress's powers under either the Commerce or Necessary and Proper Clauses and upheld the law only as taxing legislation. Thus, according to the states, when Congress eliminated the mandate's capacity to raise revenue, it rendered the mandate unconstitutional. A district court in Texas not only accepted this argument but also used the severability reasoning of the *NFIB* dissenters to invalidate the ACA as a whole.[25] There is, however, a substantial difference between the severability analysis that applies in the context of an initial challenge to a statute and that which applies to a single amendment that passed while efforts to repeal the Act as a whole repeatedly failed. Put differently, if Congress initially enacted the ACA with an individual mandate unaccompanied by a tax penalty, the logic of the Chief Justice's opinion would suggest that the mandate was unconstitutional and the dissenters' logic would suggest that the entirety of the ACA would fall because Congress did not intend to have an ACA without an individual mandate. But it does not follow that a Congress that repeatedly rejected efforts to repeal the ACA could accomplish that same result indirectly by eliminating the penalty provision.

Narrower Challenges

Although the broad challenges to the ACA have failed to persuade the Supreme Court, more targeted challenges to specific provisions of the ACA have fared substantially better. In *Hobby Lobby*, for example, the Supreme Court found that the Obama administration's interpretation of the women's health mandate ran afoul of the Religious Freedom Restoration Act when applied to employers with religious objections to funding contraception.[26] The effect of the Court's ruling was to limit the applicability of the contraceptives mandate to employers with sincere religious objections, but the suit never posed a broader existential threat to the statute as a whole. In a similar vein, religious organizations like the Little Sisters of the Poor were able to secure an exemption from the contraceptives mandate in a series of decisions culminating in the Supreme Court's *per curiam* decision and a subsequent regulatory change by the Trump administration. Challenges to the validity of that regulatory approach remain ongoing in multiple courts.

The Supreme Court will have another opportunity this year to address a specific provision in the ACA and its implementation by Congress and the executive branch in a series of recently granted cases in which I am involved as counsel for some of the insurance companies addressing the so-called risk corridors program. When drafting the

ACA, Congress recognized that the viability of the exchanges depended on private insurers' willingness to offer qualifying plans at reasonably affordable rates. Congress further recognized that one deterrent to participating in the exchanges was the uncertainty of the risk profile of the new insureds. To help address that concern, Congress adopted a number of provisions to incentivize participation on the exchanges, including the so-called risk corridors program. The program provided that during the first 3 years of the exchanges' operation, if insurers' premiums exceeded their projected costs, insurers would pay a portion of the excess to the federal government, while if costs exceeded premiums, the government would cushion the blow by covering a portion of the excess costs.

In actual operation, due in part to late-breaking changes by the executive branch that allowed a large number of relatively healthy individuals to keep their existing policies and not participate in the exchanges, a large percentage of participating insurers had excess costs. As a consequence, the government's obligations to make risk corridor payments out to participating insurers vastly outstripped the payments in by insurers with lower-than-anticipated costs. Indeed, over the 3-year life of the program, the federal government's obligations to make payments out outstripped payments in by some $12 billion. In response, Congress (by then Republican controlled) enacted a series of appropriations riders that purported to limit the government's ability to use Health and Human Services (HHS) appropriations to satisfy the government's obligations. The Supreme Court will consider whether those appropriations riders were sufficient to negate the government's obligation to make payments to insurers who responded to the government's incentives by participating in the exchanges.

The stakes of the risk corridor cases underscore the ACA's outsized impact. The Supreme Court decides many of the most contentious and significant issues facing the nation, but even the Supreme Court does not get many $12 billion cases. Similarly, it is a rare statute that occupies as much of the Supreme Court's time and attention as the ACA. And the ACA litigation has had a profound effect on Supreme Court litigation more generally.

The Supreme Court has not dedicated 3 days of argument to any case since the arguments in *NFIB*, but efforts by politicians and other interested parties to continue to litigate cases in blogs and opinion pages after the oral arguments—a practice largely pioneered in the *NFIB* litigation—have grown increasingly common. The successful challenge to the Medicaid expansion by 26 states was likewise the precursor to a series of high-profile constitutional challenges by states against major federal-government initiatives. First, a number of red states challenged Obama administration initiatives concerning immigration, and now blue states have challenged a wide range of Trump administration executive orders. And the Chief Justice's vote on the individual mandate has shaped the perception that he is the new "swing justice" on the current Court. For example, when the Chief Justice cast the decisive vote to keep a citizenship question off the census form, a number of commentators likened his handling of the census case to the individual mandate.[27] At this juncture it seems like the ACA will be as important to the Chief Justice's legacy as it is to President Obama's. But given the comprehensive and controversial nature of the ACA, the current round of cases is highly unlikely to be the last ACA cases that the Roberts Court will decide.

CHAPTER 10

FEDERALISM UNDER THE ACA
Implementation, Opposition, Entrenchment

Abbe R. Gluck and Nicole Huberfeld[1]

Whether to include the states as key implementers of the new national health care law was a fight from the beginning. In the end, the states were given a major role in ACA implementation—a role that generated not only resistance and policy inequality across states, as critics feared, but also some surprising collaboration and even resilience for the ACA's reforms. The law creates complex and shifting boundaries between state and federal control over health care policy and, in turn, reveals both the benefits and the drawbacks of health care federalism.[2]

The ACA's use of a national-state governance structure is nothing new. Despite cries that the ACA was a federal takeover of a health care system traditionally governed by states, the federal government has been involved in health care since the United States was founded, when it intervened to assist veterans of the Revolutionary War. Since then, federal regulation has grown steadily but incrementally—every president since the Great Depression has overseen a significant federal intervention in health policy. By the time the ACA was drafted, the question was not whether the federal government should be involved in health care at all but rather how far any intervention should go.

Decades of incremental national interventions had deeply fragmented health care governance, however. Different swaths of the

Abbe R. Gluck, JD, is professor of law and founding faculty director of the Solomon Center for Health Law and Policy at Yale Law School and professor of internal medicine at Yale Medical School.

Nicole Huberfeld, JD, is professor of health law, ethics, and human rights and professor of law at Boston University.

population—the elderly, veterans, employees, low-income individuals—were covered by different programs with different legal and financial regimes and different mixes of state and federal control. Although this fragmentation was widely criticized during the debates leading up to the ACA and was one commonly cited argument for health reform, the ACA did not simplify the system. Wiping the slate clean and creating a unified national health care system was neither politically feasible (the failed Clinton attempts in 1993 provided a memorable lesson in 2009) nor, in the views of some, desirable for health policy.

This is not to say that the ACA did not establish some significant national standards. The most important were setting uniform baselines for health insurance coverage and access to care for previously excluded populations. Medicaid was to be expanded nationwide, eliminating what had been each state's choice of whether to cover those beyond Medicaid's mandatory populations—children, pregnant women, very poor parents, the disabled, and the elderly—to include childless, nonelderly adults. The ACA also nationalized and profoundly changed the rules for private health insurance—an area of law traditionally under state control—establishing new quality controls and patient protections, including basic affordability standards, minimum categories of coverage, and annual and lifetime caps as well as forbidding price discrimination based on health status and coverage exclusions based on preexisting conditions.

But when it comes to *governance*, the ACA largely left control where it was before—with the states. Nationalizing Medicaid—eliminating state control—was never on the table. The House of Representatives, however, would have created a national health insurance marketplace. But in the Senate, traditionally the more state-oriented chamber of Congress, efforts (that ultimately failed) to attract Republican votes produced a plan that retained the default state-led structure for insurance regulation too. The Senate plan, which became the ACA, directed the new insurance reforms to be implemented through state-run insurance "exchanges" (a model largely innovated by Massachusetts) unless states declined the option. In another move rejecting a more nationalized model, the ACA also barely touched the private, employer-sponsored health insurance market, which covered just over half of the population in 2009.

Critics argued that these governance compromises undermined the ACA as effective reform. They worried that state-led structures opened the ACA's new protections to unequal and inequitable implementation across the country, which has been Medicaid's experience. But leaving the insurance markets under state control and using a policy model pioneered and tested in states themselves—even with the new national standards—seemed less of a federal "takeover" and, thus, more politically palatable.

It turns out that the ACA's critics were partly right and partly wrong. The ACA's federalism—meaning its structure of state-national relationships—did indeed bring instability and some inequality to health policy. It also further cemented the health care system's fragmented and complex regulatory structure. But the ACA's federalism also had some surprising benefits. Perhaps most importantly, the ACA's state-federal structure has helped to entrench the law and its core value of universal health care coverage in the face of unprecedented political and legal opposition.

States took ownership behind the scenes of health reforms they publicly opposed. The choices the ACA put to the states—whether to expand Medicaid or to operate their own health insurance exchanges—made access to health care the focus of public debates, elections, state ballot initiatives, and congressional and presidential showdowns. This public engagement elevated the ACA's national salience and fed its resilience. More recently, the autonomy the ACA gives to the states has allowed states to shore up the ACA's insurance reforms against attacks by a new presidential administration hostile to the law.

Beyond these practical and political benefits, however, it is harder to determine whether the ACA's federalism was actually good for health policy. Medicaid has been expanded in 37 states (including DC) thus far, but with varying degrees of generosity. The mix of state- and federally run insurance markets fared well enough under the Obama administration, but under the Trump administration some states' markets have fared well while others have fallen victim to or cooperated with the administrative efforts to sabotage ACA insurance reforms.

To be sure, policy variation will occur in any regulatory scheme decentralized across 51 governments. But the ACA's particular federalism brought *unexpected* variation and, with it, instability because the political winds changed forcefully with the ACA's enactment. From the moment the law passed, it met with opposition from Republican-controlled states. The same party that at the federal level demanded the ACA's new insurance markets be left in state control refused, at the state level, to implement the law and acted to undermine it. The Supreme Court amplified the political chaos in its first ACA decision, giving states unexpected control over Medicaid expansion.[3]

Perhaps a fully nationalized model would have achieved simpler, more complete, and more stable reform. But it is also possible that, without state involvement, the ACA would not have proved as resilient as it has. Ten years in, a statute that was decried at the outset for being insufficiently transformative and inadequately national has come to stand for the core value of nationwide universal coverage, largely because of the ways in which the ACA has persisted in implementation, survived unprecedented challenges, and driven near-constant intergovernmental negotiation and public conversation. This trajectory—one enabled at least in part by the ACA's federalism—also seems to have paved the way for a new national debate on health reform that may realize more completely the ACA's goal of nationalized, universal coverage.

The ACA's State-Federal Design, Flipped on Its Head

The ACA's principal goal was near-universal health insurance coverage, which was to be accomplished through its federalism architecture for Medicaid and the exchanges, the law's 2 key structural mechanisms that relied heavily on the states and are the focus of this chapter. First, as noted, the ACA would have expanded Medicaid eligibility to all nondisabled, childless adults under age 65 earning up to 138% of the federal poverty level (FPL). Before the ACA, states were required to cover only the categories of low-income individuals who were historically the "deserving poor"; others were excluded unless states used their own funds to cover them or obtained a federal waiver. Many states chose to cover just the very poorest members of optional populations; Texas, for example, only covers childless, nonelderly adults earning up to 17% of the FPL, about $2,123 per year.

Second, the ACA introduced new supports for individual and small-group health insurance markets—for those who cannot secure insurance through a government program or a large employer—by creating the one-stop-shop health insurance exchanges. Exchanges ensure that all plans offer a minimal level of coverage, including 10 essential health benefits, within a prescribed rate structure; make the options transparent; and determine tax subsidies to make purchasing insurance more affordable.

Although both pillars of the ACA rely heavily on states, their governance structures were designed differently. The Medicaid expansion was intended to be more national in the sense that the ACA required the new category of eligibility to apply nationwide; any state's failure to cover this new group would end its entire Medicaid program. The private insurance reforms embraced more state choice: states were expected to run their own insurance markets but had some flexibility in how the exchanges were to be designed. Further, if states chose not to or failed to operate their own exchanges, the federal government would do so for them, creating a federal fallback that does not exist for Medicaid.

But the ACA's federalism as implemented was the mirror image of its federalism as drafted. The exchanges became more nationally governed than expected, and Medicaid expansion became more state driven. This flip occurred because states destabilized the law in unforeseen ways; in particular, the states became the primary drivers of litigation-based resistance: 26 states brought the first major Supreme Court challenge to the ACA, the constitutional challenge in *NFIB*. States again brought the second major Supreme Court challenge to the ACA, the statutory question in *King v. Burwell*, which, as discussed in Chapter 8 of this volume, challenged the legality of insurance subsidies on federal exchanges. In the 2014 challenge to the ACA's contraceptive mandate 20 states also filed friend-of-the-court briefs. And 20 states launched the fourth and latest major battle, *Texas v. United States*, also discussed in Chapter 8, challenging the existence of the entire ACA on the ground that the law cannot function without an enforceable insurance mandate.

The effects of these state-led legal challenges on implementation cannot be overstated. The courtroom strategy—not only the victories but also the messaging and instability that accompanied them—handed the states unforeseen and significant leverage that upended the ACA's design. For the 2 years *NFIB* took to reach the Supreme Court, the ACA's future was uncertain. Many states had started planning for exchanges but halted those plans when the litigation gained momentum. Eventually, resistance to implementation became a litmus test for loyalty to the Republican Party. Republican-controlled states faced enormous pressure to refrain from implementing the law, and most succumbed to that pressure. Nine states passed laws requiring legislative approval for any state implementation of the ACA, and 18 states passed laws stating that they would not implement or enforce the individual or employer mandates.[4]

Regarding Medicaid, the Supreme Court's 2012 decision in *NFIB* largely upheld the ACA, but it ruled that the mandatory Medicaid expansion was unconstitutional. The Court's remedy was to render the expansion optional for each state, a major change in the ACA's design that handed the states dramatic new negotiating power vis-à-vis the federal government.

States took advantage of these unexpected developments. States interested in expanding Medicaid negotiated concessions to which many Medicaid experts objected, including premiums, tiered coverage and benefits, enforceable co-payments, limitations on nonemergency medical transportation, limited retroactive eligibility, and (under the Trump administration) even work requirements. States also worked with the Obama administration to innovate new forms of insurance exchanges that allowed them to retain control but still publicly appear to be resisting.

The Obama administration, as we have previously documented, said it was playing a "long game."[5] It wanted to see the ACA implemented, even if controversial concessions to the states were necessary to get there. The administration also needed the states as a practical matter because the federal government did not anticipate and could not have handled implementing all aspects of the ACA alone. HHS Secretary Kathleen Sebelius—a former governor—negotiated with each state individually when it came to Medicaid and the exchanges, a strategy that many credit with getting numerous states on board. Former federal officials stated that "federalism was everything we did."

Negotiating Medicaid

The Medicaid expansion has occurred in waves, each with unique federal-state dynamics. The first wave began even before *NFIB*. Led by Minnesota, 7 states took advantage of ACA provisions allowing early expansion at a state's usual federal funding match before the ACA's increased match took effect in 2014.

The second wave came after *NFIB*. Democrat-led states opted into Medicaid expansion as drafted in the ACA, anticipating the January 1, 2014, implementation date. Governors of split and even Republican-led states also stepped up, as states like Kentucky (Democratic governor, split legislature); Ohio, North Dakota, and Arizona (Republican governor and legislature); and Nevada (Republican governor, Democrat-majority legislature) expanded, sometimes despite recalcitrant legislatures. The National Governors Association's annual meeting one month after *NFIB* was a turning point, galvanizing states to explore their new leverage. HHS fed their interest soon after that meeting, issuing guidance and indicating that the door was open for expansion negotiations. HHS also informed states that Medicaid expansion could occur any time, a totally different timeline from the ACA's design.

The third wave introduced "red-state" policies into Medicaid expansion. It began in September 2013, when Arkansas became the first state to obtain a demonstration waiver for ACA expansion, pioneering privatization of expansion by funneling the newly eligible population into private insurance available through the exchange rather than enrolling beneficiaries in traditional Medicaid. After Arkansas, states learned to wait out other states' negotiations, seeing that they could benefit from others' efforts.

The fourth wave saw the new phenomenon of states *re*negotiating expansion after witnessing HHS's new concessions to other states. It also saw the transition to a new administration that was hostile to the ACA and eager to make even more novel Medicaid concessions, including work requirements never before approved in Medicaid's history. The Obama administration surely knew that the waiver concessions it was granting set a precedent. As one former federal official told us: "Anything you give to another state you have to assume the next state will come in and ask for that and more. There was a sense among states that . . . it was best to be last in line for the next negotiation."

Kentucky led this trend in 2016 with a waiver application, which was held over from the end of the Obama administration into the Trump administration, requesting work requirements and other coverage limitations. In January 2018, after Congress failed to repeal the ACA, the Trump administration issued a policy encouraging work requirements, and Indiana, Arkansas, New Hampshire, Arizona, Michigan, Ohio, and other states quickly applied. As of fall 2019 the Trump administration had approved work requirements in 10 states, 7 more had requests pending, and lower federal courts had struck down Kentucky's, Arkansas's, and New Hampshire's waivers, with litigation in those states and others continuing. Notably, even *non*expansion states, including Alabama, Mississippi, South Carolina, and Wisconsin, have sought work requirements and other limitations in waiver negotiations, such as Tennessee's proposal for a modified block grant. On the other hand, after the 2018 election some states may be reversing course, another example of the dynamic landscape.

Throughout, Medicaid expansion became the focus of democratic engagement. State governments fractured over the decision. Republican governors, bombarded by stakeholders, broke with their own party-controlled legislatures to find ways to expand. (State legislators, in contrast, often focused on the short-term political gains of opposing "Obamacare.") Litigation ensued over some governors' attempts to bypass recalcitrant legislatures.

Medicaid also has been on the ballot in 5 states, all red (or purple) at the time of the referendum. In 2017 Maine had the first successful voter initiative, created to defeat an antiexpansion Republican governor who vetoed expansion legislation multiple times. Three of the 4 states that voted to expand Medicaid in 2018 were red states (Utah, Idaho, and Nebraska). Montana's expansion was up for renewal with tobacco tax funding and was defeated by Big Tobacco pouring in ad money (Montana renewed anyway but added new work requirements). Some state governments, whose resistance was trumped by their voters, have implemented voter initiatives narrowly—for instance, by seeking demonstration waivers with work requirements, limited retroactive enrollment, and spending caps.

Perhaps most surprisingly, Medicaid expansion became the focal point of the 2017 congressional battle to repeal and replace the ACA. Although the ACA itself embraces a somewhat ambivalent mix of private-market and government-provided models for health insurance, Medicaid expansion embraces the public insurance model. During 2017 repeal-and-replace fights, swing-state senators and a coalition of bipartisan governors repeatedly emphasized the importance of retaining the ACA's Medicaid expansion. Coverage losses from any potential repeal were also a focal point. Medicaid's core value—a government guarantee of universality in coverage—became a symbol of what protecting the ACA meant. No one could have predicted after *NFIB* that Medicaid would later get credit for saving the ACA from repeal.

So was the ACA's federalism, as implemented post-*NFIB*, good for the health policy goals the statute aimed to accomplish through Medicaid? As detailed in Chapter 12, the states committed to the program have experienced the ACA's intended improvements, with more than 300 studies showing expansion is a plus for health policy goals.[6] For example, expansion states have increased coverage, with gains for historically vulnerable populations, including minorities, people with low education, and the poor; improved access to care; and decreased maternal and infant mortality. Expansion decreases health disparities and improves social determinants of health such as financial stability.[7] Some evidence indicates that Arkansas-style premium assistance waivers experienced little difference in coverage as compared to traditional Medicaid expansion. But states that implemented waivers imposing premiums (like Indiana) have created barriers to enrollment that decrease coverage.[8] Arkansas showed immediate effects from work requirements, with more than 18,000 people disenrolled within 3 months in 2018 and no increase in employment or employer-sponsored insurance.[9] Health care providers in expansion states report improved financial stability, fewer uninsured visits, and less uncompensated care, especially significant for states with high rates of uninsurance before the ACA. Since 2010 more than 100 rural hospitals have closed nationwide, almost none in expansion states.[10] And expansion states experience budget neutrality or savings and economic growth. Expansion also has been linked to lower insurance premiums in non-Medicaid marketplace plans.

The ACA as drafted—with its unequivocal, nationwide Medicaid expansion—was likely the best available choice from a health policy perspective. Even optional expansion fared well enough under an administration committed to Medicaid, allowing policy tradeoffs as part of its strategy to cover as many people as possible. But the situation is different with an administration hostile to the law. Medicaid's flexibility has enabled new attempts to undermine the program. This is not to say that a strong federal baseline—like the ACA was supposed to have—that allowed for some state tailoring would necessarily be undesirable. And nevertheless, Medicaid under the ACA now insures a population that had been excluded from coverage for decades and now covers nearly ¼ of the population.

Conversely, even though optional Medicaid expansion has been inferior to mandatory expansion from a health-outcomes perspective, that structure has brought unexpected political and instrumental advantages. By putting the choice to each state, the Supreme Court unwittingly made Medicaid the subject of constant public deliberation. Americans were compelled to engage in democratic processes to defend Medicaid. Negotiated waivers also have invested state bureaucrats more deeply in their Medicaid programs and opened lines of communication with federal administrators, which have been public under the ACA.

As such, whether the ACA's federalism was good for the law depends largely on what role federalism is supposed to play in health policy. Do we rely on the states for better health outcomes? Or merely for political or governance reasons? Does state implementation achieve either goal? We return to this point at the end of the chapter.

Strategic Adaptivity and State-Federal Structures in the Exchanges

Insurance exchange implementation likewise encountered obstacles within the unexpected flipped state-federal dynamics of the ACA. Every state except Alaska received exchange planning grants shortly after the ACA became law. But after *NFIB* only 12 states plus Washington, DC—all controlled by Democrats—had decided to establish their own exchanges.

On the surface, a red vs. blue state divide emerged between federally operated exchanges and state-operated ones. Ironically, in refusing to implement their own exchanges, the resisting states triggered the ACA's mandated fallback of a federal exchange within their borders. Douglas Holtz-Eakin, a prominent Republican economist and former head of the Congressional Budget Office, opined that inviting the federal government to operate a state's exchange would be a "Trojan Horse" that would pave the way for a full-scale federal takeover of state insurance markets. But the hot politics of the opposition turned the ACA's federalism expectations on its head. Republican-led states—which had fought hard in Congress for the ACA to have a state-led structure in the first place—effectively nationalized the ACA within their borders, while most Democrat-led states were the ones that chose a state-led structure.

Below the surface, however, the exchange governance structures were more complicated. Congress's initial structural allocation was more of a starting point than an endpoint in terms of the exchange-design options that emerged. States worked with HHS to develop a variety of different models and moved among them. Some federal-exchange states became state-exchange states and vice versa. Mixed models emerged. It became difficult to deduce merely from a state's political leaders or even from the type of exchange structure a state adopted how much policy control any state exerted over its exchange. In other words, the way a state's exchange operated had less do with the formal governance structure of the exchange and more to do with the policy choices made within each state and its engagement with the Obama administration.

Some Democrat-controlled states, like Oregon, wanted to implement their own exchanges but met technical challenges that led them to fail and to rely on the federal exchange. Those "blue" states appeared to be "red" in the sense that the federal government operated their exchange; however, their insurance commissioners closely cooperated with federal officials to manage the exchange. Other exchanges that *looked* red—where the federal government took over exchanges after states publicly refused to implement them—actually have a great deal of engagement through their own insurance commissioners. Almost all states review their own rates and plans, regardless of exchange structure.

Throughout, state officials anxious to keep control over their insurance markets were worried about appearances. They needed to look resistant to "Obamacare" to save face with the Republican Party even as they secretly sought guidance and cooperated. The Obama administration enabled these subterfuges and more. It allowed new forms of exchanges to develop and kept collaboration under the radar as needed.

HHS proved remarkably adaptive. In 2011, when it seemed that the strict binary choice between a state or federal exchange that the ACA appeared to offer would lead very few states to establish their own exchanges, HHS developed a hybrid model, the partnership exchange, which was attractive to some red states because they remained federal exchanges (and therefore they still appeared to be resisting) but gave states significant control. Partnership exchanges left important decisions such as consumer assistance, plan management, and insurer oversight to the states. One official called this the "secret boyfriend model" of federal-state implementation: states treasured their relationships with the Obama administration but were ashamed to reveal them.

And, as with the Medicaid expansion, exchange implementation often divided state governments controlled by a single party. Four of the 7 states that adopted a partnership exchange model used purely executive authority to do so, avoiding the need for legislative approval. In some states insurance commissioners anxious to retain market control but unable for political reasons to sign onto a written agreement for "partnership" with the federal government worked with HHS to get around these obstacles. HHS facilitated their efforts with another new exchange model, the "plan management" exchange, which specifically allowed insurance commissioners, rather than governors, to set up federal exchanges that gave states policy control and deleted any symbolic mention of partnership. Yet another type of exchange, the State-Based Marketplace-Federal Platform, emerged soon thereafter to allow states that needed support from the federal government's Healthcare.gov technical platform to receive it but to continue running their own exchanges.

Some states copied other states' exchange designs rather than reinventing the wheel. The classic federalism vs. nationalism—"1 or 51"—policy models choice in which Congress usually engages when structuring new federal programs seemed too extreme; ACA implementation suggested a middle ground instead. As Connecticut's Exchange Chief Kevin Counihan (later chief executive officer of the national exchange) said in 2014: "We don't need 50 of these things, but we may need 8."

As for health policy outcomes, for the first few years of ACA implementation the particular governance structure of any state's exchange did not appear closely linked to any particular health outcomes. What mattered more was a state's engagement with the ACA. Many such states, even without their own exchanges, made their own policy decisions on matters, including conducting plan management; setting geographic rating areas, reinsurance, and risk adjustment formulas; and running rate reviews and medical-loss ratio. Those states that engaged with the ACA generally performed better across metrics like premium prices and number of insurers than those that did not, even if the state did not operate its own exchange.

But as with Medicaid, under a new administration hostile to the ACA, choice of governance structure has become much more significant. Under the Obama administration states with federal exchanges received as much if not more federal support as states with their own exchanges. But the Trump administration has tried to destabilize the ACA. It has attempted to splinter and refragment the insurance markets, permitting states to offer cheaper short-term and association-based health plans that are not subject to the same protections as exchange plans. It also has tried to depress enrollment, shortening the period for open enrollment, decreasing advertising, and defunding personnel ("navigators") charged with connecting people to plans. Federally operated exchanges are more susceptible to these hostile efforts simply because the federal government has control over those exchanges. And states that wish to undermine the ACA are enabled by an administration with similar goals.

However, states running their *own* exchanges can choose to forego these new options, continue to aggressively enroll, and undertake other efforts to strengthen their own markets.[11] These choices make a difference. For 2019 open enrollment, in federal-exchange states enrollment declined while state-exchange states and state-based-federal-platform states had increased enrollment. States running their own exchanges have also had lower marketplace premiums,[12] more insurers offering exchange plans in that state,[13] more plan selections, and increased Medicaid enrollment.[14]

State-based exchanges also implemented other policies to maintain insurer participation in the face of federal uncertainty surrounding the ACA. California, for example, modified insurer contracts to allow carriers that incurred losses in 2018 due to federal policy or enrollment changes to recover those lost funds in future years.

More generally, regardless of exchange structure, the ACA's federalism gives states significant policy flexibility, and this has proven helpful for states interested in stabilizing their insurance markets.[15] Creative state administrators have used the choices the ACA offers across plan structures to shift more of their populations into the middle level plan—the silver plan—because under those plans individuals pay only a fixed percentage of their income, with tax credits absorbing the rest.[16] By shifting the increased costs due to ACA sabotage to silver-plan premiums, a practice known as silver loading, the federal government paradoxically winds up picking up most of the tab for its own undermining actions because the federal government provides the subsidies.[17] One recent study found that silver loading increased enrollment by 8% in exchange plans among individuals with incomes over 200% of FPL, "largely offsetting the effects of other, simultaneous federal changes in policy and practice that depressed participation levels."[18] Somewhat ironically, the vast majority of federal-exchange states also have engaged in silver loading because that decision remains in the hands of state insurance commissioners regardless of exchange structure. States with both types of exchanges—including Maine, New Jersey, Maryland, Wisconsin, Oregon, Alaska, and Colorado as of this writing—also have pursued reinsurance waivers to stabilize their markets and to lower premiums.

Legal Entrenchment Through the States

States' legal actions to implement the ACA also directly furthered the law's entrenchment and resilience. States had to pass numerous laws and adopt regulations to implement the new insurance reforms, especially states running their own exchanges. States worked furiously to implement essential health benefits packages, bans on discrimination based on preexisting health conditions, new rating standards, and more—and often customized those reforms for their specific markets. In the context of Medicaid many states had to enact new laws to authorize, fund, or otherwise implement expansion, and some states also had to implement pro-Medicaid ballot initiatives.

Perhaps even more significantly, at least 18 states to date—some Republican controlled—have enacted aspects of the ACA's reforms into their *own* laws. For example, states have enacted their own state-law versions of protections for people with preexisting conditions, community-rating requirements, and insurance-purchase mandates, giving those reforms legal permanence even if the ACA is repealed at the federal level. Similarly, Washington and Colorado have enacted legislation creating state-based public insurance options that build on each state's Medicaid expansion and exchange. A handful of other states are considering comparable Medicaid-based reforms.

That space for states to exercise policy control and, with it, to legally entrench the ACA's reforms would not have existed had the ACA nationalized the entire insurance market—because a nationalizing law would have legally preempted and prevented states from legislating on the same topics. This is another practical and political benefit of the ACA's federalism structure that has mattered more in the face of persistent opposition.

Conclusion: What Is Federalism in Health Care For?

Was the ACA's state-federal structure a benefit or a detriment? We are more confident that the ACA's federalism was pragmatically beneficial in terms of passing and entrenching the law, and in retaining an important role for states in health care policy, than that it benefitted health policy outcomes, especially in the context of Medicaid expansion. Federalism's predictable variability raises moral questions about inequities across states when we know states make different policy choices, especially if strong federal baseline rules do not guide those choices. Those moral questions are heightened when medical care is on the line.

ACA implementation also deconstructs traditional assumptions about the benefits of federalism. Common reasons why policymakers turn to federalism in statutory design—including a desire to advance intergovernmental cooperation, state autonomy, and policy experimentation—do not seem to rely on "federalism" in the ACA at all. Especially in the context of the exchanges, formal federalism architecture mattered much less to generating policy variation and state control than did each state's interactions with HHS, its engagement with policy, and its resulting choices. We saw all of the traditional federalism values through all kinds of exchanges, whether federally run, state run, or hybrid.

Finally, it is impossible to know whether the ACA would have "done better" without its federalism. That counterfactual scenario—fully nationalized health care reform without a key role for states—was not politically feasible when the ACA was drafted in 2009. It is plausible that a fully nationalized ACA might have achieved more complete and more stable reform more quickly and with fewer constitutional questions.[19] But it also could have occasioned less state and public buy-in and been more susceptible to later executive branch attempts to undermine it.

Today, even as some states continue to fight the law, others have taken on ACA stewardship in the face of federal hostility, not only in savvy administrative, financial, and policy decisions that have stabilized the law but also in litigation: more than 20 state attorneys general are currently defending the ACA and its goals of universal coverage in court. The enduring fights over the law, largely enabled by the choices that the ACA's federalism puts to each state and its citizenry, have kept health care policy front and center for more than a decade. The debates and policy decisions that have emerged from those fights may ultimately be responsible for paving the way toward even more comprehensive, universal—and, ironically, *national*—reform. Proposals for some form of universal health care, such as Medicare for All, are being debated in ways not seen since the end of World War II. The national conversation the ACA generated, often through its state-oriented, negotiated implementation, is largely responsible for that.

CHAPTER 11

EXECUTIVE POWER AND THE ACA

Nicholas Bagley

As with any law of its complexity and ambition, the Affordable Care Act (ACA) vests in the sitting president broad implementation discretion. The law is not a blank check: in many ways both large and small, the ACA shapes and constrains the exercise of executive power. But Congress has neither the institutional resources nor the attention span to micromanage the rollout of a massive health program. It has no choice but to delegate.

Naturally, both President Obama and President Trump have drawn on their authority to tailor the ACA to their policy preferences. Neither president, however, has been able to turn to Congress for more sweeping changes to the law. Stymied in Congress and buffeted by the partisan combat over Obamacare, they have come under enormous pressure to ignore legal constraints that stand in the way of their political objectives. The story of the ACA's implementation is thus a story of two presidents who have tested—and at times exceeded—the limits of their legal powers.

Yet Obama and Trump have committed very different legal sins. President Obama's lawbreaking reflected his efforts to cope with the ambiguities, omissions, and outright mistakes that are common in any massive law and were especially common in the ACA. To implement the bill in the face of congressional resistance, the Obama administration cut corners. President Trump, however, exploited his position as

Nicholas Bagley, JD, is a law professor at the University of Michigan.

the head of the executive branch to mount an unconstitutional campaign to sabotage the very law he is charged with faithfully executing.

It would be comforting to treat these legal violations as aberrant responses to particular features of the ACA or to the intensity of debate over health reform. But they cannot be so easily dismissed. The ACA is the most assertive effort in 50 years to make good on the claim that health care is a right, not a privilege. That is another way of saying that the have-nots have a moral claim to the resources and privileges of the haves. The campaign against the law is the reactionary counter-mobilization of those who believe that the principles animating the ACA pose an incipient threat to the established order. No wonder that health reform provoked the most rancorous battle over a piece of domestic legislation since the adoption of the Civil Rights Act in 1964.

The fight over the ACA may therefore offer a disquieting preview of what may come if Congress moves to address the nation's other yawning inequalities. Like the ACA, future laws will delegate wide authority to the president. They too will contain unanticipated flaws. And they will also be subject to implementation by hostile presidents. Legal constraints on the executive branch buckled in the white-hot heat of the battle over the ACA. They could melt away altogether in the next war.

President Obama

In November 2010, a scant eight months after the ACA's adoption, Republicans took control of the House of Representatives. Spurred by a Tea Party that saw Obamacare as its principal grievance, the restive House majority committed itself to dismantling the law. Without Congress to help it iron out implementation difficulties, the Obama administration was on its own.

The Delays

In July 2013, Valerie Jarrett, a senior adviser to the president, announced that the administration would temporarily suspend enforcement of the so-called employer mandate. Technically, the name is a misnomer: the law imposes no mandate but instead exacts a tax on larger firms that do not offer health insurance to their workers. That tax serves a dual purpose: it encourages employers to offer coverage and, failing that, generates revenue to offset the costs of the ACA's coverage expansion.

Under the law, the employer mandate was supposed to go into effect in 2014. But the administration, under intense pressure from business groups, said that it would not collect the tax that year. "In our ongoing discussions with businesses," Jarrett explained, "we have heard that you need the time to get this right. We are listening."[1] Later, the administration announced additional suspensions of the mandate for midsize firms.

These were not the only delays. In pressing for the ACA's adoption, President Obama repeatedly promised that "if you like your health care plan, you can keep it."[2] But that was not exactly true. The ACA imposed stringent new rules on privately sold insurance—including limits on out-of-pocket spending and a mandatory suite of benefits—that rendered most existing policies unlawful. (The law did include a grandfather clause, but it was too narrow to save most plans.) As 2013 came to a close, thousands of people began receiving cancelation notices in the mail.

Republicans pounced. As the political heat rose, moderate Democrats in Congress began to clamor for legislation. The administration, however, feared that any law that could make it through a Republican-controlled House would damage the ACA on the eve of its implementation. President Obama called for an administrative fix, one that entailed another delay. In a letter, the Department of Health and Human Services (HHS) invited state insurance commissioners to waive, for one year, the ACA's new rules for existing plans.[3] More than 30 states did, and four subsequent letters have extended the administrative fix through 2021.[4]

Was it legal for the Obama administration to delay parts of the ACA? In general, the executive branch has the discretion to choose when and how to enforce a particular law against particular offenders. As the Supreme Court has said, a federal agency knows best "whether agency resources are best spent on this violation or another."[5] In the Obama administration's view, delaying the employer mandate and the

ACA's insurance rules amounted to a routine and temporary exercise of enforcement discretion.

The ACA delays were unusual, however, because they were not efforts to target limited enforcement resources at the worst offenders. Instead, they were blanket policies adopted for reasons of political expedience—in this case, the perceived need to mollify employers and Congress in an effort to minimize threats to a fledgling statute. The delays were also unusual in that they were announced publicly. The federal government usually keeps its enforcement policies secret because it wants people to comply with the law even if it does not wish to prioritize its enforcement. Here, however, the publicity was necessary to relieve employers and insurers of their legal obligations. As the courts have explained, "An agency's pronouncement of a broad policy against enforcement poses special risks that it has consciously and expressly adopted a general policy that is so extreme as to amount to an abdication of its statutory responsibilities."[6]

In short, President Obama lacked the power to prospectively license large groups of people to disregard one of Congress's laws.[7] Doing so violated his constitutional obligation to "take Care that the Laws be faithfully executed."[8] The delays may also embolden future presidents to delay laws that they dislike. Indeed, early in his presidency, President Trump toyed with suspending enforcement of the individual mandate—which, like the employer mandate, was also a tax.[9]

The Cost-Sharing Payments

To make individual health plans affordable, the ACA offers generous subsidies to cover the costs of monthly premiums. Those subsidies, however, do not cover out-of-pocket payments, which can be extravagantly large: deductibles for an exchange plan in 2019 averaged $4,375.[10]

To address the problem, the ACA requires insurers to give their lowest-income customers a large discount on their out-of-pocket payments. In exchange, the ACA promises to pay insurers to make up for the lost revenue. Without those promised cost-sharing payments, premiums for health plans on the exchanges would skyrocket (or so the thinking ran at the time of the law's adoption). With the payments, coverage would remain affordable.

There was a hitch, however. The Constitution says that "no Money shall be drawn from the Treasury, but in Consequence of Appropriations made by Law."[11] Although Congress specifically appropriated the money for premium subsidies, the ACA did not include an express appropriation for the cost-sharing payments. Its absence was apparently an oversight—one that would probably have been addressed had the ACA passed through a House-Senate conference committee for a final clean-up, as was the original plan. As detailed in Chapter 7, however, the death of Senator Ted Kennedy and Republican Scott Brown's subsequent victory in the Massachusetts special election foreclosed that possibility.

In the normal course, Congress would have promptly appropriated the money necessary to make good on its promises. But the ACA was not a normal statute, and a Republican-controlled House of Representatives was unlikely to supply an appropriation to fund a law that it had voted dozens of times to repeal. As the 2014 date for fully implementing the law drew near, the Obama administration was in a bind. It could either adhere to the Constitution—and watch the ACA collapse—or it could find some way to make the payments anyhow.

The Obama administration took the latter approach, offering a paper-thin legal rationale for the claim that Congress had implicitly appropriated the money. In the administration's view, the premium subsidies and the cost-sharing payments were both essential parts of a common scheme to defray the cost of health plans. Congress must therefore have wanted the appropriation for premium subsidies to do double-duty as an appropriation for the cost-sharing payments.

The argument, however, does not hold together. To appropriate the money for premium subsidies, Congress amended a portion of the tax code allowing the IRS to return tax refunds to individuals. That made sense: the premium subsidies are, in fact, tax credits. Cost-sharing payments, in contrast, are direct payments to insurers. It is a big stretch to read an appropriation governing refunds for individual taxpayers to also cover payments that have nothing to do with the tax code. And federal law prohibits the executive branch from reading a law to appropriate money unless the law "specifically states that an appropriation is made."[12]

An angry House of Representatives filed suit to challenge the payments. Two years later, it won its case in federal court in Washington, DC.[13] Although the court put its opinion on hold to allow for an appeal, President Trump was elected before that appeal could be heard. As congressional Republicans moved to repeal the ACA, President Trump tried to force Democrats to the bargaining table by threatening the cessation of the cost-sharing payments. When repeal legislation stalled out, the president unceremoniously terminated the payments. Only a clever workaround (so-called silver loading, discussed in Chapter 10) has allowed the states to avoid the feared deterioration of their insurance markets.

In some respects the Obama administration's decision to ignore appropriations law was an understandable—if regrettable—response to the kind of statutory problem that arises when a complex bill passes through an unconventional legislative process in a sharply divided Congress. But the decision has unsettling implications. Will future presidents likewise misconstrue appropriations measures when necessary to achieve their policy objectives?

Again, the question is not hypothetical. When Congress refused to appropriate $5 billion that Trump requested for the construction of a wall at the southern border, the administration declared a "national emergency" and interpreted an existing law to allow him to reprogram funds appropriated for military purposes.[14] The statutory argument was weak, but no weaker than the argument President Obama advanced to make cost-sharing payments.

The point is not that one bad act leads to another. Trump would still have reprogrammed the wall funding even if Obama had been more scrupulous about appropriations law. The point, instead, is about presidential incentives. Confronted with an uncooperative Congress, both presidents broke the law, betting that the American public would not punish them for doing so in the next election. They were probably right about that: in a country riven by a stark partisan divide, elections are unlikely to turn on a president's adherence to the finer points of appropriations law. There is thus reason to worry that our next president will exercise even less self-restraint than either Presidents Obama or Trump.

President Trump

President Trump's first act as president was to sign an executive order telling his agencies to "take all actions consistent with law to minimize the unwarranted economic and regulatory burdens of the act."[15] These were to be temporary measures, lasting only until the president secured the ACA's repeal. When the repeal effort faltered in Congress, however, Trump was put into the awkward position of implementing a law he hated.

Trump could have embraced his constitutional duty to "take care that the laws be faithfully executed." Instead, he has used his authority to sabotage the ACA at every turn. Inured as we are to the hardball of partisan politics, it would be easy to overlook just how irregular this is. A president is not obliged to exercise his discretion in a manner that his political opponents would prefer, but the Constitution places out of bounds actions that aim to undermine an act of Congress in order to pave the way for its elimination. Not since Reconstruction has a president worked so systematically to subvert a major congressional initiative.

The still-unfinished story of Trump's sabotage may set a template for what is to come. One party gains temporary control of Congress and the White House and adopts an ambitious new policy, only to watch a subsequent president from the other political party move to dismantle it through executive action. Guarding against that kind of abuse may prove difficult. The ACA, for example, contains more than 40 provisions contemplating rulemaking from federal agencies, which is not at all unusual for major legislation.[16] Though Congress could try to bulletproof future laws by narrowing the discretion they afford to the executive branch, those laws might then be too rigid to achieve the legislature's goals. In any event, no law of any complexity can be implemented without the aid of the executive branch, meaning that every significant reform will be subject, to some degree or another, to presidential tampering. In this bitterly divided country, sabotage may become the new normal.

The Exchanges

Immediately after taking office, the Trump administration moved to destabilize the insurance exchanges. Its first act was to cut 90% of the $100 million that Healthcare.gov had used for advertising in 2016. The administration paired that cut with a 41% cut to the navigator program, which pays for in-person guides to help people buy insurance. Still deeper cuts to navigator funding were announced in July 2018. None of these cuts was likely to discourage sick people from enrolling; they would, however, depress enrollment by healthy people, unbalancing the risk pool and driving premiums higher.

In 2018 the Trump administration proposed two rules that would have much the same effect. The first offered a new definition of what the ACA calls "short-term, limited duration insurance." Because short-term plans are meant to cover only brief gaps in coverage, they are exempt from most of the ACA's rules. Short-term plans can reject unhealthy people, decline to cover preexisting conditions, and exclude benefits like maternity care or drug coverage. The only advantage of short-term plans is that they are cheap, at least for healthy people. But the ACA's insurance exchanges will struggle to spread risk if too many healthy people buy short-term plans instead of conventional insurance.

Nonetheless, the Trump administration proposed defining short-term insurance to include plans that lasted 364 days in the year and could be renewed for up to three years. The interpretation is controversial: Is a health plan that covers you for 99.7% of the year really "short term"? Nonetheless, the administration has moved forward and hopes to make short-term plans a realistic long-term option for healthy people. Many of those same people will be in for a surprise when they discover just how stingy those short-term plans are.

The second rule relaxed restrictions on association health plans. Under federal law, small businesses are allowed to join together to buy insurance for their employees. When they do, the law treats them as large employers and exempts them from rules requiring insurers to sell health plans at much the same price to everyone. In the past, only businesses in the same line of work were allowed to create association health plans—all the bakeries in town, for example. The Trump administration, however, sought to relax that obligation and enable small businesses in any line of work—and even self-employed individuals—to form association health plans.

As with the rule governing short-term plans, the goal was to allow healthier-than-average people to flee the exchanges. Both rules would therefore drive up the costs of insurance for the sicker-than-average people left behind. Among stakeholders, the rules were wildly unpopular: "More than 95% of health care groups that have commented on President Trump's effort to weaken Obama-era health insurance rules criticized or outright opposed the proposals," reported the *Los Angeles Times*.[17] In the summer of 2018 the Trump administration finalized the rules anyway.

There is nothing unusual about an administration issuing rules to interpret an ambiguous law. What is unusual, however, is for an administration to adopt legally dubious interpretations in a deliberate effort to thwart the law altogether. Predictably, both rules have been challenged in court. In March 2019 one judge in Washington, DC, invalidated the rule governing association health plans because it "was intended and designed to end run the requirements of the ACA."[18] Not long after, a different judge on the same court upheld the rule governing short-term health plans, reasoning that Congress did not impose hard-and-fast limits on the length of plans and that the court "cannot simply ignore the legislature's choice to use indefinite, flexible phraseology."[19] As of this writing, both cases have been appealed.

There is more. Under the ACA's risk-adjustment program, insurers with relatively healthy enrollees are required to transfer some of the premiums they receive to health plans with relatively unhealthy enrollees. By balancing risk, the program is supposed to discourage insurers from competing with one another to attract the healthiest people. Risk adjustment is not controversial and is used in both Medicare Advantage and Medicare Part D. In February 2018, however, a court in New Mexico decided that the HHS rule governing the program was invalid because it had not been adequately explained.[20] The Trump administration could have issued a new rule to address the court's concerns. Alternatively, it could have appealed and asked that the court's decision be placed on hold. Instead, without warning, the Trump administration abruptly suspended risk-adjustment payments, sending shockwaves through the insurance industry.[21] The political blowback was so intense that the administration quickly backtracked. But the signal was clear: the exchanges were in the crosshairs.

The latest blow to the exchanges came in a highly technical rule, released in April 2019, that increased the amount that the ACA requires people to pay toward their insurance. The details of the new rule are less important than the bottom line: according to the Trump administration's own estimates, 100,000 people are expected to lose coverage on account of the price hike.[22] Nothing in the ACA demanded the change, and leaked documents indicate that HHS recommended against it because it "would cause coverage losses, further premium increases, and market disruption."[23] But these were virtues, not vices, to a White House bent on sabotage.

All told, the Trump administration's actions are estimated to have increased annual premiums on the exchanges by an average of $580.[24] So far, however, the exchanges have survived, mainly because of how the ACA structures its premium subsidies. For people earning less than four times the federal poverty level (just under $50,000 for an individual in 2019), the ACA caps their premiums at just less than 10% of their income. No matter how high premiums go, most people will pay the same. The biggest losers, instead, are people earning more than four times the poverty level who need to cover every dollar of those increased premiums.

Republicans may come to rue their support for the Trump administration's sabotage campaign. The exchanges are the types of public-private partnerships that they have long endorsed as an alternative to bloated government bureaucracies. The more dysfunctional the exchanges become, the less defensible these sorts of partnerships appear. It is no accident that the Trump administration's attacks on the exchanges have coincided with an increase in support for reforms like Medicare for All that do not depend on private insurance. Such programs may also be less vulnerable to tampering by an unfriendly executive branch.

Medicaid

As Chapters 10, 12, and 18 explained, the ACA transformed Medicaid from a welfare program for the "deserving" poor into a social-service program for *all* the poor. The Trump administration, however, has tried to use its executive power to undo that transformation—most significantly, by granting waivers allowing nine states to impose work requirements on the expansion population. Nine more requests are pending.

A number of lawsuits have been filed challenging the waivers. As of this writing, a district court in Washington, DC, has struck down work requirements in three states: Arkansas, Kentucky, and New Hampshire.[25] The court's reasoning is straightforward. By law, any waivers must be "likely to assist in promoting the objectives" of the Medicaid program. And Medicaid's central objective, the judge found, is to extend medical care to needy people. The Trump administration never adequately explained how waivers that would force tens of thousands of people off Medicaid could possibly be consistent with that objective.

In so doing, the court brushed aside the Trump administration's argument that the point of Medicaid is not just to provide medical care but also to improve *health*. "Were that the case," the court reasoned, "nothing would prevent the Secretary from conditioning coverage on a special diet or certain exercise regime."[26] Even if work requirements might promote health for some people, the administration never weighed those health benefits against the harms arising from the loss of coverage. The court found that such a failure of explanation made the waivers arbitrary and capricious.

Taken together, the court's rulings reflect the view that the Trump administration cannot use work requirements to thwart the ACA's changes to Medicaid. Whether those rulings hold up on appeal is another question. In the past, the courts have generally not been moved by the argument that Medicaid waivers cannot be used to make fundamental changes to Medicaid.

Texas v. United States

Perhaps the Trump administration's most audacious move against the ACA has been its support of a lawsuit seeking to invalidate it altogether. As discussed in Chapters 8 and 9, Republican attorneys general from 20 states brought a case in February 2018 claiming that the individual mandate—the same mandate that the Supreme Court had previously sustained as a proper exercise of Congress's power to tax—is now unconstitutional, and that the entire ACA must fall with it.

In late 2017, after several failed attempts to repeal and replace the entire ACA, Congress passed the Tax Cuts and Jobs Act, which included what President Trump characterized as "the Repeal of the highly unpopular Individual Mandate."[27] The Republican attorneys general, however, noticed that Congress did not formally repeal the ACA's command to buy insurance. Instead, Congress zeroed out the penalty for going without coverage. Functionally, it was a distinction without a difference: only the penalty gave the mandate any force and effect. Without a penalty, the mandate was defunct.

The attorneys general, however, seized on the formal distinction. When it upheld the individual mandate as a tax, the Supreme Court had also reasoned that it would exceed Congress's powers under the Commerce Clause to order people to buy coverage. Now that the tax penalty had been repealed, the attorneys general argued, the naked mandate that remained on the books could not be defended as a tax. It was simply a command and must therefore be unconstitutional.

From that premise—that the zero-dollar mandate is unconstitutional—the attorneys general built the astonishing argument that the entire ACA must fall. When Congress passed the ACA in 2010, Congress adopted findings saying that the individual mandate was essential. Because those findings remain on the books, Congress in 2017 must still have thought that the mandate was essential—even a mandate backed by no penalty. And because this mandate is so intertwined with the law as a whole, the entire law must be invalidated.

The consensus among legal scholars on both sides of the aisle is that the argument is frivolous. Congressional Republicans had a chance after Trump's election to repeal the ACA. They did not have the votes. Zeroing out the mandate penalty was a consolation prize. As such, there is no need to speculate on whether Congress preferred the ACA without a mandate to no ACA at all. It made that choice by repealing the only mechanism for enforcing the mandate while leaving the rest of the law intact. The very same Congress did not harbor the secret belief that a zero-dollar mandate was vital to the law's continued operation.

The Trump administration saw a chance, however, to achieve in court what it could not achieve in Congress. The Justice Department has a long tradition, adhered to across Republican and Democratic administrations, of defending acts of Congress if any reasonable argument can be made on their behalf.[28] Otherwise, the Justice Department could pick and choose which laws remained on the books by declining to defend when a lawsuit is brought challenging a law it dislikes. Refusing to defend can thus do violence to the principle that Congress makes the law, not the president.

Nevertheless, the Trump administration's Justice Department threw its support behind the lawsuit. Initially, it argued that the individual mandate's supposed constitutional defect required invalidation of those portions of the ACA requiring insurers to sell to all comers at more or less the same price—in other words, the protections for people with preexisting conditions. But it has since decided that the entire Act must fall and is now pressing that view in the federal courts.

By filing suit in Fort Worth, Texas, the challengers were able to channel their case to one of the most conservative judges in the country, one who had already invalidated prior Obama-era rules implementing the ACA. In December 2018 the judge declared the individual mandate unconstitutional and the entire ACA invalid.[29] On appeal, a conservative panel of the US Court of Appeals for the 5th Circuit agreed that the mandate could not be sustained. But it asked the judge to reconsider whether there might be some portions of the law that could be salvaged.

As of this writing, most close observers believed the lawsuit is unlikely to succeed. Nothing is certain, however, especially where the ACA is concerned. And the sheer irresponsibility of the lawsuit is breathtaking. The ACA is now part of the plumbing of the US health care system and ripping it out would inflict untold damage on the economy. Yet the Trump administration has publicly committed itself to a legal position that would do just that.

More worrisome still, the duty to defend is a close cousin to the president's constitutional duty to faithfully execute the law. If the ACA really is so unconstitutional that the Trump administration can make no argument in its defense, the law's continued implementation must likewise violate the Constitution. It is not hard to see that as an incipient justification for refusing to enforce any law that the president believes to be unconstitutional, however preposterous or partisan that belief might be.

Conclusion

One president broke the law to save it. The next abused his power to savage it. Each in his own way violated his constitutional duty of faithful execution.

It is tempting but wrong to chalk up the legal violations to these presidents' particular psychologies: an arrogant Obama, an unprincipled Trump. The truth is bleaker. In high-stakes battles where partisan lines have been drawn, the incentives to adhere to the law—the fear of political fallout, concerns about judicial review, some ingrained sense of morality—may not be robust enough to keep the president within bounds.

After all, the public's ability to censure a lawbreaking president depends on knowing when censure is warranted. But the legal experts who might object to illegal executive actions are not immune from partisan tribalism. Few lawyers who support the ACA criticized Obama when he broke the law. Those who complained loudest about Obama's lawbreaking have mostly fallen silent under Trump. As claims of lawbreaking come to be seen as partisan gripes, the American public grows numb to arguments that the president is flouting the law.

And so the rule of law decays. All major statutes—the ACA included—assign vast responsibilities to the executive branch; indeed, broad delegations are an ineradicable feature of the modern administrative state. But that makes any substantial legislative reform vulnerable to abuse from the very executive branch charged with overseeing it. If we are indeed entering an era marked by the steady erosion of legal constraints on the president, Congress's authority to chart the country's course will diminish over time—a development with consequences for American governance that are hard to predict but likely pernicious.

The adoption of the ACA marked a progressive victory. The story of its implementation, however, offers a cautionary tale.

Part IV

ASSESSING IMPACT

CHAPTER 12

INSURANCE ACCESS AND HEALTH CARE OUTCOMES

Katherine Baicker and Benjamin D. Sommers

One of the primary purposes of the Affordable Care Act (ACA) was to expand health insurance coverage to previously uninsured Americans. A greater share of the US population is uninsured than in any other developed nation—50 million people at the time the ACA was passed in 2010.[1] The ACA took a multipronged approach to extending coverage. Unlike Medicare, in which coverage is essentially automatic when individuals turn 65, the ACA's multiple coverage options all required people to actively enroll. Evaluating the law's impact requires answering 3 key questions. The first is: Who got covered? In other words, how many people signed up for the different insurance options under the ACA? And perhaps just as importantly: Who did *not* get coverage? Second: Once the dust settled, what were the effects of these gleaming new insurance cards? Could newly insured Americans afford their health care? Could they find providers willing to see them? Did they get more primary care, crowd the nation's emergency departments—or both? And the third question is: After billions of dollars spent, were Americans any healthier?

Katherine Baicker, PhD, is a health economist and the dean of the University of Chicago's Harris School of Public Policy.

Benjamin D. Sommers, MD, PhD, is a professor of health policy and economics at the Harvard School of Public Health and associate professor of medicine at Harvard Medical School. He served as a senior adviser in the US Department of Health and Human Services (2011–2012).

These critical questions have been the subject of nearly a decade's worth of research.[2] In this chapter we sift through studies by economists, physicians, policy experts, and others to answer these questions. We will not be able to touch on every study of the ACA—a number that, as of spring 2019, had topped 8,500![3] Rather, we synthesize the literature and focus on some of the most prominent studies with strong research designs that provide a representative look at what we know about the ACA's effects.

The ACA's coverage expansions came through multiple avenues, including the option for young adults to stay on their parents' plans; the creation of health insurance marketplaces (or exchanges), where lower- and middle-income families could receive premium tax credits to make that coverage more affordable; and a large expansion of Medicaid eligibility to low-income adults. Each of these types of health insurance potentially has short- and long-term impacts on health care and health outcomes. Our chapter explores how the ACA affected health insurance coverage; how insurance affected health care affordability, access to and use of health care services, and the quality of care; and ultimately whether this translated into changes in health outcomes.[4] Fundamentally, this chapter seeks to answer the question: Did the ACA's coverage expansions work?

Coverage Effects: Projections, Website Malfunction, Navigators, and More

October 1, 2013, marked the long-awaited beginning of the ACA's first open enrollment period for the law's new health insurance marketplaces, where people could sign up for policies that would take effect in 2014. Newspapers ran "how to sign up" articles, cable news stoked the longstanding debate over the law, and many Americans looked forward to their first opportunity to sign up for coverage. But almost immediately it was clear that something was amiss. The *New York Times* front page declared, "Opening Rush to Insurance Markets Hits Snags."[5] The words "trainwreck" and "website malfunction" became common parlance. At the same time, news of insurance cancellation notices dominated discussion of the ACA, as several million consumers received notification that their insurance plans were shutting down because they did not meet the law's new coverage requirements. The fate of the marketplaces garnered much of the attention around the law, but it was neither the first nor the largest component of the ACA's coverage expansions. In this section we review the evidence on each of the law's main coverage provisions.

Young Adults' Coverage

In late 2010 one of the first ACA provisions to take effect required most health insurers to let young adults stay on their parents' plans until their 26th birthday. This policy, often called the "dependent coverage provision," was designed to remedy a longstanding problem of low coverage rates among young adults. Too old for the Children's Health Insurance Program (CHIP), often in school or entry-level jobs without insurance, and sometimes just because they were healthy and thought they did not need coverage (leading to the label "young invincibles"), nearly 1 out of 3 adults between 19 and 25 had no insurance prior to the ACA, the highest uninsured rate among any age group in the United States.[6]

The dependent coverage provision was implemented smoothly— many young adults enrolled, and coverage rates climbed rapidly in this age group. By 2012, 2 to 3 million more young adults had health insurance (representing as much as 10% of this age group), a change demonstrated in several studies comparing insurance trends for the 19- to 25-year-olds affected by this policy to patterns for slightly older adults who were not affected by the change.[7]

Health Insurance Marketplaces and Insurance Market Reforms

Meanwhile, with plan cancellations and website malfunction dominating the news in late 2013, what actually happened to coverage in the marketplaces? Despite the troubled roll-out, marketplace enrollment grew steadily the first few years of the program—climbing from 8 million in 2014 to 12.2 million by 2017.[8]

Although the hubbub over plan cancellations (directly related to the law's new requirements for nongroup insurance plans—i.e., private plans not offered through employers) attracted political attention and created real difficulties for some of the estimated 2.5 million people whose plans were canceled, research indicates that most individuals in this population were eligible for newly subsidized and more comprehensive marketplace insurance, and the cancellation rate was not far from the historical norms in this market.[9] Thus, few people actually lost coverage on net (vs. having to change plans) because of cancellations.

But despite the steady enrollment growth, total marketplace enrollment fell far short of the original projections, with the Congressional Budget Office (CBO) having projected in 2012 that 23 million people would obtain coverage via the marketplaces by 2016; the actual total was only half that number.[10]

There are multiple potential reasons for this gap. One important factor is that analysts had predicted that several million individuals would switch from employer coverage to the marketplaces. This would not have represented a net increase in the number of Americans with insurance—just a shift in who provided coverage. But this shift never occurred, as overall rates of employer-sponsored insurance remained stable after the ACA's implementation.[11] Another factor was that the marketplaces in some areas of the country experienced significant premium growth year to year and high-profile departures by several large insurers, which likely dampened consumer interest.[12]

Overall, about 25% of Americans without insurance in 2017— roughly 7 to 8 million people—were thought to be eligible for subsidized marketplace coverage but had not enrolled.[13] One of the main barriers for this group was affordability: more than half described feeling that the coverage options—even with subsidies—were unaffordable.[14] Subsidies were thus a major determinant of take-up. Of the 12.2 million people enrolled in marketplace policies in 2017, 83% (10.1 million) received premium subsidies, with the average annual subsidy of $4,600 covering 78% of the total premium.[15] Marketplace premium affordability is likely an even larger barrier for those with incomes just above 400% of the poverty level who are not eligible for any subsidized coverage under the ACA, though 85% of individuals in this income group receive coverage through an employer.[16]

Information challenges and difficulties with the enrollment process also were important factors. For instance, 40% of uninsured adults in 2017 reported that they had not even heard of the marketplaces.[17] Enrollment was substantially higher in states that ran their own marketplaces (even though a fair number of these states also experienced technological growing pains as they got their websites up and running).[18] This is likely due to several factors, including that most states running their own marketplaces were more engaged in outreach efforts, with political leaders expressing support for the law as well as the ACA's navigator program, which was designed to assist consumers' efforts to understand their options and sign up for coverage. In contrast, other states passed laws restricting community organizations' ability to help with enrollment (on either state or federal marketplaces) or outlawing the use of state funds to advertise the marketplaces.[19] Given evidence that advertising was an important driver for marketplace signups[20] and that many low-income individuals in particular benefited from navigators and application assistance,[21] these state and local policy choices likely played an important role in total enrollment.

Medicaid Expansion

The last of the major aspects of the ACA's coverage expansion to take effect—Medicaid expansion—had the largest coverage impact. The changes to Medicaid envisioned by the ACA were sweeping. Prior to the law, only certain low-income populations could qualify for Medicaid coverage—primarily children, pregnant women and parents, individuals with disabilities, and the elderly. Millions of low-income Americans, particularly childless adults, could not qualify for Medicaid either because they did not fit into one of these categories or because their incomes were still too high to qualify in their states. For instance, in Arkansas prior to the ACA low-income parents in a family of 4 had to have an income less than $4,000 annually to qualify for Medicaid— just 17% of the federal poverty level (FPL).[22] The ACA aimed to make Medicaid available starting in 2014 to all US citizens or qualifying legal residents with income below 138% of the FPL—just over $17,000 for a single person or $35,000 for a family of 4 in 2019—not just those in particular categories of eligibility. However, as noted in Chapters 8 and 9 of this volume, the Supreme Court's 2012 ruling effectively made this expansion optional for the states, which had profound impacts on Medicaid.

The result is that on January 1, 2014, only 26 states (including Washington, DC) were participating in the Medicaid expansion. By March

2019, 34 states had expanded, and 3 more had passed 2018 ballot initiatives in favor of expansions that their state legislatures had yet to implement. All told, over 16 million more people were enrolled in Medicaid in 2017 than in 2013—most of them in expansion states, but not all. In fact, the Medicaid rolls grew by more than 2 million in nonexpansion states.[23]

To understand why coverage increased even in nonexpansion states, we need to dive into the details of Medicaid enrollment. Coverage in the program is not automatic—people who are eligible for the program need to sign up in order to be covered, and once they do, they need to actively renew their enrollment annually to stay in the program. Because of these factors, combined with confusion about eligibility and a substantial dose of red tape, researchers estimated that only about ⅔ of eligible adults with no other coverage were enrolled in Medicaid prior to the ACA.[24] Media coverage around the ACA, additional spending on outreach efforts, a streamlined application process, and possibly the influence of the individual mandate all combined to increase enrollment in Medicaid even among groups who were eligible all along. This "welcome mat" or "woodwork effect" led millions of already-eligible adults—as well as nearly 1 million children—in both expansion and nonexpansion states to sign up for Medicaid starting in 2014.[25] That said, coverage gains from Medicaid were largest in those states that did choose to expand eligibility and among individuals who were not previously eligible.[26]

Overall Effects on Coverage

All told, by the end of 2016 the US uninsured rate stood at its lowest recorded level, with 90% of the population having coverage.[27] The Obama administration estimated that the number of US residents without health insurance had dropped from 50 million before the ACA to 30 million (which includes roughly 5 million undocumented immigrants who do not have coverage, while another 6 million in this population have non-ACA-related health insurance).[28] Research attributed roughly 60% of this coverage gain to Medicaid and 40% to subsidized private insurance via the marketplaces.[29]

Why did 10% of the population remain uninsured, particularly in contrast to the 97% coverage rate attained in Massachusetts after its 2006 health reform, which was in many ways the model for the ACA? In part, this reflects the lack of Medicaid expansion in more than a dozen states as well as less generous premium subsidies for lower-income adults in the ACA's marketplace than in the Massachusetts model (individuals with incomes below 300% of the poverty level in Massachusetts receive additional state subsidies to cover a larger share of premiums and co-pays than under the ACA). Greater political opposition to the ACA in many states than was seen in Massachusetts likely played a role as well.[30] Finally, Massachusetts began with a much lower uninsurance rate before its health reform (and a higher average household income) than the country as a whole.[31]

Research examining the overall effects of the ACA on insurance coverage rates has shown that coverage gains were substantial in all geographic parts of the country—urban, suburban, and rural.[32] Although insurance rates increased in essentially every major demographic group, not everyone benefited equally. The first wave of coverage expansion, the dependent coverage provision, benefited young adults whose parents had private coverage—a group who were, on average, higher income and disproportionately white.[33] But the 2014 expansions increased coverage particularly among lower-income households and racial and ethnic minorities.[34] Figure 12.1 shows changes in insurance coverage from 2010 to 2017 by race/ethnicity, using national survey data.[35] The share of nonelderly US residents without any insurance decreased dramatically starting in 2014 for all groups, but the largest changes occurred for those groups that started with lower rates of coverage—racial and ethnic minorities. By 2017 the historic gap between Asian Americans and whites had been eliminated entirely, while the largest absolute changes in coverage occurred among Latinos and blacks. The ACA thus substantially reduced disparities in coverage by race and ethnicity—but large gaps remain.[36]

What about coverage related to employment—and employment itself? Was the ACA a job killer? Some critics were concerned that the ACA's new coverage options, combined with a new employer mandate requiring larger firms to provide workers with insurance or else pay a fine, would lead to job losses and the erosion of employer-based insurance. However, multiple studies have found no evidence of changes in overall employment or part-time vs. full-time employment as well

Figure 12.1 Coverage Changes by Race/Ethnicity, 2010–2017

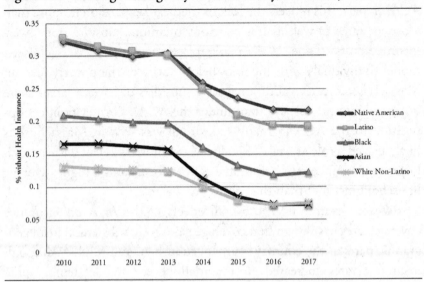

Source: From authors' analysis of survey data from the US Census Bureau of US residents aged 0 to 64.

as no reductions in employer-sponsored insurance.[37] Indeed, among workers the largest coverage gains under the ACA occurred among the self-employed and those with blue-collar jobs, the groups of workers who were least likely to have access to affordable insurance coverage through their jobs prior to the ACA.[38]

Since 2016, coverage rates have plateaued and, according to some analyses, begun to decline again. Several studies have found an erosion of coverage rates in 2017–2018, including the most recent estimates from the US Census Bureau.[39] Why coverage may have declined—despite a booming economy—is difficult to determine with certainty, but some analysts have pointed to several changes in the implementation of the ACA under the Trump administration starting in 2017.[40] These changes include reduced spending on outreach and advertising, a shortened open enrollment period, and uncertainty over payments to insurers designed to reduce the risk of high-cost patients and to subsidize lower-income families' co-pays.

Moving forward, Congress's elimination of the individual mandate through zeroing out the tax penalty, effective in 2019, may also have important effects on future coverage, though some studies suggest that the mandate played only a limited role in increasing insurance enrollment.[41] Finally, new requirements in several states that Medicaid beneficiaries must work (or participate in other qualifying "community engagement" activities) to remain eligible may lead to additional reductions in coverage.[42] These trends remain an important area of ongoing evaluation.

Affordability of Care and Health Care Use: What Can You Do with an Insurance Card?

Having health insurance is just one factor affecting access to health care. As one policymaker put it, insurance expansion without improvement in health care affordability and access would be a "hollow victory of numbers covered."[43]

There are several reasons—varying by type of coverage—that insurance might have limited effects on health care use. First, there have been longstanding concerns about provider acceptance of Medicaid, which is lower than Medicare or private insurance.[44] Several states have also implemented higher levels of cost sharing and premiums in Medicaid, which may present a particular challenge given the low incomes of those enrolled in the program.[45]

Second, marketplace plans vary even more widely than Medicaid in their cost-sharing requirements and provider networks, which can have important implications for access. The ACA created different metal-named tiers for marketplace plans, which vary in their "actuarial value"—that is, the percentage of a typical enrollee's medical expenses that the plan will pay for (with the enrollee responsible for the remaining share): bronze plans cover 60% of expected costs, silver 70%, gold 80%, and platinum 90%. In addition, those with incomes below 2.5 times the poverty level (numbering roughly 60% of marketplace enrollees in 2017) qualify for cost-sharing reductions to cover a portion of their required co-pays.[46] Overall, silver plans have proved the most popular, accounting for 71% of enrollees in 2016 and 74% in 2017; 21% picked bronze in those years, and less than 10% picked gold or platinum.[47] Most of these plans included deductibles, with an average silver-plan deductible of approximately $3,000 and bronze deductible of \$5,800 in 2016.[48] These features are responsible in part for the finding that, though the uninsured rate has declined sharply under the ACA, there has been a simultaneous increase in the share of Americans who are "*under*insured"—typically defined by having to spend a high proportion of income on health care out-of-pocket payments or delaying needed care due to cost.[49] This has occurred despite ACA provisions requiring certain preventive services to be covered without any cost sharing.

Cost sharing is not the only potential barrier to obtaining care in marketplace plans. Although the ACA explicitly outlawed denying coverage based on preexisting conditions, studies and case reports suggest that some plans have taken steps to avoid high-cost patients through overly restrictive formularies (e.g., not covering any HIV medications)[50] and extremely narrow provider networks, in some cases having no physicians in certain subspecialties within 100 miles.[51] The Trump administration has issued regulations (now under legal challenge) allowing for greater availability and duration of short-term plans that are exempt from several ACA coverage and rate provisions[52] and has encouraged greater availability of association health plans, which may provide cheaper, less-comprehensive coverage than ACA plans.

Given concerns about high cost sharing, skimpy insurance plans, and limited provider availability, how has the ACA actually fared in terms of making affordable health care available?

Despite their reputation as young invincibles who felt they did not need health care, the 19- to 25-year-olds who gained insurance via the dependent coverage provision did use their new insurance to get more care. Surveys indicate fewer young adults delayed needed medical care due to cost, while their average out-of-pocket spending on health care declined by 18%.[53] An analysis of emergency department visits showed that the policy had collectively covered more than \$147 million per year in costs of emergency care for serious conditions such as appendicitis and major fractures.[54]

Dozens of studies have examined the effects of the Medicaid expansion. Figure 12.2 highlights just a few of these findings, including significant improvements in affordability of care[55] and financial security.[56] Medicaid expansion also led to a wide range of changes in health care utilization. Low-income adults were more likely to have a primary

Figure 12.2 Changes in Health-Care Access and Affordability in States Expanding Medicaid under the ACA Relative to States that Did Not

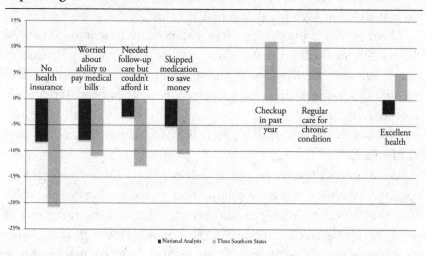

Source: From published studies comparing outcomes among low-income adults in Medicaid expansion versus nonexpansion states. All estimates refer to the percentage-point change in outcomes for this population. National analysis is from Sarah Miller and Laura R. Wherry, "Health and Access to Care during the First 2 Years of the ACA Medicaid Expansions," *New England Journal of Medicine* 376 (2017): 947–956, https://doi.org/10.1056/NEJMsa1612890. No estimates were available in this study for "check in past year" and "regular care for chronic conditions." Three-state analysis (Arkansas and Kentucky, which expanded, compared to Texas, which did not expand) is from Benjamin D. Sommers et al., "Three-Year Impacts of the Affordable Care Act: Improved Medical Care and Health among Low-Income Adults," *Health Affairs* 36, no. 6 (2017): 1119–1128, https://doi.org/10.1377/hlthaff.2017.0293.

care provider or personal doctor, and they increasingly received preventive services such as an annual checkup, HIV testing, mammograms, cholesterol tests, and screening for diabetes,[57] though the expansion did not appear to increase rates of preventive dental care[58] (notably, paying for dental care for adults in Medicaid is still optional for states). Overall, estimates indicate that Medicaid expansion led to a 6 to 16 percentage-point increase in the share of low-income adults obtaining primary care.[59]

How about appointment wait times, a perpetual concern in Medicaid and especially so with millions of new people entering the program? The evidence is mixed: one study showed an increase in patients experiencing long delays in obtaining appointments,[60] while another found better availability of appointments after expansion—in part attributable to a provision in the ACA that temporarily boosted Medicaid primary care payment rates in 2013–2014.[61]

Other studies using patient surveys showed that Medicaid increased the use of medications and reduced patients' skipping pills due to cost.[62] An analysis of national pharmacy data showed that the largest increases in medication use occurred among treatments for chronic conditions such as diabetes and cardiovascular disease as well as contraception—though with smaller effects in states charging higher co-pays in Medicaid.[63]

What about the emergency department (ED)? Many advocates of coverage expansion voiced the hope that giving people health insurance that increased access to primary care would keep them out of the ED—and even save money in the process. However, there is little evidence that this occurred. Some studies of the ACA have shown reduced use of the ED among young adults gaining private coverage and among low-income adults in 2 Medicaid expansion states,[64] while another study found stable ED rates after the Medicaid expansion in Maryland.[65] However, the strongest evidence on the effect of Medicaid on ED use comes from a pre-ACA randomized controlled evaluation of Medicaid coverage in Oregon that showed that Medicaid increased ED usage by 40%.[66] Taken as a whole, it is far from clear that expanding insurance reduces ED use—and even if it does in some contexts, the modest reductions in ED use would not be nearly enough to cover the added costs of the other types of health care utilization that increase when people gain insurance. Thus, the economist's refrain that "there's no such thing as a free lunch" applies in health care too: the benefits of gaining health insurance come with a substantial price tag.

What about the effects of marketplace coverage? Here there is far less evidence than for Medicaid—mostly because it turns out to be more difficult to study. Medicaid expansion created a natural experiment to study its effects by comparing expansion vs. nonexpansion states, but the marketplaces extended coverage simultaneously in all 50 states, leaving researchers without an obvious group for comparison. Nonetheless, a few studies offer insights. One study compared middle-income individuals without employer coverage prior to the ACA to people who did get coverage through their employers. For the group without employer coverage, the ACA led to significant gains in marketplace insurance in 2014 that were associated with an easier time affording medications and more office visits.[67] Another recent analysis looked at people just above and below the income cutoff for receiving premium subsidies for marketplace coverage and found that receiving the subsidies led to a 25% reduction in the risk of being behind on housing payments.[68]

Finally, at the population level—despite general concerns over affordability and whether the system could absorb 20 million more people with health insurance—national survey trends suggested that the ACA increased access overall. Data from 2012 to 2015 on over half a million US adults showed that Americans have been less likely to report putting off needed care due to cost and are better able to access primary care and prescription medications since 2014, thereby reversing the negative trends from before the law took effect.[69]

Quality of Care and Health Outcomes: Did Anyone Get Better?

Clearly, the expansion of coverage led to real changes in how millions of Americans interacted with the health care system, how they paid their bills, and how often they saw the doctor. But at the end of the day, was the care they received any good, and were they any healthier?

For the first group to gain coverage under the ACA, young adults, serious health problems are fortunately relatively uncommon. But studies indicate that some of the first young adults to sign up for coverage on their parents' plans were ones with more serious health problems,[70] and they reported feeling that their health had improved after the policy took effect.[71] Young adults suffering from acute appendicitis went to the hospital earlier on in their symptoms, which reduced rates of perforation.[72] Meanwhile, pregnant women in this age group gaining coverage had better maternal outcomes, with small but significant increases in prenatal care and fewer premature births.[73]

For the law's much larger Medicaid and marketplace coverage expansions, there are also some signs of improved health care quality. Several studies have found increased rates of diagnoses of chronic conditions such as diabetes and high blood pressure, a necessary first step to getting treatment.[74] Hunger and poor health outcomes often go together, and another study found that Medicaid expansion led to lower levels of food insecurity, meaning adults were less likely to go hungry due to lack of money.[75] As a fairly crude measure of whether people diagnosed with chronic conditions are actually getting better care, surveys show that among adults who know they have a chronic medical problem, Medicaid expansion led to much higher rates of obtaining regular care for those conditions and improvements in the reported quality of care.[76] In more detailed examinations of chronic-disease care, there is evidence of improved care for some conditions—with better blood pressure control among community health center patients and higher quality of care for patients about to start dialysis for kidney failure.[77] Patients presenting to the hospital with acute surgical conditions like appendicitis, life-threatening aneurysms in their aorta, and poor limb circulation experienced improvements in the quality of surgical care and health outcomes—with fewer perforated appendices, fewer ruptured aneurysms, and fewer limb amputations.[78] At the same time, studies of patients in the hospital with cardiac disease have not found any improvements in quality.[79]

But here, too, it is challenging to gather persuasive evidence because the kind of detailed clinical data needed for these analyses are generally only available on the patients who are already engaged in the health care system. If one of the effects of expanding coverage is to bring new patients into contact with care, these studies may yield biased conclusions. For this reason, the Oregon health insurance experiment mentioned earlier is still some of the strongest evidence we have on this front. In that study, gaining Medicaid did not lead to any statistically significant improvement in blood pressure, diabetes control, or cholesterol over the first 2 years of coverage, though patients did experience substantially lower rates of depression.[80]

But one striking finding in both the Oregon study and several ACA studies is that giving people health insurance leads them to *feel better*. A broad, population-level survey showed improving trends in self-reported health since 2014,[81] while assessments of the Medicaid expansion have found improved quality of life and overall well-being,[82] reduced psychological distress,[83] and better self-rated health[84]—though not all studies show these results.[85]

And that brings us to what is literally the final health outcome—mortality. Perhaps no question has motivated fiercer debate about the ACA than whether it has saved lives. If assessing the law's impact on chronic diseases and health care quality is challenging, the difficulties in doing so related to survival are even greater and the evidence more uncertain. Several studies of hospitalized populations have not found significant mortality changes, but this approach is somewhat hard to interpret because gaining health insurance is likely to alter who comes to the hospital in the first place.[86] Two papers incorporating broader populations have come to different conclusions. One study found that among 19- to 25-year-olds, despite their general good health, the ACA's coverage expansion reduced disease-related mortality from conditions like heart disease and cancer, compared to slightly older adults not affected by the policy.[87] Another study looked at the population of nonelderly US residents (under age 65) who had end-stage kidney disease and were starting dialysis. In this very high-risk population Medicaid expansion led to improved dialysis care and an 8.5% mortality reduction, amounting to 1 death prevented per 18 individuals gaining Medicaid coverage.[88]

Mortality changes and health improvements—if they occur at all—also may not be evident for several years, both because they represent the potential long-term impact of cumulative improvements in access to care and because it sometimes takes several years for detailed data on these outcomes to become available. In this context it can be helpful to look at some of the long-term studies from before the ACA as a potential guide. Two large population-based assessments of survival that we conducted—one after 3 states expanded Medicaid in 2002–2003 and the other after Massachusetts implemented its statewide health reform law in 2006 that extended insurance to more than 95% of the state—found significant reductions in death rates in the 4 to 5 years following the coverage expansions, particularly related to deaths potentially preventable with timely health care.[89] But it is unclear whether similar assessments under the ACA will produce similar results—or even whether this study design is practical. The challenge for researchers looking at the effect of the ACA on population-level mortality is that, unlike these prior state-based evaluations, there is no group in the United States unaffected by the law to serve as a comparison group. Based on this, some scholars have argued that it may not be feasible to tease out the impact of the ACA on population mortality.[90] More targeted studies of high-risk populations like those described above may thus be our best indication as to whether the ACA has saved lives. However, even with these limitations, 2 recent studies do find suggestive reductions in cardiovascular[91] and all-cause mortality[92] related to the ACA's Medicaid expansion, and future work will continue to explore these issues.

Final Thoughts: Did the ACA Work?

We opened our chapter by posing the question: Did the ACA work? Having highlighted dozens of studies from a large body of research about the law's coverage expansions, there is no simple answer. If we had to give our best cocktail party reply, we would say, "On the whole, yes. But in some ways, not as well as hoped. And in many ways, it's still too soon to know."

Undoubtedly, the ACA succeeded in bringing health insurance coverage to about 20 million Americans who would otherwise be uninsured. On average, those gaining coverage have experienced major improvements in access to affordable care, have obtained more care to treat their acute and chronic conditions, and, by several important measures, are feeling better and perhaps even living longer.

But the ACA fell short of total enrollment targets, expanding coverage to fewer than half of the nation's uninsured population, and it is possible that some of the law's early coverage gains are already waning. And the health care that was delivered to newly covered populations might not have produced as much health improvement as it could have. At its 25th anniversary, should the law survive that long, we will have a much clearer sense of which changes implemented by the ACA have stood the test of time and what long-term effects on health care use and health outcomes it has produced. In the meantime researchers will continue working to expand our understanding of the effects of this complex and far-reaching law.

CHAPTER 13

DELIVERY-SYSTEM REFORMS

Evaluating the Effectiveness of the ACA's Delivery-System Reforms at Slowing Cost Growth and Improving Quality and Patient Experience

Ezekiel J. Emanuel and Amol S. Navathe

Some commentators claimed that the Affordable Care Act (ACA) was 90% about coverage and not much about cost, quality, or transformation. Is that claim true? How effective were the ACA's efforts at transforming the delivery system to higher quality and lower cost?

The delivery-system reforms (DSRs) developed or implemented via the ACA have been arguably as impactful—if not more impactful—than the insurance market and regulatory changes in curtailing the upward trajectory of cost growth. Although the ACA stimulated technical policy innovations meant to adjust payment rates, reporting requirements, and other matters related to the actual delivery of care, its success in changing health care delivery is as much psychological and cultural as it is about specific policy changes.

At the center of the ACA's approach to DSR is the philosophy that fee-for-service (FFS) payment is a major cause of overuse of medical

Ezekiel J. Emanuel, MD, PhD, is the vice provost for Global Initiatives, Diane and Robert Levy University Professor, and codirector of the Healthcare Transformation Institute at the University of Pennsylvania. He was a special assistant in the Office of Management and Budget in the Obama administration (2009–2011).

Amol S. Navathe, MD, PhD, is an assistant professor of health policy and medicine, codirector of the Healthcare Transformation Institute, and associate director of the Center for Health Incentives and Behavioral Economics, University of Pennsylvania. He led the Comparative Effectiveness Research Program in the Obama administration (2009–2011).

services and poor quality. Inherent in the FFS payment model is the incentive to do more to get paid more, and because fees do not vary based on the quality of care, they do not encourage efforts to improve quality. This contrasts with how prices are set for most products and services outside of health care, where higher quality yields a higher price (think about an iPhone compared to a generic, other phone). Hence, the idea underlying the ACA reforms was that changing payment was necessary—but *not sufficient*—to incentivize physicians and hospitals toward medical practice that is more cost effective and higher quality.

Beyond initiating a change in the financial model for care delivery, the ACA likely had a deeper impact on the culture of health care delivery. Enactment of the ACA convinced clinicians and health care organizations that the current system was changing—payment change was inevitable and was going to alter care practices. And the payment change would require considering both quality and cost—that is, the value of health care—when making clinical decisions. This mental and cultural change encouraged physicians, hospitals, and others to adopt value-based payments—payments linked to the cost and quality of services—in place of traditional FFS, even if they were not immediately and obviously financially beneficial. In turn, they would begin to change how they cared for patients—such as by changing their office scheduling practices, attending to gaps in care such as immunizations, introducing more chronic care coordination, and integrating mental health care into primary care—and to address the social determinants of health. This psychological change can be observed through the rapid ramp-up in participation in many value-based payment programs, many of which did not actually have strong financial incentives to reduce FFS spending. For example, Model 2 of the Bundled Payments for Care Improvement Initiative (BPCI) grew from 304 participants in 2013 to 432 in 2018, and the Medicare Shared Savings Program grew from 114 accountable care organizations (ACOs) in 2012 to 518 as of July 2019 (see Tables 13.2–13.3). Similarly, because of the government's payment changes, commercial insurers seized the opportunities to introduce analogous, value-based payment programs, which amplified the impact of the ACA.

In these programs, clinicians and health care systems changed practice patterns. For example, many participants reduced hospitalizations or use of expensive nursing home care after hospitalization. Conse-quently, savings and quality gains increased over time.[1] This reflects well on the provider community, demonstrating strong intrinsic moti-vation to improve because extrinsic incentives, both financial and non-financial, were not terribly strong.

These broader psychological and cultural changes have implica-tions for the evaluation of the ACA's DSRs. Inevitably, research fo-cuses on the financial and quality outcomes of a single model. And ironically, the broad cultural changes may have made it more difficult to prove the benefits of each new single payment model the ACA spawned. This is because each model gets vetted against the underly-ing trend of a system that is moving toward greater value. In critical assessment of the policy evaluation literature, we observe this under-lying trend: the control group of "health care as usual" in the United States itself has been dynamically moving toward greater efficiency and health care value. This is likely one reason why single-model eval-uations understate the ACA's true impact on health care quality and spending growth. DSR initiatives, even if not included in the actual ACA, spurred many other secular trends. For example, in response to value-based payment models, many providers have begun sharing resources and data and collaborating on patient care together as well as contracting with insurers jointly.[2] Although this may have ripple ef-fects on increased prices in the commercial sector, this has likely had a positive impact on Medicare because of its regulated prices.[3] Another example is the growth in participation in Medicare's managed care program, Medicare Advantage.

This underlying trend may be one critical reason why financial sav-ings for individual programs may be lagging behind an otherwise ob-viously positive sign—overall health care spending as a percentage of gross domestic product (GDP) has roughly plateaued since the ACA's enactment. Spending remains below 18% of GDP despite authoritative predictions that it would exceed 20%.[4]

Another important consideration in evaluating the ACA's DSRs is the timeline of change. The literature on change management in business demonstrates that transforming the culture and practices of organizations is a 7- to 10-year process, with the most active and clear signs of change beginning in the fourth year.[5] Making judgments on the success or failure of DSR after just a few years of each individual program may be premature and lead to erroneous conclusions.

Ultimately, however, the quantitative evidence we have to date comes from single-model evaluations of the many programs that the ACA spawned directly or were initiated by the Center for Medicare and Medicaid Innovation (CMMI). The ACA contained many important provisions that attempted to improve quality and reduce costs, including Section 3021, which established the CMMI. The CMMI was given $10 billion over 10 years and was charged with developing new payment and care-delivery models aimed at reducing costs without compromising—and hopefully improving—quality. Although these models directly affected payment and care for Medicare beneficiaries, CMMI also pursued coordination with commercial payers as part of multipayer arrangements in select programs.

Section 6301 established the Patient-Centered Outcomes Research Institute (PCORI) as an independent, nonprofit, nongovernmental organization to conduct clinical effectiveness research and improve the evidence base supporting patient, caregiver, and clinician decisions.

These individual reforms span hospital care (the HRRP), primary care (the Comprehensive Primary Care [CPC] and CPC Plus programs), global budgets models centered around primary care that provide incentives to reduce the total cost of care for Medicare beneficiaries (shared savings ACO programs), and specialty care (bundled payments). We summarize the data on each of these programs.

One overall conclusion is clear: although definitive long-term effects on national spending growth and quality are still required, it is clear that the shift to value-based payment under the ACA has not produced worse quality or outcomes than the previous FFS system. Although this is not the goal, it is important that the shift away from the old payment system is not harming patients during the transition to a more sustainable one. This allows us to take the long view, particularly in light of the time it takes to transition payment and physician and hospital practices. Thus, the data on DSRs initiated by the ACA provide a good rationale for targeting and refining the most promising programs, with an aim of increasing cost savings and quality.

Hospital Care

Section 3025 created the Hospital Readmissions Reduction Program (HRRP), a program targeted at reducing rehospitalization within 30 days after an initial hospitalization (called readmission). The HRRP penalizes hospitals by reducing Medicare payments if they have excessive readmissions within 30 days of initial hospitalization for 6 conditions/procedures: acute myocardial infarction, chronic obstructive pulmonary disease, heart failure, pneumonia, coronary artery bypass graft surgery, and elective primary total hip or knee arthroplasty. In 2019 the penalty was 3% of hospital revenue from Medicare—not a small number, considering hospital margins. It is considered a value-based program because excessive readmissions to hospitals are likely avoidable and, thus, low value. Starting in 2012 HRRP applied to 2,213 hospitals nationwide, excluding critical access hospitals and mental health institutions.[6]

Before considering the data on the impact of HRRP, it is important to note that there is no true control group. Mandating a nationwide program without a preceding evaluation period or a staggered roll-out makes it difficult to disentangle the program's true impact from secular changes in the dynamic landscape of US health care. This makes strong, definitive inferences on program success or failure impossible to ascertain and strongly suggests that future implementation of new programs should be designed with an eye toward ensuring rigorous evaluations.

Overall, HRRP policy seems to have modestly improved quality via small decreases in readmissions without a rise in mortality. However, it may have adversely impacted hospitals treating a high proportion of low-income patients.

There are 4 distinct findings related to HRRP. First, most evidence suggests an overall decrease in readmissions from roughly 21% to 18%—that is, a reduction of about 3% on an absolute level and 17% on a relative level.[7] Hospitals subject to penalties under the HRRP had greater reductions in readmission rates compared with those at nonpenalized hospitals, supporting the idea that the penalties were the reason for the declines in readmissions.[8] Even in communities with declining hospital admission rates as HRRP ramped up, 30-day readmission rates seemed to decline further. This was despite the fact that patients needed to be sicker to get hospitalized because more patients were being managed out of hospitals.[9]

However, some studies challenge the claim that HRRP actually reduced readmissions. One concern was whether hospitals simply substituted hospitalization with observational stays, in which relatively less-sick patients are kept in the hospitals but technically remain as outpatients for monitoring.[10] This means either that the types of patients eligible for readmissions changed during the HRRP period or that readmissions were directly avoided by using observation status instead—both alternate explanations for positive results. Other studies suggest that half of the reductions in readmissions were an artifact of risk-adjustment changes arising from a greater number of diagnosis codes on claims forms starting in 2011.[11] Nonetheless, the data do suggest a modest decline in readmissions.

Second, there was a modest spillover effect for patients who were not directly targeted by HRRP. These benefits in the form of reduced readmissions occurred for Medicare patients admitted with non-HRRP-covered conditions and non-Medicare patients (e.g., Medicaid patients).[12]

Third, there is some evidence that certain hospitals may have been unfairly penalized because they cared for sicker patients. For instance, financially poorer patients or hospitals may have been disproportionately penalized. The penalty burden was greater in hospitals that were large, urban, academic medical centers that treated larger shares of Medicaid or socioeconomically disadvantaged patients. This was true even when those hospitals did better on another measure of quality—risk-adjusted mortality rates.[13] However, as with all things HRRP, there is also conflicting evidence that hospitals caring for large proportions of patients of low socioeconomic status had similar readmission rates to other hospitals.[14]

Finally, and most importantly, there is controversy about whether HRRP increased Medicare mortality rates. Critics contend that the policy could have increased mortality by discouraging medically necessary readmissions. At the heart of this debate are seemingly contradictory results between 3 articles published in 2018, with 2 that pointed to increases in 30-day mortality after hospitalization for congestive heart failure (CHF) after HRRP started[15] and 1 that stated the trends predated HRRP.[16] How can we make sense of these conflicting conclusions? Much depends upon the methods used and the details of which hospitals and patients were included in the studies.

Peter Orszag points out 2 fundamental flaws in concluding that HRRP increased mortality. First, mortality should be assessed from the time of admission rather than exclusively for patients who survive to hospital discharge.[17] Thus, postdischarge rates fail to capture improvements in in-hospital mortality, and if improvements cause fewer patients to die in the hospital, patients surviving to discharge may be sicker and more likely to die on average. Of the 3 articles consulted, 2 actually found evidence consistent with this hypothesis.[18]

The second flaw is that the underlying trend in mortality is difficult to establish in the context of simultaneous improvements in hospital care. Such improvements, like the introduction of new drugs (e.g., Entresto for patients with congestive heart failure, which improves survival and reduces hospitalizations), make it important to examine different time windows to verify that findings are not one-off results. The 2 articles concluding that HRRP led to higher mortality did not do this, but the article showing no increase in mortality did make this adjustment.[19]

Maybe most importantly, even the articles showing an increase in 30-day mortality found *no* increase in 45-day mortality. Differences in mortality that depend upon small differences in the time of observation bring into question the validity of the increased mortality finding and also suggest that even if there were a change in 30-day mortality, it was unlikely to have been clinically meaningful.

Indeed, the Medicare Payment Advisory Commission (MedPAC), a nonpartisan agency that advises Congress on Medicare policy, conducted its own report on HRRP.[20] MedPAC concluded that readmission rates decreased modestly because of HRRP and that there was no evidence that mortality increased.

Primary Care

Initially launched in October 2012, the Comprehensive Primary Care (CPC) Initiative was a 4-year collaboration between CMS and 32 commercial and state health insurance plans to enhance primary care. It

Table 13.1 Primary Care Models

Primary care initiatives	Years	Number of participants at program start	Number of participants at program end	Number of commercial payers involved	Distinct design features	Results	Lessons and implications
CPC	2012–2016	502	442	26	• Prospective monthly care management fee with potential retrospective shared savings • Focus on providing 5 comprehensive primary care functions[a]	• No changes in total cost or quality of care • Reduction in emergency department visits • Improved access, including decreased wait times, extended hours, and use of telephone and telemedicine	• May improve care delivery and reduce emergency department visits • Not enough to create measurable changes in cost and quality
CPC+	2017–2022	2876	2881	62	• Prospective monthly care management fee with potential retrospective shared savings • Focus on providing 5 different comprehensive primary care functions[b]	• Participants mostly small physician practices • Practices from high-income areas more likely • Preliminary results still pending	• Program may not be serving the populations most in need

[a]Risk-stratified care management, access and continuity, planned care for chronic conditions and preventive care, engagement of patients and caregivers, and coordination of care across the medical neighborhood.

[b]Access and continuity, care management, comprehensiveness and coordination, patient and caregiver engagement, and planned care and population health.

included 442 practice sites, 2,188 clinicians, and 2.7 million patients across 7 geographic regions.[21] The innovative feature of the model was a $15–$20 per beneficiary per month care-management fee paid to participating practices, with requirements to focus on 5 strategies related to "comprehensive" primary care: (1) longitudinal management of chronic conditions and social needs; (2) access and continuity; (3) planned care for chronic conditions and preventive care; (4) engagement of patients and caregivers; and (5) coordination of care across sites of service. CPC also incorporated financial incentives by allowing Medicare to share any financial savings—net of care management fees—with the participating practices.

Overall, CPC did not reduce the total cost of care and did not generate savings for Medicare, nor did it lead to quality or patient care improvements. Rather, CPC's main achievement was a small reduction in emergency department visits.[22]

However, primary care practices did seem to change how they were delivering care, despite researchers' inability to detect quantitative changes in cost or quality. For example, 2 years into the 4-year program practices reported in a survey that they had substantially transformed their delivery of care by increasing access through lower wait times, staying open after hours, and using more remote visits like telephone or telemedicine.[23] The main results were replicated in a 2018 study, which found that although quality was beginning to improve as a result of care transformation, with a 2% decline in emergency department visits, these improvements still did not lead to overall savings that offset care management fees. They also did not improve either physician or beneficiary experience.[24] Importantly, however, there is evidence that participation in CPC has not led to an increase in patient dismissal, showing that doctors are not feeling pressured to alter their patient panels—"cream skimming" or "lemon dropping"—in order to meet quality targets.[25]

The CPC+ program built upon the design of CPC. Begun in 2017, it is a 5-year collaboration between CMS and commercial and state health insurance plans to enhance primary care. It expanded the geographic regions of participation from 7 to 18,[26] extending reach to include 2,881 clinicians and 62 commercial and state insurers.[27] Like CPC, it offered per-person care management fees and opportunities for participating practices to share in savings. Thus far, CPC+ has mostly attracted small physician practices. In addition, practices located in areas with high incomes were more likely to join the program, indicating that it may not be serving the population most in need.[28] In addition, federally qualified health centers (FQHCs) and rural health clinics are not eligible for CPC+.[29] Preliminary program results are still pending.

Global Budget Models—
Accountable Care Organizations (ACOs)

Section 3022 of the ACA required CMS to fund the creation of accountable care organizations (ACOs). An ACO is a physician-led organization that convenes and partners with other health entities, such as physician groups and hospitals, and is responsible for the overall quality and cost of at least 5,000 Medicare beneficiaries. By creating accountability for a population of patients, ACO programs can stimulate improved care coordination that reduces wasteful practices, increases preventative management, and shifts care out of the hospital in order to generate cost savings.

Overall, ACOs have modestly improved quality and reduced spending growth. The most effective ACOs at improving quality and reducing costs are physician-based without an administratively or financially affiliated hospital, promote evidence-based medicine, coordinate care, monitor and evaluate the quality and cost of care, and foster patient engagement and patient-centered care.[30] Such physician-based ACOs have improved quality and reduced costs by 4.9% over 3 years.[31]

Since its inception, Medicare has continually evolved the ACO program, going from the Medicare Shared Savings Program (MSSP) (January 2012), Advanced Payment Model ACOs, and the Pioneer ACOs to newer "risk-bearing" tracks of MSSP and the Next Generation ACOs (January 2016) (see Table 13.2). Despite many ACOs terminating their participation, there has been a growth in the overall number of ACOs over time. There are 3 important points about ACO programs.

First, the incentives in upside-only ACO models (like MSSP) are weak. ACOs can earn bonuses if they save money but do not get penalized financially if they do not. The modest savings are a testament to the cultural and psychological change described earlier; however, to more robustly catalyze behavior change, ACOs will need to face much larger financial penalties and rewards—up to 20% of revenue. That said, we must also remember that most physician groups and hospitals were not operationally or financially ready to be at risk in 2012. Hence, the early "upside-only" ACOs played an important role in initiating the transition to full financial risk.

Second, ACOs that tended to do well in cutting costs were more likely to be physician only, without affiliation with a particular hospital.[32] A main source of cost savings for ACOs is likely to be shifting care out of the hospital to home or other lower-cost facilities, such as ambulatory surgery centers or skilled nursing facilities (SNFs). This is bad for hospitals, lowering their bed-occupancy rates and using non-hospital-affiliated outpatient facilities. Hospital-based ACOs are likely to have a harder time making this practice change. In other words, the incentive for hospital-based ACOs to keep beds full or use higher-cost hospital-affiliated outpatient services is stronger than the incentive to reduce hospitalization by shifting the site of care.

Third, the complexity of the ACO program may have been an impediment to behavior change. There were many challenges identified in the ACO program as initially implemented. One of the most important was the issue of the attributed population—the patient population for which the ACO is clinically and financially responsible. Initially this was retrospective, meaning that the patients the ACOs were responsible for were determined *after the fact* based on which primary care or specialty care groups predominantly provided care services to the patients. Not knowing at the start of a year which patients should be targeted for enhanced care activities, such as chronic care coordination, is a problem for a practice trying to improve care and lower costs.

Overall, ACO participation within the MSSP has been associated with modest but increasing improvements in cost and quality. In the first year of the contract, MSSP contracts were associated with early reductions in Medicare spending. By 2014, the third year of the program, spending reductions exceeded bonus payments—meaning there were real cost savings to Medicare and the taxpayer.[33]

There is mixed evidence of whether all the savings came from true changes in practice versus finding ways to treat healthier patients. For

Table 13.2 ACO Care Models

ACOs	Years	Number of participants at program start	Number of participants at program end	Number of commercial payers involved	Distinct design features	Results	Lessons and implications
MSSP	2012–ongoing	114	518	N/A	• No downside risk • Shared savings beyond cost reductions of 2–3.9%	• Greater savings for physician-led groups than hospitals • Increased savings over time for participants that stay in the program	• May be an effective model for targeting high-risk patients, but will require greater financial risk passed to ACOs
Advanced Payment Model	2012–2015	20	35	N/A	• Designed for physician-based and rural providers • Prospective up-front and monthly payments to invest in care-coordination infrastructure • CMS recoups advanced payments through shared savings	• Lower-than-expected spending in 2012 and 2013, but higher-than-expected in 2014. No significant differences in quality. After the program ended, most participants continued to participate as either the same or a new MSSP ACO in 2016	• AP ACOs may need more time for investments to produce lower spending and higher quality

Program	Years			Design	Findings	Conclusions
Pioneer ACOs	2012–2016	32	9	N/A	• Designed for ACOs with experience coordinating care • Participants assume downside risk	• Early reductions in Medicare spending for 2012 entrants but not 2013 entrants • Little difference in patient experience compared to nonparticipants • Pioneer ACOs generally improved in quality across the years	• Savings and quality improvements are achievable with downside risk
Next Generation ACOs	2016–ongoing	18	41	N/A	• Designed for ACOs with experience coordinating care • Participants assume downside risk	• Overall 1.7% decrease ($18.20 per beneficiary per month) in Medicare spending relative to a comparison group, with significant variation across NGACO	• Some ACOs have the capability to assume and succeed under a downside risk arrangement

example, there is some evidence that ACOs avoided areas with larger populations of low socioeconomic status individuals, while other data suggests that physician-only ACOs cared for similar or more clinically and socially vulnerable patients.[34] Further, some studies suggest that ACOs may have influenced the risk of their patients, either by avoiding high-risk patients or the physicians who care for them.

The smaller Pioneer ACO program, which began in 2012 and ended in 2016, was designed for ACOs that included clinicians and health care organizations with experience managing populations and engaging in financial risk. In other words, the Pioneer program made its ACOs financially accountable for the cost of its patient, not just eligible for bonuses. While the Pioneer program started with 32 ACO participants, this dwindled to 9 ACOs by the conclusion of the program. Despite the considerable dropout, the Pioneer program has been viewed somewhat favorably. Over the first 2 years of the model, Pioneer ACOs exhibited modest reductions in Medicare spending, reductions in low-value services, and reductions in utilization of different health services, with little difference in patient experience compared to general Medicare FFS beneficiaries.[35]

The Pioneer program was reincarnated as the Next Generation ACO program. An analysis by Medicare contractors reported that among 18 ACOs responsible for the care of 477,197 beneficiaries in year one of the program, there was a 1.7% decrease ($18.20 per beneficiary per month) in Medicare spending relative to a comparison group, though there was significant variation across the different Next Generation ACOs.[36] In the same analysis qualitative evaluations highlighted care management as a key focus area, with emphases on care transitions, end-of-life care, and beneficiary engagement.

Specialty Care

To complement the population-based payment approaches of the CPC programs and ACOs, Medicare introduced bundled payments for specialty care. Under bundled payments, a provider entity, such as a hospital or physician group, is held financially responsible for the quality and costs across a clinically defined episode of care. The episode of care starts with a clinical event and extends for a predefined duration. Participating organizations are eligible for shared savings if they hold spending below an episode-specific financial benchmark, which corresponds to a fixed, bundled payment referred to as the target price. To receive financial bonuses, however, providers must maintain or improve quality. Unlike ACOs and existing population-based models, from the start Medicare's large bundled payment programs involved 2-sided financial risk, thereby creating the potential for financial losses alongside the potential for financial gain.

Bundled Payments for Care Improvement (BPCI)

From 2009 to 2012—prior to the enactment and implementation of the ACA—the Acute Care Episodes project involving 5 hospital systems demonstrated savings for orthopedic bundles and some cardiac bundles.[37] CMMI used these findings to implement the Bundled Payments for Care Improvement (BPCI) initiative nationwide. BPCI was a 5-year voluntary program initiated in October 2013.[38] BPCI allowed 4 participation options (models). In Model 2 the episode began with an initiating hospitalization and extended to 90 days after discharge from the hospital. It garnered the greatest participation and served as the basis for subsequent bundled payment programs. In Model 2 payment was made after an episode of care based on the difference between actual expenditures and set target prices. Overall, 402 participants proposed their bundle, what condition(s) they would participate in (of 48 possible choices), and which quality metrics they would report. BPCI's 48 conditions ranged from medical conditions, such as managing hospitalization for congestive heart failure exacerbation, to surgical conditions, such as hip replacement and heart bypass surgery.

Overall, BPCI showed savings for surgical procedures but no savings for medical procedures. There was no evidence that bundles increased utilization or induced practices to avoid sicker patients. There are 3 important findings on bundled payments.

First, BPCI has been associated with decreases in costs for surgery. In the first 21 months of the BPCI initiative Medicare payments declined more for lower-extremity joint replacement (LEJR, or hip and knee

Table 13.3 Bundled Payment Models

Bundled payments	Years	Number of participants at program start	Number of participants at program end	Number of commercial payers involved	Distinct design features	Results	Lessons and implications
BPCI Model 2	2013–2018	304	432	N/A	• Retrospective payments for 48 possible episodes of care • Covers hospitalization to 90 days postdischarge	• Statistically significant cost reductions for hip and knee replacements • No significant changes for medical conditions • No quality change	• Bundled payments may be better suited to surgery than to medical treatments as currently designed
CJR	2016–2020	800	471	N/A	• Retrospective payments for an LEJR episode • Covers hospitalization to 90 days postdischarge • Originally mandatory, now voluntary in some areas	• Participants achieved nearly $1,000 lower cost per episode compared to controls in first 2 years • Some lower-performing participants dropped out in voluntary areas	• Overall success that justifies scaling up • May need changes to ensure that less-resourced hospitals are able to benefit as well

| OCM | 2016–2021 | 190 | 175 | 10[a] | • Monthly care management fees with retrospective bonus payments for cost reduction and quality improvement
• Covers 6-month episodes of care beginning with a chemotherapy claim | • No statistically significant changes in cost or quality yet, though OCM episodes saw a reduction in use of hospital-based services and $173 lower cost relative to control groups
• Participants report using extended hours and patient navigation to reduce hospitalizations and emergency department visits | • While results are not definitive, there are signs of potential improvements in costs and practice redesign |

[a]Aetna; Blue Cross Blue Shield of Michigan/Blue Care Network; Blue Cross Blue Shield of South Carolina; Cigna Life & Health Insurance Company; Health Care Services Corporation; Highmark, Inc.; Priority Health; SummaCare; the University of Arizona Health Plan; UPMC Health Plan.

replacement) episodes provided in BPCI-participating hospitals than for those provided in comparison hospitals.[39] These results, reporting approximately 4% savings, were corroborated in longer-term evaluations up to 3 years after the program initiation.[40] Outstanding hospitals achieved savings as high as 20%. Two studies of Baptist Health System, a continuous participant in Medicare LEJR bundles since 2009, found that there were substantial savings and reduced Medicare payments for LEJR episodes, even at a time when Medicare payments overall for LEJR episodes increased by 5%.[41] The chief drivers of hospital cost savings were reductions in artificial joint costs. Medicare payments dropped primarily through the reduced use of expensive posthospital institutional care, such as rehabilitation facilities. Importantly, Medicare savings in BPCI reflected a shift from expensive, high-intensity services after discharge toward more cost-efficient, home-based physical and rehabilitation care.[42]

Second, these results do not appear to be the result of gaming of the system. There appears to be no net increase in surgical procedures nor evidence of selecting healthier patients for surgery instead of those who are sicker or more complex. Further, shifting care patterns to more cost-effective care sites was not associated with any reported untoward effects on patient health. The evidence refutes some experts' worries that BPCI would lead to increases in the number of surgeries performed that offset savings to Medicare.[43]

Third, bundles for medical conditions do not appear to save money or substantially change practice patterns. Evidence to date suggests that patients admitted to hospitals participating in BPCI for common medical conditions—including pneumonia, congestive heart failure, acute myocardial infarction, sepsis, and chronic obstructive pulmonary disease—did not experience significant changes in Medicare payments for their care, clinical complexity, length of stay, emergency department use, hospital readmission, or mortality.[44] This may suggest that bundled payments are better suited to surgery than to medical treatments. This may also suggest that the design of bundled payments for medical conditions needs to be changed. That said, it is also important to note that these results were very preliminary, based on limited data, and have been challenged by CMS itself. Clearly, longer-term, rigorous data are still required before making definitive inferences.

Comprehensive Care for Joint Replacement (CJR)

Using the financial savings from BPCI as proof of concept, in April 2016 CMMI announced the Comprehensive Care for Joint Replacement (CJR) model. CJR focuses exclusively on LEJR and enforced bundled payment as the required method for paying certain hospitals for the surgery and up to 90 days of postsurgical care. CJR is important for several reasons. First, LEJR is the second most common surgical procedure for Medicare beneficiaries, with over 510,000 per year.[45] Second, CJR participation was *mandatory* for hospitals located in about a quarter of US health care markets. To enhance the rigor of the data and enable a robust evaluation of program, CMS used randomization to select the markets in which it would pay using the mandatory bundles. Unfortunately, the Trump administration cut the program in half at the start of year 3, making participation voluntary in 33 of the 67 health care markets and allowing low-volume hospitals to drop out, compromising the ability to produce robust, long-term results.

CJR is supposed to conclude in 2020. Preliminary evidence suggests that CJR achieved savings of a similar magnitude to that in BPCI. For example, in one analysis of the first year of CJR, patients treated by hospitals participating in CJR had a lower percentage of discharges to institutional postacute care, but hospitals did not actually save money per episode.[46] However, a later study examining hospital-level findings established that after 2 years, there was a modest reduction in spending per episode, and it attributed this reduction to the decrease in discharges to postacute institutional care.[47] This is consistent with broader research suggesting that hospitals participating in bundled payments for LEJR are reducing spending through 2 principal strategies: either by reducing SNF referrals as much as possible or by enhancing integration with SNFs in order to exert influence over the costs and quality of their service.[48]

Although CJR has driven savings for Medicare, some concerns remain about equity. Hospitals that left the CJR program when it became voluntary served more lower-income, nonwhite, and Medicaid-enrolled patients and were more likely to be safety-net hospitals than were those that remained in the program. The hospitals that left tended to perform poorly and may have left because they would be more likely to sustain financial losses by remaining in the program. However, patients at these hospitals may have the greatest need for improvements in care coordination.[49] A 2019 study corroborated these findings when it reported that, compared to other hospitals, safety-net hospitals were 42% less likely to receive rewards in year one of CJR, and their rewards were 39% smaller per episode. This suggests that in future years safety-net hospitals will be less likely to receive rewards, more likely to pay penalties to CMS, and may drop out of the program entirely.[50] Some types of hospitals—larger, higher-volume, more integrated hospitals—may be better situated to succeed in this program than others.[51] But overall there is still an argument that the early success of the program justifies scaling the program up nationwide, although it may require altering the design.[52]

Oncology Care Model (OCM)

CMS also instituted a bundled-payment program for cancer care, the Oncology Care Model (OCM), which began in July of 2016. Unlike other bundled-payment models that have largely focused on hospital care, in OCM 190 physician practices serve as the key accountable entity for 6-month episodes of care for cancer patients initiated by chemotherapy administration. This is also an example of a multipayer model in which CMS is partnering with 10 commercial insurers to align incentives facing physician practices across patients with differing insurance coverage. OCM provides $160 per patient per month ($960 for 6 months) for enhanced oncology services that include care coordination, care navigation, and adherence to national treatment guidelines. OCM also affords the opportunity for participants to earn a portion of savings on the overall episode cost as a financial bonus, but they must also meet quality benchmarks.

Overall, preliminary results demonstrate no measurable impacts of OCM on quality or costs.[53] That said, given the 4 or more years it takes to change organizations, it is not surprising that preliminary results do not show savings yet. Further, OCM practices did report engaging in practice redesign such as extended hours and patient navigation that may be harbingers of future positive results.

Conclusion

Delivery-system reform is hard and takes longer than many people think. Enactment of the ACA initiated important reforms, and this is an ACA success story. In addition, as we see, these various value-based payment reforms have not made the system worse either in terms of quality or cost. At this critical juncture, abandoning value-based payment programs would be shortsighted, ignoring harbingers of longer-term benefits and the totality of evidence supporting a large national shift in the mindset and approach to care delivery from health care organizations and clinicians.

The pace of change is also accelerating, with Medicare announcing, with bipartisan support, new models such as Primary Care First and Direct Contracting for primary care. These come on the heels of earlier multipayer efforts initiated under Medicare Advantage and the ACO investment model. These may serve as building blocks of alignment, shifting health care organizations beyond a tipping point of risk bearing that enables them to invest more fully in infrastructure and process innovation supporting value-based models.

Table 13.4 Summary Table

Reform type	Model/program	Years	Description	Results	Conclusions and implications
Hospital care	Hospital Readmissions Reduction Program (HRRP)	2012– ongoing	Penalizes hospitals by reducing Medicare payments by up to 3% of hospital billings if they have excessive readmissions for 6 conditions/procedures[a]	• Significant decrease in readmissions (from 21% to 18% for targeted conditions; from 15% to 13% for nontargeted conditions) • Hospitals subject to penalties under the HRRP had greater reductions in readmission rates • Penalty burden was greater for hospitals with larger shares of low-income patients • No conclusive evidence of increased mortality	• HRRP policy seems to have improved quality by modestly lowering readmissions without increasing mortality • May adversely impact hospitals with high numbers of lower-income patients
Primary care initiatives	Comprehensive Primary Care (CPC)	2012– 2016	Provides primary care practices with a $15–$20 per-beneficiary per-month care management fee as well as the opportunity to share in financial savings, with requirements to focus on 5 strategies related to comprehensive primary care[b]	• No changes in total cost or quality of care • Reduction in emergency department visits • Improved access, including decreased wait times, extended hours, and use of telephone and telemedicine	• May improve care delivery and reduce emergency department visits • Not enough to create measurable changes in cost and quality

Comprehensive Primary Care Plus (CPC+)	2017–2022	Provides participating practices with a monthly care management fee as well as retrospective performance-based payments on measures of patient experience, quality, and utilization. Like CPC, has 5 practice requirements[c]	• Participants mostly small physician practices • Practices from high-income areas more likely • Preliminary results still pending	• Program may not be serving the populations most in need
ACOs				
Medicare Shared Savings Program (MSSP)	2012–ongoing	• No downside risk • Shared savings beyond cost reductions of 2–3.9%	• Greater savings for physician-led groups than hospitals • Increased savings over time for participants that stay in the program	• May be an effective model for targeting high-risk patients, but will require greater financial risk passed to ACOs
Advanced Payment Model	2012–2015	• Designed for physician-based and rural providers • Prospective upfront and monthly payments to invest in care-coordination infrastructure • CMS recoups advanced payments through shared savings	• Lower-than-expected spending in 2012 and 2013, but higher-than-expected in 2014. No significant differences in quality. After the program ended, most participants continued to participate as either the same or a new MSSP ACO in 2016	• AP ACOs may need more time for investments to produce lower spending and higher quality

(continues on next page)

Reform type	Model/program	Years	Description	Results	Conclusions and implications
	Pioneer ACOs	2012–2016	• Designed for ACOs with experience coordinating care • Participants assume downside risk	• Early reductions in Medicare spending for 2012 entrants but not 2013 entrants • Little difference in patient experience compared to nonparticipants • Pioneer ACOs generally improved in quality across the years	• Savings and quality improvements are achievable with downside risk
	Next Generation ACOs	2016–ongoing	• Designed for ACOs with experience coordinating care • Participants assume downside risk	• Overall 1.7% decrease ($18.20 per beneficiary per month) in Medicare spending relative to a comparison group, with significant variation across NGACOs • Increase from 18 participants in 2016 to 41 in 2019	• Some ACOs have the capability to assume and succeed under a downside risk arrangement
Bundled payments	Bundled Payments for Care Improvement (BPCI) Model 2	2013–2018	• Retrospective payments for 48 possible episodes of care • Covers hospitalization to 90 days postdischarge	• Statistically significant cost reductions for hip and knee replacements • No significant changes for medical conditions • No quality change • No evidence that bundles increased utilization or led to avoiding sicker patients	• Bundled payments may be better suited to surgery than to medical treatments, as currently designed

Comprehensive Care for Joint Replacement (CJR)	2016–2020	• Retrospective payments for an LEJR episode • Covers hospitalization to 90 days postdischarge • Originally mandatory, now voluntary in some areas	• Participants achieved nearly $1,000 lower cost per episode compared to controls in first 2 years • Some lower-performing participants dropped out in voluntary areas	• Overall success that justifies scaling up • May need changes to ensure that less-resourced hospitals are able to benefit as well
Oncology Care Model (OCM)	2016–2021	• Monthly care management fees with retrospective bonus payments for cost reduction and quality improvement • Covers 6-month episodes of care beginning with a chemotherapy claim	• No statistically significant changes in cost or quality yet, though OCM episodes saw a reduction in use of hospital-based services and $173 lower cost relative to control groups • Participants report using extended hours and patient navigation to reduce hospitalizations and ED visits	• While results are not definitive, there are signs of potential improvements in costs and practice redesign to improve patient access

[a] Acute myocardial infarction, chronic-obstructive pulmonary disease, heart failure, pneumonia, coronary artery bypass graft surgery, and elective primary total hip or knee arthroplasty.

[b] Risk-stratified care management, access and continuity, planned care for chronic conditions and preventive care, engagement of patients and caregivers, and coordination of care across the medical neighborhood.

[c] Access and continuity, care management, comprehensiveness and coordination, patient and caregiver engagement, and planned care and population health.

CHAPTER 14

HAS THE ACA MADE HEALTH CARE MORE AFFORDABLE?

Carrie H. Colla and Jonathan Skinner[1]

Introduction

The primary goal of the Patient Protection and Affordable Care Act (ACA) of 2010 was to expand health insurance coverage, but a key secondary goal was to lower spending growth—indeed, given its title, to make health care affordable for all Americans. Clearly, providing insurance coverage to people previously uninsured makes health care more affordable to them. But we address a closely related question: How successful was the ACA in making health care more affordable to society as a whole by reducing the growth of health care spending?[2] For some the ACA was the obvious cause of the health care spending slowdown in the early 2010s[3] or at least the slowdown in real per-enrollee Medicare cost growth.[4] Others point to the evidence on weak cost saving from accountable care organizations (ACOs)[5] or other delivery reforms and the current prices in the exchanges as evidence that the ACA was much less effective.

A decade after the ACA was enacted, we critically evaluate the evidence of health care cost growth. We use 2 approaches based on micro-level policy estimates and macro-level trends to address this

---

Carrie H. Colla, PhD, is an associate professor at the Dartmouth Institute for Health Policy and Clinical Practice, Geisel School of Medicine.

Jonathan Skinner, PhD, is the James O. Freedman Presidential Professor in Economics at Dartmouth College and a professor at the Geisel School of Medicine's Institute for Health Policy and Clinical Practice.

question. First, we use a disaggregated approach that relies primarily on original budget scoring of individual policies included in the ACA by the Congressional Budget Office (CBO), the most reliable non-partisan adjudicators of changes to federal spending.[6] Although the CBO projections were not uniformly accurate (and not all of the ACA cost-saving policies were implemented), we use these as a starting point to assess the micro-level impact of the ACA on overall health care costs.

Recognizing the limitations of budgetary projections, we also consider the macro evidence of trends in health care spending that capture any factors missing from the CBO analysis but where we also acknowledge that at the macro level it is more difficult to identify causal factors affecting health care spending trends or a counterfactual for health care spending absent the ACA. In this macro approach we account for the dramatic increase in spending that naturally occurs when 20 million additional people become newly insured[7]—whether through provisions of the ACA or because of the gradual increase in Medicare enrollment as uninsured baby boomers reach 65, by considering how the introduction of the ACA was associated with (inflation-adjusted) health spending *per enrollee* for Medicaid, Medicare, and commercially insured insurance coverage.

To summarize our overall findings: At the micro level we find a modest estimate of cost saving, on the order of about $52 billion annually, or 1.4% of total spending; over 10 years this translates to a reduction in the *growth rate* of health care spending of about 0.14% annually. On the macro level we find a quite divergent path of spending for Medicaid, Medicare, and commercially insured enrollees. Like Amitabh Chandra, Jonathan Holmes, and Jonathan Skinner,[8] we find that even with more recent data through 2017, real (inflation-adjusted) spending per Medicaid enrollee has been flat since 2001—that is, spending per enrollee has not budged for nearly two decades. Medicare spending was rising rapidly during the early 2000s, particularly after Medicare Part D (prescription drug coverage) was introduced in 2006, but since 2009, one year before the passage of the ACA, real Medicare spending per enrollee has been flat as well. The exception to this trend is spending per enrollee for commercial health insurance, which rose prior to 2010, moderated between 2010–2013, and has since reverted to a higher growth rate.

What we do not believe has been captured in CBO projections or in the general discussion of the ACA was a temporary *pause* in growth rates from 2010–2013 as the ACA became a reality and health care institutions began to focus on rationalizing care; real (inflation-adjusted) spending per capita grew at just a 1.1 percentage-point rate during this period, slightly below the corresponding growth rate in GDP. Despite these early promising signs, the optimism has been crushed by the continued pressure of market consolidation, leading to higher prices, continued technological developments, and, importantly, the uncertainty around and weakening of the ACA. Since 2014, real per-capita spending has reverted back to a more rapid growth path of 2.6% after adjusting for population growth and inflation (based on author analysis of Altarum Institute data).[9] Nearly 400,000 jobs have been added in the past 12 months, 21% of all new US employment.[10]

Thus, the micro-level calculations may have missed a longer-term effect of the ACA captured by the 2010–2013 "great pause" in health care spending: it laid the foundation for a shift away from uncoordinated fee-for-service (FFS) payment systems and toward a future environment of alternative payment contracts, global budgets, scaled-back reimbursement rates, and public pricing options. Of course, a foundation is only useful if built upon; for the investment in the ACA to pay off, there must be continued commitment to a transition to sustained cost reductions—which, because every dollar of cost saving is some interest group's dollar of income—has proven to be an ongoing political challenge.

Micro-Evidence on the ACA and Cost Saving

The ACA experienced a bumpy legislative road and, unlike earlier legislation such as Medicare and Medicaid in 1965, ended up squeaking through Congress along party lines.[11] The goals of increasing the number of people with health insurance through the expansion of Medicaid coverage and insurance exchanges as well as improving the quality of care were matched by an interest in reducing costs.

The ACA proposed multiple revenue streams aimed at offsetting the spending needed for coverage expansion. The provisions fall into 3 main categories: (1) changes in Medicare and Medicaid payment rates or policies, (2) new policies to allow flexibility for innovation in government health care programs, and (3) increased taxes. We consider each in turn.

Changes in Medicare and Medicaid Payment Rates or Policies

One way in which the ACA clearly saved was by cutting payments or reducing updates or subsidies for Medicare Advantage (MA),[12] health care providers, and high-income Medicare beneficiaries. A direct reduction in federal spending growth and likely overall spending growth arising from the ACA was payment cuts to MA. MA enrollment has grown significantly, from 10 million in 2009 to 22 million in 2019, with MA plans serving 36% of all beneficiaries.[13] Prior to the ACA, federal payments to MA plans per enrollee were 14% higher than the cost of covering similar beneficiaries under the traditional Medicare program, according to the Medicare Payment Advisory Commission (MedPAC).[14] The ACA changed the benchmark payment methodology to align more closely with traditional Medicare payment, reducing payments to MA plans over time and providing bonus payments to plans receiving high quality ratings.[15] By most accounts, these payment reductions have not caused beneficiary harm, nor have they made the MA program less attractive. Initial estimated savings were $136 billion over 10 years (2010–2019);[16] given the growth in MA enrollment in the past decade, this is likely an underestimate of the impact of the change in payment methodology. In discussions about repeal of the ACA in June 2015, the CBO estimated that repealing the MA payment changes from the law alone would cost an additional $358 billion over 10 years.[17] We updated our micro estimate of savings to include half of this larger amount because of the caveat that this estimate was for the time period beginning in 2015 rather than 2010.

The ACA reduced updates in Medicare payment levels to hospitals, SNFs, hospice, home health, and other providers, for a projected savings of $196 billion.[18] Similarly, Medicare's Competitive Bidding Program for durable medical equipment, prosthetics, orthotics, and supplies was implemented in 2011 and was projected to save the federal government $25.7 billion from 2013 to 2022, with beneficiaries estimated to save an additional $17.1 billion;[19] however, since January 2019 the program has been suspended. All of these policies cut payments to payers and providers with little or no evidence of harm to patients. In 2015 the CBO estimated that the Medicare FFS reimbursement changes totaled approximately $358 billion over the 2015–2025 period, which we adopt for our saving calculations (taking half for the 2015–2020 period).[20] Other planned reimbursement cuts have not yet been implemented and may never be. For example, the Medicaid disproportionate share cuts in payments to hospitals have been delayed—with large cuts looming in late 2019, absent action from Congress.[21]

Policies to Allow Flexibility for Innovation and Reducing Costs and Utilization

Other reforms included a policy to guide reimbursement for biosimilars, encouraging competition to reduce premiums on health insurance exchanges, ACOs, bundled payments, value-based hospital purchasing (hospital readmissions reduction program [HRRP], penalties for hospital-acquired infections), and the Independent Payment Advisory Board (IPAB). We consider each in turn.

The Biologics Price Competition and Innovation Act, which provides a regulatory pathway for generic biologics, was passed as part of the ACA. Specialty biologics are currently the biggest driver of pharmaceutical cost growth, but thus far, biosimilars have failed to gain widespread traction. While 11 are FDA approved, only 3 have launched, with relatively small market shares.[22] The CBO estimated that this program would save $7 billion, but actual savings are likely much less (we estimate less than $1 billion based on the market share of the 3 biosimilars launched). To the extent that new biosimilars are added, the program has been estimated to reduce direct spending on biologic drugs by $54 billion from 2017 to 2026, or about 3% of total estimated biologic spending.[23]

Another objective of the ACA was to encourage competition among insurers for new enrollees on the insurance exchanges. However, the hoped-for price competition leading to lower premium costs does not appear to have reduced aggregate prices.[24]

Similarly, ACOs have failed to save more than modest amounts, with recent studies estimating savings of 1% to 4% in Medicare spending,[25] largely offset by shared savings bonuses paid to providers.[26] The HHRP, which was initially lauded as a success as readmissions appeared to decline by 6% to 17%,[27] has recently been called into question because of how coding changes were managed in reporting reductions in readmissions[28] and concerns about observed improvements simply reflecting reversion to the mean.[29] Nor has the Comprehensive Joint Replacement bundled-payment program delivered significant savings after subtracting out the bonus payments the federal government paid to qualifying hospitals.[30]

Some ACA cost-control measures were designed to respond dynamically to changes in the health care system, such as the IPAB.[31] The innovation in the structure of the IPAB was, because of prespecified conditions under which it would trigger spending cuts, that politicians could avoid blame for unpopular coverage or reimbursement decisions. Yet political pressure against it was strong, and it was repealed in 2018. That said, it would not have been triggered to date, owing to low Medicare spending growth.

Increased Taxes

We ignore most tax increases designed to pay for enrollment expansion, such as the Medicare tax supplement, because they were not designed to have any impact on health care spending, only to raise revenue to fund new expenditures. An exception is the Cadillac tax on high-cost employer-sponsored health plans, which was anticipated to reduce the generosity of health insurance plans over time rather than to raise tax revenue *per se* and, thus, to help bend the cost curve. But this provision was delayed until 2022, and the House of Representatives voted to repeal it in July 2019. However, a longer-lasting legacy of the Cadillac tax may have been to encourage the introduction in the early 2010s of high-deductible plans as employers sought to avoid triggering the tax by placing more onus on employees through greater premiums, deductibles, or co-insurance.[32]

For our micro-level cost saving, we estimate a combined $524 billion overall for the 10-year savings, based on taking half the original CBO estimates for the first 5 years (subtracting major offsets not implemented) and half of the CBO's 2015 estimate for the second half of the past decade.[33] This translates to a reduction of about 1.4% in total health care spending annually between 2010 and 2019, or a reduction of roughly 0.14% in growth rates per year.[34] In sum, taking the CBO estimates at face value, we would not have predicted much progress in bending the cost curve.

Macro Evidence on the ACA and Cost Saving

In a discussion of the ACA and health care spending it is important to differentiate changes in spending due to expansions in coverage from changes in spending per insured American, with the latter better capturing the idea of bending the cost curve. For this reason we initially consider spending per insured individual in Medicaid, Medicare, and commercial insurance and, thus, abstract from secular changes in health insurance *enrollment* since 2010, including the 20 million people newly insured through the implementation of Medicaid expansions and the establishment of insurance exchanges under the ACA or because of the "aging in" of baby-boomers into Medicare.

Figure 14.1 shows the changes over time in inflation-adjusted per-enrollee spending.[35] The first thing to note is that since 2001, real Medicaid spending per enrollee has actually declined slightly, by 3%, as of 2017. This may partially reflect the expansion of Medicaid to people who are healthier (e.g., for those up to 138% of the poverty line rather than those who are eligible because of severe illness), but it is still notable that spending per enrollee has been so stable. Presumably, states face more stringent budget constraints and impose restrictions or reimbursement cuts to Medicaid during recessions or in the face of expanding demand.

The second quite distinct pattern arises in Medicare, where real spending per enrollee rose between 2001 and 2009, caused in part by a large jump in 2006 when prescription drug coverage was introduced under the newly enacted Part D coverage. Since 2009, just before the passage of the ACA, the real (inflation-adjusted) annual growth rate in per-enrollee Medicare has flattened; the annual growth rate between 2009 and 2017 was -0.12%. Some of the decline is likely the consequence of younger baby boomers aging into Medicare, a secular decline in inpatient admissions, and, in particular, a decline in surgical and medical hospital admission rates, which have fallen by nearly a third

Figure 14.1 Real Health Spending Per Enrollee by Payer, 2001–2017

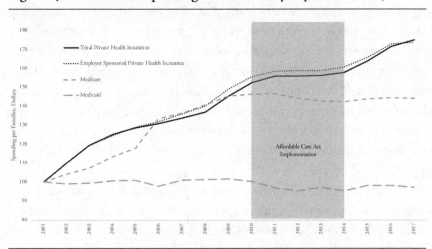

Source: Centers for Medicare & Medicaid Services, Office of the Actuary, National Health Statistics Group. Real values are deflated using the GDP deflator published by the Federal Reserve.

since 2006.[36] In an analysis for the CBO, Michael Levine and Melinda Buntin found that the recession had no effect on beneficiary demand for services and, therefore, had little to no effect on the slowdown in spending growth for Medicare beneficiaries through 2010.[37]

The third distinct pattern is for commercial health insurance costs, which rose prior to 2010, exhibited a distinct pause during the implementation of the ACA, and, after 2014, resumed nearly its pre-ACA growth rate, as shown in Figure 14.1. Why the pause? The optimistic view would be that much of this was because of efforts by health care systems to take the ACA seriously by considering new models of care delivery. For example, in congressional testimony in 2013 Len Nichols stated,

> A good metaphor for the US health care system today is the opening sweeping panorama [in *The Sound of Music*] followed by the crescendo of Julie Andrews' voice singing "The Hills are Alive" with the sound of care process redesigns and incentive changes designed to make better outcomes sustainable at lower total cost.[38]

There is also evidence that, as noted above, employers had begun to respond to the incentives in the Cadillac tax and interest in passing costs along to employees more generally by reducing the generosity of health benefits.[39] This sequence of events corresponds with the patterns we observe; the implementation of new cost-saving innovations, combined with the continued growth in high-deductible plans, could have helped to slow spending growth. High-deductible plans have been shown to reduce spending (at times at the expense of quality);[40] over the 2013–2018 period, the average general annual deductible for workers increased by 53%.[41]

A number of studies have tried to parse out the contribution of different factors to the pause in spending; the portion of the reduction in health care spending growth attributed to the Great Recession varies from the relatively high proportions of 77%[42] and 70%[43] to lower estimates of 37%.[44] We do not think that the pause can be attributed entirely to the recession, as it ended officially in June 2009,[45] but we acknowledge that the slow economic recovery since 2009 could have contributed to scaling back health benefits in commercial health insurance. Additional research has attributed the slowdown to reductions in Medicare payment rates, less-rapid development of imaging technology and new pharmaceuticals, increased patient cost sharing and less generous benefits in private insurance, and greater provider efficiency.[46]

The causes of the reemergence of spending growth in 2014 are not difficult to find. These include rising prices (both for new and existing drugs and treatments),[47] newly developed medical technologies, and the realization that many aspects of the ACA had been delayed or threatened, introducing further uncertainty surrounding the implementation of cost-saving mechanisms.

The pause in health care cost growth during this early period of the ACA took health care actuaries by surprise, leading to a subsequent scaling back in future spending predictions. For example, in January 2010, just before the ACA passed, projected Medicare spending for 2020 was $1.038 trillion.[48] As of January 2019 projected Medicare spending for 2020 was $821 billion (Figure 14.2).[49] Similarly, CMS actuary 2010 projections for total US spending on health care have changed from a projection of $4.14 trillion per year in 2017 (20.2% of GDP)[50] to actual 2017 estimates of $3.5 trillion (17.8% of GDP, Figure 14.3).[51] It is on this

Figure 14.2 Changes in 10-Year Congressional Budget Office Projections of Medicare Spending, 2010–2019

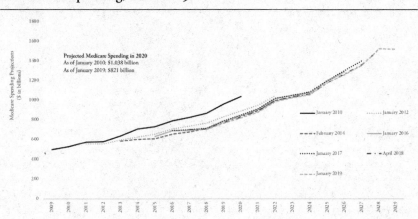

Source: Congressional Budget Office, https://www.cbo.gov/about/products/budget-economic-data.

Figure 14.3 Changes in Projected National Health Expenditures, 2011–2018

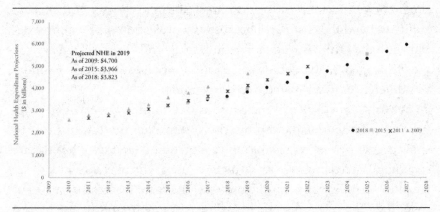

Source: CMS Office of the Actuary, https://www.cms.gov/Research-Statistics-Data-and-Systems/Statistics-Trends-and-Reports/NationalHealthExpendData/downloads/NHE_Extended_Projections.pdf; https://www.cms.gov/Research-Statistics-Data-and-Systems/Statistics-Trends-and-Reports/NationalHealthExpendData/Downloads/Proj2012.pdf; https://www.cms.gov/Research-Statistics-Data-and-Systems/Statistics-Trends-and-Reports/NationalHealthExpendData/Downloads/ForecastSummary.pdf; S. Keehan, J. Poisal, G. Cuckler, A. Sisko, S. Smith, A. Madison, et al., "National Health Expenditure Projections, 2015–25: Economy, Prices, and Aging Expected to Shape Spending and Enrollment," *Health Affairs* 2016, 35(8): 1522–1531.

Figure 14.4 Growth in per Capita Health and Non-Health Spending, 2001–2019 (2001 = 100)

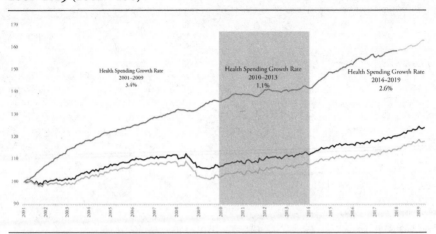

Source: Altarum analysis of monthly Bureau of Labor Statistics price data, FRED population data, and monthly GDP data.

basis that Ezekiel Emanuel suggested that the ACA could claim some credit for helping to save more than \$2 trillion in spending.[52] Yet one should be cautious in reading too much into these views of the ACA's ability to bend the cost curve because any projection of spending a decade into the future is speculative, and small errors in predicted average growth rates over the decade can easily compound into large cumulative differences in estimated overall spending.

We can see evidence of the pause as well in the aggregate data. Figure 14.4 relies on data (and projections) from the Altarum Institute to show overall per-capita real health care spending (and non–health care spending) since January 2001 (which we use as the reference month set equal to 100). As shown in Figure 14.4, there are (at least) 3 phases of spending. There is a discernable pause in growth rates between 2010 and 2013, despite the aging population and the expansion of insurance exchanges; the real per-capita annual growth in spending dropped from 3.4% during January 2001 through December 2009 to just 1.1% between January 2010 and December 2013[53] before resuming a 2.6% growth rate from January 2014 onward. The corresponding health care cost growth rates relative to GDP were 2.7% between 2001 and 2009, -0.3% between 2010 and 2013, and 0.8% from 2014 to 2019. (Perhaps a preferred approach to measuring change relative to GDP is the use of potential GDP, which nets out business-cycle fluctuations; these were 2.0%, 0.4%, and 1.4%, respectively, for the 3 time periods.) Although this new growth rate since 2014 is still lower than the rate in the early 2000s, it seems highly likely that the health care sector will continue to expand its share of the national economy for the foreseeable future.[54]

The Next Ten Years

Looking forward to the next 10 post-ACA years, we expect that more policies will be considered to constrain health care spending growth. Commercial prices, particularly for hospital care, have increased rapidly between 2007 and 2014,[55] and surprise bills—or bills for out-of-network providers when at an in-network facility—have exposed the American public to (at times absurd) medical service prices.[56] Recent polls found availability and affordability of health care at the top of potentially worrisome issues for the 5th straight year[57] and that the public wants lower prices but not a lot of changes to how—or how much—they consume health care.[58]

We are not altogether sanguine about containing future spending growth. Health care employment growth is a bellwether for health care expenditures because salaries and wages account for an average 55% of operating expenses for hospitals, physician offices, and outpatient care[59] as well as nearly 70% of hospital expenses.[60] In 2017, for the first time in history, health care surpassed manufacturing and retail to become the largest source of jobs in the United States.[61] Although the Bureau of Labor Statistics projects that the rate of growth in jobs in health care settings will decrease slightly in the decade from 2016 to 2026, the projected growth of jobs in health care settings (18%) is expected to outpace the remainder of the economy (6% projected growth).[62] It is unlikely that health care cost growth will moderate without a corresponding moderation in the growth of health care employment.[63]

More generally, we fear that the greater a policy's capacity to limit spending growth, the smaller its chances of political adoption, and our fragmented political institutions give opponents multiple chances to defeat or weaken proposals to limit spending.[64] Cost containment means containing medical providers' income and profits, and that triggers opposition from influential interest groups,[65] something we already see with alliances of hospitals, health insurance companies, and pharmaceuticals seeking to prevent single-payer, or Medicare for All, insurance reforms.

With the aging of the baby boomer generation, the Medicare Trust Fund faces a current expiry date of 2026.[66] After the ACA, stakeholders across the health system perceived broad changes coming—a burning platform for FFS medicine and operating as usual. This has since dissipated, and while the administration and lawmakers on both sides of the aisle tinker around the edges of health spending, looking to lower high drug prices, fix surprise medical bills, and implement value-based or shared-saving programs—all programs that could yield longer-term savings—these incremental reforms are unlikely to significantly bend the cost curve in the long run.

Conclusion

We have considered the question of whether the ACA has made health care more affordable. In one sense, the answer is yes—by expanding subsidized coverage to millions of people, a larger fraction of the American population can visit a physician or be admitted to hospital without being faced with overwhelming financial disaster. Yet from both a micro and macro perspective, the evidence suggests that the ACA has not been entirely successful at bending the cost curve. Cuts in Medicare reimbursements to providers and changes in the calculation of Medicare Advantage payments accounted for most of the federal cost saving; based on some empirical evidence, these may also have spilled over to commercial spending.[67] These changes, along with a growing sense that the shift away from FFS was permanent, employer response to the impending Cadillac tax, and reductions in inpatient stays and surgeries, may have contributed to the "great pause" in health care spending between 2010 and 2013. Yet we end on a somber note, observing that real aggregate per-capita spending has again picked up, along with a continued growth in health care jobs that is predicted to continue through at least 2026.

It is, of course, difficult to disentangle the effects of the ACA from broader economic forces and technological trends. Historically, technological innovation has been the largest contributor to cost growth.[68] Although there is some evidence that in the past 10 years there has been a slowdown or "exnovation" in the use of surgical procedures,[69] there is little evidence of a slowdown in the pipeline of new technology. Health care spending varies based on many factors influencing prices and quantity consumed; demographics, pricing power, reimbursement schemes, and coverage provisions all play important parts. The ACA touched each of these, and the role each plays in affecting health care spending continues to evolve. Overall, spending growth reflects policy and personal health care choices and how well policy choices are implemented.

In sum, there are several notable spending wins arising from the ACA that have stood the test of time, mostly related to reimbursement (price) reductions rather than reductions in low-value care. But 10 years post-ACA, many provisions designed to affect spending growth have been changed or repealed through regulation or legislation. Certainly in its weakened state, the ACA has not been successful in bending the cost curve over the long term. Still, the move away from FFS medicine continues, albeit at a slower pace. In the longer term this could create an environment where provider prices and quantities are more easily influenced—whether through global budgets, price regulation, alternative payment contracts, or public pricing options. Whether the ACA in its current form survives to celebrate a twentieth anniversary in 2030 is not entirely clear, but the long-lasting legacy is that it laid a foundation for future reforms to make health care more affordable for consumers and taxpayers alike.

CHAPTER 15

HEALTH CARE MARKETS A DECADE AFTER THE ACA
Bigger, but Probably Not Better

Leemore S. Dafny[1]

Love it or hate it, the Affordable Care Act (ACA) embraced and extended the role of private markets in financing and delivering health care in the United States. The ACA's commitment to markets is underscored by 3 key components of the Act: (1) the requirement that individuals purchase coverage (enforced by a penalty between 2014 and 2018) purchased from a *private* insurer unless the individual qualifies for public insurance (and public insurance expansions were limited—i.e., no Medicare for 50+ nor even a public option to compete alongside private plans); (2) the creation of new individual insurance *market*places with substantial federal needs-based subsidies; and (3) the encouragement of risk sharing by *private* provider groups through accountable care organizations (ACOs), the signature delivery-system innovation enshrined in the ACA.

Ten years after the ACA's passage, it is unclear whether health care markets are better (along a range of dimensions, including delivering health per dollar spent), but there is no doubt that they are *bigger*. Although growth in the share of US GDP devoted to health care has slowed since the ACA was passed, the absolute level has risen from 16.3% in 2008 (before the ACA had taken shape) to 17.9% in 2017,

Leemore S. Dafny, PhD, is the Bruce V. Rauner Professor of Business Administration at the Harvard Business School and served as deputy director for health care and antitrust in the FTC's Bureau of Economics (2012–2013).

the most recent year for which data are currently available.[2] Per-capita spending in 2020 is projected to be $12,087,[3] yielding a national total of $4 trillion, as compared to $2.3 trillion in 2008. Between 2008 and 2015 (5 years following the ACA) the S&P 500 Health Care Index more than doubled. By comparison, the S&P 500 Index (spanning all sectors) increased only 45% during the same period, notwithstanding its greater sensitivity to the economic recovery following the 2009 recession. The differences between 2008 and July 2019 (nearly 10 years following the ACA) are even starker: the Health Care Index increased by 175%, far outpacing growth in most sectors, including financials and industrials, and overshadowed only by frothy valuations in the tech sector.[4]

Although researchers have not performed a comprehensive study decomposing the various sources of market growth (e.g., running a horse race among specific components of the ACA, general economic expansion, and technological progress in various areas), the patterns suggest that either the ACA fueled the growth or that it did not impose constraints upon it. To put it colloquially, the ACA "has not been bad for business," notwithstanding the trepidation of various industry stakeholders—or perhaps owing to concessions negotiated as a result of that trepidation on the eve of its passage. But although this growth has been good for business, it has not been accompanied by more robust competition to serve patients' needs, the much-vaunted benefit of market-based systems.

After growth, the second most important phenomenon in health care markets during the post-ACA years is consolidation. By consolidation, I am referring to the increasing role of large suppliers in a range of health care subsectors, due both to structural changes (e.g., mergers and acquisitions) and nonstructural changes (e.g., changing market shares of existing industry participants). I will primarily discuss consolidation in the health insurance industry and among providers of health care services (especially hospitals and physicians), as these are sectors where research and antitrust enforcement has been particularly active. However, consolidation has occurred in virtually every corner of the health care industry, including pharmaceuticals, outpatient facilities such as dialysis clinics and ambulatory surgery centers, pharmacies, health care IT, and intermediaries like pharmacy benefit managers (PBMs) and wholesale drug distributors. I will also set aside the health insurance marketplaces (HIMs); although the ACA significantly improved the performance of the individual insurance market, the HIMs are discussed elsewhere in this volume[5] and are a relatively small component of the health care industry.

Consolidation does not necessarily mean that markets become less competitive as a result; the outcome depends, of course, on a variety of demand-side, supply-side, and regulatory factors in the market at issue. However, there is a good deal of academic research suggesting that consolidation in various health care sectors—whether horizontal (same product and service market) or nonhorizontal (e.g., mergers of hospitals across distinct geographic markets or mergers of physician practices and hospitals)—has tended to lead to price increases and little to no evidence of concomitant quality improvements. Particularly as the wave of post-ACA consolidation shows few signs of slowing, it is constructive to document what has happened and to consider how it can inform policy going forward.

Post-ACA Consolidation in Commercial Insurance Markets

Commercial health insurance is offered to several distinct customer segments, including Medicare and Medicaid enrollees in states that have contracted with private insurance carriers to administer Medicaid benefits. Although enrollment in these plans has increased markedly since the ACA's passage, in this section I focus on comprehensive insurance coverage for nonelderly individuals (off and on exchanges), fully insured small groups, and fully insured large groups, which jointly account for approximately 45% of the nonelderly, commercially insured. The ACA required insurers to report data for each of these segments by state; the key omitted category—self-insured groups—is also reported, but the allocation of lives across states is inconsistent. Figure 15.1 utilizes data from 2011 and 2017, the most recent year available.[6]

The figure shows that the market share for the largest insurer in each segment state was quite high in 2011 (median share was 40% or higher in all segments) and increased for all but the individual insurance market, where the median weighted share of the largest insurer declined

Figure 15.1 Distribution of Market Share of Largest Insurer by State and Insurance Segment, 2011 and 2017

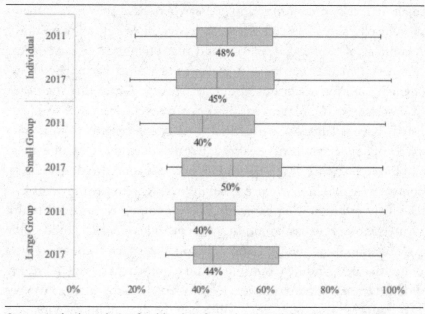

Source: Author's analysis of public data from the Center for Consumer Information and Insurance Oversight. The unit of observation is the state-year. Each observation is weighted by the number of covered lives.

slightly. Data for the Herfindahl-Hirschman Index (HHI), a common index ranging from 0 to 10,000 that is used to measure the degree of concentration in a market, corroborates the patterns evident in Figure 15.1. All segments are highly concentrated (median HHI > 2,500 in both years), and concentration increased for the group segments but remained roughly constant for the individual segment. Overall the ACA propelled more people to purchase insurance in highly concentrated markets.

Noteworthy is the fact that these figures reflecting market concentration would have been higher had the Department of Justice not blocked 2 mega-mergers proposed in July 2015: Aetna and Humana, and Anthem and Cigna.[7] A second noteworthy fact is that there were few sizeable insurance mergers during this period, implying that most of the observed changes in market concentration in the small- and large-group markets were due to nonstructural changes—that is, due to growth in the share of large incumbents.

The most convincing research on the effects of insurer-market concentration is based on structural shocks (i.e., mergers, entries, and exits)
to those levels of concentration. Researchers have shown that merg-
er-induced increases in concentration lead to higher group premiums.[8]
A number of studies have also found that premiums decrease as the
number of market participants increases (e.g., for the individual exchanges[9] and for Medicare Advantage [MA][10]). Given that the driver
of post-ACA consolidation within the commercial insurance segments
listed above is largely nonstructural (i.e., caused by growth in market
shares of large incumbents), existing research does not speak directly to
it. However, studies of the association between concentration and outcomes reveal that more concentrated insurers tend to pay providers less.
The high and increasing bargaining power among commercial health
insurers is often cited as a motivation for provider mergers.[11] Indeed, the
pace of announced mergers among hospitals—which account for 40%
of health care spending (counting hospital outpatient services)—nearly
doubled from around 50 per year in 2005–2009 to around 90 to 100 per
year by 2012.[12] As I discuss next, although the data on hospital mergers
is most readily available, sources suggest significant consolidation has
occurred across a range of provider sectors, including physicians.

Post-ACA on Consolidation
in Hospital and Physician Markets

The post-ACA era has seen a great deal of hospital mergers, physician
mergers, and hospital-physician mergers. We have also seen a variety of
other combinations—including among providers for various postacute
care services and between PBMs and insurers—but in the interest of
space I will focus on the more common combinations. The data on
hospital mergers shows a pronounced lull during the period preceding the ACA. This coincided with the Great Recession that began in
2008, but providers were also holding their collective breath in anticipation of a potentially momentous change. Once passed, the merger
floodgates opened—so to some degree the flurry of consolidation that
followed passage of the ACA was likely pent-up demand. In addition,
the design of the ACA relied upon robust, competitive markets. As

Professor Tim Greaney testified in a 2015 subcommittee hearing for the US House of Representatives,

> The Affordable Care Act depends on and promotes competition in provider and payor markets. . . . Excessive concentration in hospital, physician, insurance, pharmaceutical and medical device markets undermines the pro-competitive policies of the Affordable Care Act. . . . It would be erroneous to claim that the Affordable Care Act is somehow responsible for anticompetitive consolidation among providers and payers when in fact such mergers and joint ventures are efforts to *avoid or frustrate* the procompetitive aspects of the Act.[13]

Nevertheless, the ACA has often been cited as a driver of consolidation, in part because ACOs encourage collaboration across (previously siloed) providers through joint accountability for total spending and patient health. The American Hospital Association (AHA) reported a total of 1,587 hospital mergers over the 7 years following the Act (2011–2017),[14] as compared to 936 in the preceding 7 years (2003–2009).[15] Cory Capps, David Dranove, and Christopher Ody[16] as well as David Muhlestein and Nathan Smith[17] find increases in the share of physicians employed in larger practices, while others report increases in the share of physicians employed directly or indirectly by hospitals.[18] In 2018, for the first time, the number of physicians who reported that they were in employed relationships was greater than those who reported employment in private practice. The days of hanging up a shingle or joining a practice with a short ladder to partnership after graduation from medical school are long gone. Among physicians under age 40, the share who report being employees is now 70%, as compared to 38% among those age 55 and up.[19] However, there is no evidence that causally links the post-ACA consolidation to the ACA itself. The only study that systematically explores the relationship shows that physician and hospital consolidation predated the ACA and finds that metropolitan areas with greater ACO participation did not experience a relatively larger increase in hospital-physician integration, physician concentration, or hospital concentration between 2011 and 2013.[20]

Although the ACA may not have caused consolidation, providers seeking to expand have certainly adopted the rhetoric around coordinated care. In the words of one CEO explaining the expansion path his hospital system, Mount Sinai Health System in New York, embarked upon: "Population health management means services must be coordinated. . . . This requires hospital systems to provide a full suite of services for their patient populations, warranting expansion through acquisitions of other hospitals, as well as physician medical practices and outpatient clinics."[21]

In short, health care leaders interpreted the call for care coordination among various health care providers serving the same patients as a call for *financial* integration, after which care coordination would hopefully follow. An unintended consequence—or benefit, depending upon one's perspective—of this approach is that financial integration could yield stronger negotiating positions vis-à-vis insurers, so even if care coordination did not follow, the combined entities might enjoy stronger reimbursement growth. Thus, in the 10 years since the ACA, the health care provider landscape has transformed, and many sectors have become less fragmented.

The effects of consolidation in general are theoretically ambiguous. To take horizontal integration as an example, there can be substantial economies of scale when providers merge—for example, from consolidating back-office functions, spreading fixed costs (be they managerial overhead or IT investments) across larger enterprises, and taking advantage of many scalable HR functions (like nurse training and management). However, when horizontal mergers involve parties that were formerly rivals for patients, the reduction in competition between them can lead not only to higher negotiated prices but also to fewer hoped-for savings due to the absence of a market imperative to cut costs so as to offer lower prices.[22]

Vertical combinations also have the potential to generate a range of benefits. These may arise through better alignment of incentives across formerly independent parties, such as different provider types, insurers and providers, health insurers and PBMs, and so on. The integrated entity may allocate patients more efficiently across sites of service and/or may price services or invest in quality in a way that considers the spillover effects on other services provided by the merged organization. For example, Kaiser Permanente, the largest vertically integrated healthplan in the country, has invested substantially in the IT infrastructure needed to supply virtual care. Kaiser can incentivize its providers to deliver virtual visits, and patients enjoy the greater convenience of such visits (which could potentially reduce spending on other services, such as ER visits). This type of innovation has to date been more limited among unintegrated providers, who cannot be assured that insurers will cover their investment costs and reimburse for virtual care in a way that leaves them financially whole (or better off). There are, however, potential harms to consumers and to competition that can arise from vertical integration. For example, if an insurer employs most providers in an area, other insurers will find it difficult to develop attractive networks, potentially leaving the area with very few insurance options. This dynamic—called "foreclosure" or "raising rivals' costs"—can give rise to anticompetitive effects that may outweigh the benefits of a vertical transaction.

The data show that greater provider consolidation during the post-ACA era has coincided with soaring commercial prices. By 2016 the AHA reported an average private-payer payment-to-cost ratio of 145%, as compared to 134% in 2009. Over the same period the payment-to-cost ratio declined from 90% to 87% for Medicare and from 89% to 88% for Medicaid.[23] Several economic studies in the general acute-care hospital sector—where data is abundant and merger volumes high—have found that mergers of providers in the same geographic area result in price increases, which then spill over to rivals.[24] Although most of these studies rely upon hospital data before the ACA, some include post-ACA mergers.[25] Two recent studies[26] also show that mergers of hospitals in *different* geographic markets can result in price increases, notwithstanding evidence that some targets in these types of transactions experience cost reductions postacquisition.[27] There is also evidence that hospital mergers reduce rather than improve quality and lead to lower wages for nursing and pharmacy workers when the change in area hospital concentration is sufficiently large.[28]

The literature on physician mergers is not more sanguine than that on hospitals. Two recent studies find that horizontal integration of physician practices leads to price increases.[29] Several studies find that vertical hospital-physician combinations result in higher prices and higher spending.[30] And a recent study has also linked horizontal physician mergers to worse patient outcomes: Thomas Koch, Brett Wendling, and Nathan Wilson[31] find that mergers of cardiology practices result in higher risk-adjusted mortality rates. In short, the evidence suggests that the post-ACA growth in commercial provider prices was caused, at least in part, by the wave of consolidation, and there is no compelling evidence that this consolidation has generated better patient outcomes.

To sum up, ten years after the ACA the US health care sector relies even more heavily on private markets than before. And those markets—although bigger—have grown increasingly concentrated and *less* likely to deliver affordable health care. In this final section I address 2 pressing questions: (1) how did this happen, and (2) what might we do about it?

The ACA Assumed Competition, but Did Too Little to Generate It

The ACA was an extraordinary accomplishment, but it had many shortcomings—some of which were known a priori and resulted from political compromises that were necessary or perceived as such. It did little to actively promote and ensure competition (outside the marketplaces) and less to restrain demand that fueled the growth of spending and profits. The ACA devoted significant attention to creating one specific marketplace (individual insurance exchanges) and to regulating one key service (health insurance) but left the defining elements of other markets largely intact. In a robust market environment an influx of spending would not only generate new products and services but also stimulate significant entry to challenge incumbents. In the long run, economic profits (the excess of revenues over accounting costs and opportunity costs of inputs) would remain stable (or decline) as markets matured.

Instead, health care industry profits soared. In competitive environments market growth often yields share-shifts—that is, firms that introduce the most novel or competitive offerings gain share and trade places with the original market leaders. However, of the top 25 US health care companies by market capitalization in 2009, 22 retained their leading positions in 2019. To be more specific, 16 were still in the top 25 in 2019, 4 had merged into a top 25 company, and 2 underwent a tax inversion so they are no longer US based but would be in the top 25 if they were.[32] Of the top 21 hospitals ranked by *U.S. News and World Report*, 16 were still on the list in 2019.[33] Although market leaders *can* be the most innovative, this sort of persistence seems unlikely in a growing industry in the absence of significant barriers to entry and growth. Health care stakeholders were protected from competition via new entrants—and engaged in relatively disciplined competition among themselves as markets grew—enabling greater profits (and relaxing budget constraints for not-for-profits).

Importantly, firms' ability to profitably charge high prices depends on buyers' willingness to pay those prices, and the ACA made limited and ultimately unsuccessful efforts to restrain Americans' willingness to pay. The "Cadillac tax" on group premiums above a fixed, inflation-adjusted threshold—which would eventually have given employers a strong incentive to adopt cost-saving measures—was deferred and seems unlikely to be implemented.[34] The Independent Payment Advisory Board, which might have limited Medicare's willingness to pay for certain products and services, was defanged before the Act was passed (and the provision authorizing its creation was subsequently repealed). The economic recovery also stymied cost-control efforts, as employers found it feasible to raise wages while paying increasing insurance premiums.[35] Employers' efforts to contain their spending primarily consisted of a shift toward high-deductible health plans, which cause enrollees to cut their spending across the board (e.g., not particularly on "low-value" health care services) and, therefore, mute any impact of consumer elasticity on prices. Moreover, the majority of spending occurs well past the ACA's ceiling on out-of-pocket maxima. These maxima, along with the ACA's ban on annual or lifetime limits to insurance spending, are important consumer protections, but they incentivize higher prices and, therefore, higher insurance premiums.

The ACA demanded relatively few significant concessions on the part of the health care industry in exchange for the largesse it heaped upon it. Absent are caps on private prices, price growth, spending growth, public spending levels, or health insurance premium growth. Absent is a public option—e.g., a health plan paying Medicare prices and accessible for an actuarially fair premium to enrollees not eligible for public insurance—thus shrinking private firms' ability to set higher, market-based prices. Absent is a requirement that all insurance be purchased via public exchanges or that employers offer insurance via a private exchange. This type of requirement might have promoted dramatic changes in health care delivery and insurance design as providers and payers scrambled to develop products and services to meet a consumer-oriented, price-sensitive marketplace.

Explicit efforts to promote entry of firms are largely absent as well, with notable exceptions including federally qualified health centers (not a threat to private enterprise) and public insurance co-ops (whose regulatory constraints were so substantial they were doomed to fail or remain small; indeed, only 4 of 23 seeded by the federal government appear to be offering coverage for 2020, and in 2019 they collectively insured fewer than 180,000 people).[36] In fact, the US hospital industry *gained* a barrier to entry, as the expansion of physician-owned specialty hospitals (a threat to incumbent profits) was (and remains) prohibited. The ACA also did not embrace initiatives to contain pharmaceutical prices nor to ensure rapid adoption of biosimilars (as has occurred and restrained prices of biologic drugs abroad).

How to Address Consolidation Going Forward

To answer the question of what should be done to mitigate the impact of consolidation and promote competition, consider 3 approaches: (1) more antitrust enforcement to ensure anticompetitive transactions are less likely to occur going forward; (2) state or federal statutes imposing binding constraints on price and/or price growth (of providers and/or insurance plans); (3) actions to promote market entry or technological innovations that heighten competition or reduce the incentive of health care firms to raise prices via consolidation.

There are several ways that antitrust enforcement could be bolstered. Beginning with the least controversial, consider the combined budget of the 2 federal antitrust enforcement agencies, the Department of Justice (DOJ, Antitrust Division) and the Federal Trade Commission (FTC). The total budget has *declined* in real terms since 2010, while the volume of transactions has increased.[37] Salaries for the attorneys and economists at these agencies are well below market wages, increasing turnover and reducing the share of experienced professionals who can support legal challenges. As opposing parties grow and become more profitable, they hire more economists and attorneys to mount their defenses, and the battles increasingly resemble David vs. Goliath.

With less capacity, enforcers make tradeoffs. There has been a reduction in enforcement activity relative to the volume of reported transactions in health care, particularly since 2014. Between 2009 and 2013 there were 287 reportable health care transactions, and 22 "second requests" initiating investigations. By comparison, the subsequent 5 years saw a 50% increase in transactions (to 424), but only 12 "second requests."[38] Although it is important to caveat these figures by noting that the more recent deals may not have raised the same degree of competitive concerns as the earlier transactions, it is also worth noting that others have observed a decline in enforcement standards in general in recent decades. Using data on a wide range of industries, antitrust scholar John Kwoka documents that enforcers rarely raise concerns about changes in market structure that used to draw scrutiny—that is, mergers that yield 5 or more market participants.[39] In addition, recent evidence suggests that "stealth consolidation"—deals too small to meet the reporting threshold and therefore not subject to mandatory review—has reduced innovation in sectors such as pharmaceuticals and technology.[40] The first stage of reporting involves minimal effort by merging parties and may deter anticompetitive transactions. Thus, higher enforcement budgets and lower reporting thresholds seem like 2 complementary quick wins for advocates of more competitive health care markets.

A bolder reform would be to require merging parties of a certain size to explain or prove how their transaction will benefit the public. Current law requires the government to prove that a transaction will harm consumers—and on a relatively tight timeline—or to allow it to proceed. Thus, mergers are likely to consummate in close or ambiguous cases. The reform would place the onus on merging parties, such that gray-area mergers would be less likely to proceed. Although shifting the burden of proof could result in some potentially beneficial transactions not taking place because the benefits are too speculative or the parties find proving their existence too costly to merit the effort, it seems like tipping the balance in that direction would be an improvement in light of the current state of health care markets. For example, if insurer Aetna and pharmacy chain/PBM CVS had to demonstrate why their postmerger plans were likely to generate benefits for consumers and unlikely to diminish competition in relevant markets (e.g., sale of insurance to MA enrollees), it is likely their plans would be more specific and more tilted toward consumer benefits, and authorities would also be better positioned to penalize or remedy postmerger harm if it arose.

Even with additional funding, reporting, and presumption-shifting, there are at least 3 reasons why bolstering antitrust enforcement is unlikely to fully address concerns arising from the ongoing wave of health care consolidation. First, antitrust enforcers rarely attempt to break up existing firms because the harm from doing so is often deemed greater than the benefit by the time all legal challenges are exhausted and/or because the evidentiary standards to prove monopolization of a marketplace are steep. Most geographic areas in the United States (i.e., commuting zones) are *already* served by a dominant provider system with a greater than 50% share.[41]

Second, antitrust enforcers and/or the courts have for many years narrowly interpreted the statutes they enforce. Enforcers rarely raise concerns about nonhorizontal combinations that are becoming increasingly common (owing in part to scrutiny over horizontal combinations, where enforcers enjoy substantial precedent affirming their arguments). For example, although insurers or dialysis providers or hospitals are often blocked from merging in areas where they overlap, they are unlikely to be blocked from merging in areas where they do not overlap. Available research on cross-market combinations suggests substantial postmerger price increases,[42] but antitrust enforcers have yet to challenge such transactions.

Third, a worrisome practice has arisen: the seeking of a state-sanctioned exemption from federal antitrust enforcement by merging hospitals. These exemptions (Certificates of Public Advantage, or COPAs), whereby a state agrees to regulate a merged entity in place of enforcing competition law, have been granted in 2 recent transactions that the FTC would otherwise have attempted to block. Evidence on the effectiveness of such regulatory oversight in containing the exercise of postmerger market power is slim, and it can be—and, in some cases, has been—time-limited. Thus, politically powerful local health care systems in some areas still have an out from federal antitrust enforcement.

The next potential set of tools omitted from the ACA but increasingly on the table is price regulation of various forms, including setting rates, capping rates, and capping rate growth for providers. Capping premium growth for health plans is another possibility, one that permits market-based negotiation of prices downstream but could expose enrollees to higher out-of-pocket spending absent detailed restrictions. One logistical challenge with capping premiums or premium growth is the bifurcation of insurance regulation—that is, fully insured plans are state regulated while self-insured plans are governed by the Employee Retirement Income Security Act of 1974 (ERISA). More important is that price regulation removes, to varying degrees, the market mechanisms that determine price, and in so doing, we lose at least some benefits of the invisible hand that efficiently allocates resources and maximizes social surplus in competitive markets.

The last set of possibilities involves changes in the way health care is purchased or produced that heighten purchasers' sensitivity to price or the competition health care producers face. Consumers' responsiveness to price could be increased by giving them a greater role in selecting their health plans—for example, by incentivizing or requiring employers to offer insurance through private exchanges, where employees select from a wider range of options but retain their employer subsidies. The goal would be for consumers to face higher marginal costs for more expensive plans, though employers should risk adjust their subsidies so as to avoid death spirals of the most generous plans. Experience from the public health insurance marketplaces suggests that consumers are likely to select plans with narrower provider networks than employers offer, and several studies document that these plans are significantly cheaper.[43] An increase in the share of consumers opting for such plans would place downward pricing pressure on more expensive providers and low-value products and services.

Although the specific mechanism of downward pricing pressure exerted by greater availability and take-up of narrow network plans can only operate in markets with sufficient provider competition, insurer competition alone could generate downward pressure on optimal

provider prices, even in areas where incumbent providers have substantial current market power. For example, faced with price-sensitive
consumers, some insurers may find it optimal to offer plans with very
specific care pathways developed with advanced data techniques; ad-
hering to these pathways could reduce spending and, therefore, premiums. Alternatively, an insurer could offer—or require—proactive
chronic disease prevention and healthy behavior programs that reduce
health care utilization.

What is lacking today is an incentive for insurers to innovate in this
way because employers have not demanded it and barriers to insurance entry are high. As noted earlier, requiring consumers to purchase
insurance through a public exchange is another approach that would
heighten their sensitivity to insurance premiums, which in turn would
squeeze provider prices. Similar logic applies to so-called "leveling" of
the tax treatment of individual and employer-sponsored insurance premiums. Regardless of the specific approach adopted, purchasers must
exert more pressure on insurers, or else insurers will continue to find it
easier and cheaper to pass provider rate increases downstream than to
undertake the more difficult and complex work of cost reduction.

Lastly, a key change that would stimulate competition in all markets
is the entry of new firms and business models that mute the role of incumbents with market power. Disruptive innovation on the part of the
technology giants may revolutionize the way we access and receive our
health care services. Regulation can help to facilitate competition as
well—for example, by favoring insurance entrants when auto-assigning
enrollees in public insurance programs.

One place where entry has occurred—and at least some benefits are
accruing to patients—is Medicare Advantage (MA). MA has been a
hotbed of delivery-system innovation, in part because individuals can
choose their plans (thus, entry is a bit easier), so carriers can tailor their
benefits and provider networks to serve distinct subsegments of the
market. MA insurers also benefit from the ability to pay government-set
prices for any out-of-network services delivered to their enrollees. For-
profit provider organizations, including Oak Street Health, ChenMed,
and Caremore, are all working to improve health and reduce costs by
increasing access to primary care and, thus, avoiding hospitalizations.

Conclusion

In the decade following the ACA, US health care markets have expanded and consolidated. This consolidation—which the ACA may not have caused but failed to prevent—has contributed to higher prices and slower delivery-system innovation. It will take many years to understand the full effects of the ACA on health care markets and to develop a clearer understanding of the characteristics of transactions that do—and do not—weaken competition in those markets. But there is a great danger in waiting and taking limited action to intervene during those years because the effects of consolidation that is undertaken to deflect competition are so difficult to reverse. The ACA sought to harness the power of markets. For that potential to be realized, we must take actions now to mitigate trends that would undermine it.

CHAPTER 16

THE ACA'S EFFECTS
ON MEDICAL PRACTICE

David Blumenthal, Melinda K. Abrams,
Corinne Lewis, and Shanoor Seervai

Any major effort to improve the health care system must necessarily affect the practice of medicine. This has certainly been true of the Affordable Care Act (ACA). It is impossible, after all, to significantly expand
access to care—while also trying to improve its quality and lower its
cost—without touching the work and lives of the health professionals
who daily lay caring hands on millions of Americans.

Nevertheless, the ACA's precise effects on practice are not easy to
pinpoint. Evaluations of the law have not attempted to directly measure its impact on physicians and other clinicians, how they deliver
care, and how patients receive care. And where changes have occurred,
they likely reflect a variety of influences, including public policies other
than the ACA and the many complex societal trends that have influenced health professionals' behavior since the time of Hippocrates.

David Blumenthal, MD, MPP, is president of the Commonwealth Fund and served
as the national coordinator for Health Information Technology (2009–2011).

Melinda K. Abrams, MS, is a senior vice president of Delivery System Reform and
International Innovations at the Commonwealth Fund.

Corinne Lewis, MSW, is a senior research associate at the Commonwealth Fund.

Shanoor Seervai, MPP, is a senior research associate and communications associate at
the Commonwealth Fund.

In this chapter we assess recent and developing changes in medical practice from several perspectives: (1) we look at how the ACA sought to directly affect the practice of medicine and what, if anything, resulted; (2) we note some other critical public policies that are affecting physician behavior; and (3) we look at forces beyond public policy that are changing medical practice now and will likely continue to do so in the future.

For reasons of space, we focus on physicians. This is not to underestimate the vital role of other health professionals in the American health care system; nurses, physician assistants (PAs), and other disciplines play critical parts in providing health care services and likewise deserve a dedicated review of the effects of the ACA and other forces on their lives and practices.

Direct Interventions by the Affordable Care Act and Their Effects

Expanding Coverage

Physicians are deeply affected by the insurance status of their patients. Treating uninsured patients imposes a range of difficult and often time-consuming choices and tasks on physicians. Though the societal cost of treatments should ideally be a consideration in all physician recommendations, the fact is that for many insured patients, doctors have the luxury of prescribing diagnostic and therapeutic regimens based largely on clinical considerations without calculating financial effects on the individuals for whom they are caring.

For uninsured patients the financial impact becomes a pressing problem that must influence physicians' clinical decisions. Lack of insurance or high out-of-pocket costs are some of the many reasons uninsured patients forgo prescribed medications (they are 3 times as likely to do so[1]), have worse clinical outcomes, and do not receive necessary preventive care. For primary care physicians—who are likely to have more long-term relationships with uninsured patients—finding specialists who will treat uninsured patients poses an additional, time-consuming burden. And nothing is more wrenching for a physician than managing a chronic illness for a patient who has suddenly become uninsured, thus requiring a modification of their treatment. Not only is the alternative treatment often suboptimal, but changing patient habits in relationship to managing their condition is also likely to lead to worse compliance and, thus, outcomes. Extending insurance to millions of Americans, therefore, has the potential to relieve some emotional strains for physicians, simplify their decision making, and enable them to take better care of patients.

Expanding Primary Care

A high-performing health system needs robust primary care. The United States has long suffered from a shortage of primary care physicians (PCPs), and the ACA sought in several ways to attract more physicians to primary care. The law increased physicians' compensation from Medicare with a 10% bonus between 2011 and 2015. In 2012, for which the latest data are available, roughly 170,000 primary care doctors received a total of $664 million in bonus payments, averaging $3,938 per participating physician.[2]

The ACA also temporarily increased Medicaid payments for primary care by an average of 73% to help reduce the discrepancy between Medicaid and Medicare reimbursement rates. The federal government covered the costs for 2 years, from 2013 to 2014, but thereafter states had the option to continue the primary care boost.

Several studies examined the early impact of the Medicaid fee increases, which yielded variable results. A *New England Journal of Medicine* study measured patients' appointment availability for Medicaid enrollees in 10 states and found a significant increase between 2012 and 2014.[3] However, a *Health Affairs* study, which analyzed physician-reported measures of their participation, found no significant increase in the percentage of primary care physicians accepting new Medicaid patients during the same period.[4] Despite varied results based on different perspectives, as of 2016, 19 states had continued the Medicaid fee increase in part or full, suggesting that state policymakers found value in the program as an approach to increase access to primary care for low-income patients. No studies have yet evaluated whether this ongoing bump has improved access to primary care on a continuing basis.

In addition, the ACA expanded the National Health Service Corps (NHSC), which forgives physicians' educational debt if they practice primary care in underserved areas for 2 to 4 years after completing their training. In 2018, 10,900 NHSC providers (physicians, nurses, and PAs) provided care to 11.5 million people at more than 5,000 sites.[5] The hope is that the NHSC experience will encourage some fraction of these practitioners to stay in primary care and perhaps even to stay in those underserved geographic locations.

To our knowledge, there have been no formal evaluations of the effects of these ACA policies on the supply of PCPs, but available data show mixed results at best. In absolute numbers, the supply of PCPs rose from 196,014 to 204,419 between 2005 and 2015. But the numbers of US PCPs per 100,000 people actually fell from 46.6 to 41.4 over the same period.[6] Projections of physician supply and demand in both primary care and other fields continue to predict shortfalls over the next several decades, though such projections are contested and have not always proven accurate in the past. Furthermore, some analysts believe that nonphysician sources of primary care—advanced practice nurses (APNs), PAs, retail clinics, and telehealth—could alter care practices and more than mitigate any PCP shortage by shifting responsibility for many care activities that do not require physician-level skills to these nonphysician clinicians. Supplies of APNs and PAs are expected to increase dramatically in the future.

It seems likely that the rather modest primary care supply policies in the ACA have not dramatically changed specialty choices among the nation's physicians or achieved a significant improvement in the nation's supply of PCPs. The availability of primary care remains a critical problem for the US health care system.

Increased Accountability for Cost and Quality of Care

A variety of ACA policies have attempted to improve the quality and reduce the cost of care through changing financial incentives so as to reward improvements in the value of health care services. These policies have been numerous and varied, ranging from penalties for the occurrence of hospital-acquired conditions and Medicare readmissions to promoting accountable care organizations (ACOs), bundled payments, the adoption of patient-centered medical homes, and others. The systemic effects of these initiatives on cost and quality are examined elsewhere in this volume. Importantly, changes in financial incentives associated with the provision of care can only achieve their objectives with corresponding changes in practice patterns by frontline clinicians as well as changes in documentation and reporting behaviors.

Here again, information on the direct effects of these ACA policies on the lives and behaviors of physicians is sparse. Claims data collected to report on quality and cost effects of such payment reforms do not capture the changes in daily work that clinicians must make to achieve improved outcomes or to document those improvements.

One of the most important ways the ACA encouraged changes in care delivery and reductions in cost is through the ACOs, which consist of combinations of doctors, hospitals, and other health care providers that accept responsibility for the total cost and quality of care of a defined population. As of 2019 there were more than 1,000 ACOs covering almost 33 million people.[7]

ACOs are implementing programs that are likely affecting the daily practice of medicine. These include improvements in medication management and support, efforts to prevent hospital use (emergency department visits and readmissions), and active management of high-need, high-cost patients. According to estimates, 95% of all ACOs are hiring care coordinators to help better manage patient services. ACO formation has also led to new initiatives in data analytics and provider education. The result—presumably at least in part through changes in physician behavior—has been high-quality scores, including some improvements in patients' satisfaction. However, cost savings have been modest, ranging from 1% to 3% among Medicare ACOs and 3% to 9% for commercial ACOs. On average, the cost savings come from multiple sources, such as reductions in utilization of emergency departments or SNFs in Medicare as well as changes in referral patterns among their commercial counterparts.

Increasingly, the federal program is requiring ACOs to assume downside financial risk on the assumption that this will more strongly incentivize changes in practices. If ACOs accept downside risk and succeed in effectively transmitting such risk to frontline clinicians—for example, through meaningful reductions in compensation when physicians either individually or in groups fail to achieve cost-containment targets—there is every reason to expect that practice will change. In one early and successful accountable care experiment, the Alternative Quality Contract in Massachusetts (which preceded the ACA), physicians referred to lower-cost specialists and facilities as one strategy. More concerted efforts to make primary care available off hours (thus avoiding emergency room visits) and to focus care on high-utilizing patients with multiple chronic conditions would also be some welcome results of more effective financial incentives. Again, targeted evaluations are needed to track these possible changes in medical practice.

Physician Burnout

Recent changes in payment and delivery approaches—from the ACA and other sources—have increased attention to the topic of physician burnout. A growing literature and a proliferation of professional conferences now focus on a perceived deterioration in the quality of practicing physicians' professional lives and the resulting threats to the quality and availability of care.[8] The ACA is thought to be contributing to this development because of its efforts to increase providers' accountability for cost and quality of care.

Physician burnout is a work-related syndrome characterized by emotional exhaustion, depersonalization, and a sense of reduced personal accomplishment. Prevalence rates among physicians and physicians-in-training are thought to be near or to exceed 50%. But although some studies find that burnout is on the rise, others find that it is stable or decreasing, depending on how the syndrome is defined.

There are multiple possible sources of burnout. Some studies indicate that physicians working with electronic health records (EHRs) were less satisfied with their work and were at increased risk for professional exhaustion. EHRs were not part of the ACA. The roots of the current crisis around burnout likely precede EHRs and the ACA—some trace this back to the 1999 publication of the Institute of Medicine report "To Err Is Human," which highlighted the prevalence of medical errors that brought new attention to and pressure on accountability.

Other explanations for high rates of burnout include loss of work-life balance as well as payment models that are purely based on incentives and/or performance, thus neglecting physicians' intrinsic motivations as professionals. In addition, physicians are increasingly spending more time on paperwork and administrative tasks, with 70% of physicians in 2018 reporting they spent 10 or more hours per week on administrative work, compared to 33% of physicians in 2012. On the whole, if burnout rates are increasing in medicine, this should be a concern for policymakers. However, the precise role of the ACA in causing the phenomenon is uncertain. It does seem likely, however, that provisions of the ACA embody and further deepen societal trends to hold physicians more accountable for decisions that contribute to exorbitant costs and shortfalls in quality within the US health care system.

Other Public Policies Affecting Medical Practice

One reason it is hard to pinpoint the effects of the ACA on the practice of medicine is that other, highly consequential public policies have been enacted separately from the ACA. Two deserve special emphasis: the Health Information Technology for Economic and Clinical Health (HITECH) Act and the Medicare Access and Chip Reauthorization Act of 2015 (MACRA).

HITECH
The HITECH Act actually became law before the ACA as part of the 2009 economic stimulus legislation responding to the economic crisis of 2008–2010. The law promoted the adoption and meaningful use of EHRs by offering incentive payments through Medicare and Medicaid to physicians and hospitals who adopted EHRs and attested to using them according to federal requirements defined through Meaningful Use regulations.

The HITECH Act was not unrelated to the ACA. Policymakers saw the adoption of EHRs as laying the groundwork for needed reforms in the delivery of health care services, reforms that could make expanded coverage more affordable and more effective by reducing the cost of care and improving its quality.

Between 2008 and 2017 the proportion of office-based physicians reporting the use of at least a basic EHR increased from 42% to 86%.

For hospitals, where many physicians practice, the proportion of facilities with EHRs increased from 9% to 97% over the same period.[9]

The effects of EHRs on practice have been controversial. The installation of EHRs has been associated temporally with a dramatic reduction in the occurrence of hospital-acquired conditions, including adverse drug events. Although this trend began before HITECH reached its full effect, studies have shown that EHRs and, particularly, the entry of medication orders in computers (a requirement of meaningful use) reduces medication errors.

Another positive effect of the adoption of EHRs has been the required implementation under meaningful use of portals that provide patients remote access electronically to their medical records. Altogether, more than a quarter of Americans reported in 2017 that they had accessed their medical records electronically in the past year, and 80% of these reported the experience was both easy and useful. More informed patients are bound to affect patient-physician relationships and the nature of medical practice. As discussed below, the sharing of electronic data with patients could be a major spur to increasing their participation in the processes of care, which consumer groups and some medical experts vigorously advocate. It seems very unlikely that physicians and hospitals would have initiated such efforts to share data with patients without requirements included in meaningful use and subsequent federal legislation.

At the same time, documentation is an important part of physicians' work, and some physicians have found recording clinical encounters in EHRs burdensome and distracting. For example, as noted, the use of EHRs is cited as a major contributor to physician burnout. Complaints about the poor usability of current software are widespread, as is the perception that data entry distracts physicians from engaging with patients during office visits. Another complaint is that exchange of data between different EHR systems has proven more challenging than expected, both for technical and economic reasons.

MACRA

Signed into law 5 years after the ACA, MACRA replaced the preceding Medicare physician-reimbursement system that paid on a fee-for-service basis with a new framework that encourages value-based compensation. MACRA presented physicians with 2 options for payment under Medicare: participation in an Advanced Alternative Payment Model (APMs) or in the Merit-Based Incentive Payment System (MIPS).

Advanced APMs are intended to spur reform in delivery of care by encouraging clinicians to take greater responsibility for health care quality and spending in their practices. From 2019 to 2024, physicians who participate in one of the CMS-designated Advanced APMs (there were 13 in 2019) and meet the necessary performance benchmarks will receive an incentive payment of 5% of their Medicare-covered professional services revenue. In 2019 (based on 2017 performance) 99,000 clinicians earned the associated incentive payment based on their participation in an Advanced APM, with accountable care organizations—NextGen or Medicare Shared Savings Program (tracks 2 and 3)—being the most popular.

MIPS is a system that calculates individual clinician-level or group-level payment adjustments based on 4 dimensions of physician performance: quality, cost, clinical practice improvement activities, and meaningful use of EHRs. Based on the clinicians' performance in these 4 areas, the Medicare payments can increase or decrease and change over time. Clinicians received their first payment adjustment in 2019 based on their performance in 2017, with 93% of those in MIPS (approximately 984,000 providers) earning a positive payment adjustment and 2% (116,000 clinicians) having a neutral adjustment. Maximum positive payment adjustments were modest, ranging from .22% to 1.88% for clinicians with exceptional performance. Early results indicate that larger, urban practices are faring better under MACRA than smaller, rural practices.

Clinicians and policymakers alike have expressed concerns about the sustainability and success of MIPS because of the inconsistency of the quality measures (a clinicians' quality score is based on 6 measures from a set of several hundred chosen by the clinician), lack of sufficient sample size in some practices to produce meaningful results, the focus on individual clinician performance rather than on team results, and the complexity and burden of reporting under MIPS. There is also ongoing debate—as there is with all alternative payment models—on the relative benefit of pushing clinicians toward taking on more downside financial risk versus allowing upside-only risk.

The changes introduced by MACRA likely affect more physicians more directly with respect to both compensation and reporting requirements than the totality of the ACA's provisions. However, it seems likely that many physicians have trouble sorting out which changes in their lives result from which new federal policies.

Secular Trends Affecting Medical Practice

Consolidation

The period since the enactment of the ACA has witnessed a dramatic consolidation among providers of medical service, a trend that started before the ACA but appears to have accelerated after the ACA and MACRA were implemented. This has included both horizontal consolidation, in which suppliers of the same services merge (e.g., hospitals with hospitals and physician groups with physician groups), and vertical consolidation, in which suppliers of different services combine (e.g., hospitals with physicians, hospitals with long-term care facilities). According to research by Professor Richard Scheffler and his group at the University of California, Berkeley, 70% of hospital markets are now highly or super concentrated.[10] This trend is associated with reduced competition among hospitals and increased hospital prices and insurance premiums, without accompanying documented improvements in quality.

Similarly, ambulatory physicians are combining both with hospitals and each other. Between 2007 and 2017, ⅓ of cardiology and oncology practices merged into hospitals. From 2013 to 2015 the percentage of physicians in practices of 100 or more increased from 30% to 35%. Conversely, small practices and the traditional solo practice are in decline. In 1994, 29.3% of physicians were in solo or 2-physician arrangements; by 2014 the figure was 17%.

The causes of these trends toward increased size among suppliers are manifold. In health care, size gives hospitals and doctors the leverage to extract better prices from insurers, and economies of scale can reduce administrative costs. The accountability demands of the ACA have undoubtedly played a role, as have other, non-ACA-instigated policy requirements. For physicians in particular, the support that large organizations can provide in helping doctors manage increasing documentation requirements and accomplish improvements in performance can be extremely attractive. As some organizations assume financial risk for services, administrative support—including improved information systems and analytic capabilities—can prove vital. Small practices and hospitals simply lack the resources and expertise to manage these new challenges.

However, it would be overly simplistic to attribute the changes in practice organization solely to the ACA. Consolidation is occurring in many economic sectors, prompting an ongoing reassessment of current antitrust law and enforcement. And not only government but also private payers and purchasers are demanding increased accountability, and this is to some degree an international movement in medicine. The Organisation for Economic Co-operation and Development (OECD) now collects comparative data on quality of care across its member nations.

The effects of consolidation on medical practice are likely to be mixed. On the positive side, the administrative support available to physicians in large organizations has the potential to simplify their professional lives and free them to focus on clinical rather than administrative functions of medicine. Peer review and peer learning are also more feasible in organizations, and the more regular hours that employed physicians generally work can assist with work-life balance and potentially reduce burnout. Organizations—especially when they employ a wide variety of health professionals—facilitate the formation of multidisciplinary care teams, which are increasingly viewed as vital to high-quality, efficient practice as medicine and patients get more complex.

At the same time, some observers worry that organizational demands for increased productivity and standardization of clinical practice may reduce physicians' ability to spend time with patients and adapt care to patients' individual needs. And available data on the comparative quality of care in large organizations and small physician practices do not show a definitive advantage to the former.

Digitization of Health Care Information

The disruption associated with the deployment of EHRs has obscured the underlying trend they exemplify: the long-delayed arrival of the information revolution in health care.

Information is the lifeblood of medicine. Without data about their patients, physicians are virtually powerless to bring the benefits of modern health care to their patients. The digitization of health data, encompassing many aspects of the patient experience, is sure to change the way physicians practice medicine—to the almost certain benefit of both patients and physicians.

This journey will not be direct, simple, or painless. The advent of EHRs has imposed new documentation requirements on physicians that are especially burdensome for doctors who are not facile with keyboards or technology, such as older doctors. Reducing that burden should be a major priority, and prospects are good that natural language processing will help improve EHRs' convenience and usability.

In the meantime the huge repositories of electronic information now available as a result of health professionals' labors at data entry have become a new "unnatural resource" that is available for exploitation in a multitude of ways. To realize their benefits, the data must be extracted, refined into useful products, and distributed to users. The process of extraction has recently been significantly advanced by a new legal requirement that all EHRs include application programming interfaces (APIs) that facilitate access to EHR data repositories by third parties (e.g., patients themselves, other clinical providers, and technology companies acting as authorized patient agents). Artificial intelligence will help turn electronic health information into useful applications. And new and existing technology companies will provide distribution channels for the applications (e.g., mobile devices of many varieties).

One of the first uses of these newly extracted, processed, and distributed data products may be a personally controlled patient information resource—let us call it a "digital health adviser"—that provides individualized assistance with patients' decisions. Such an application could have major and as yet unexplored implications for medical practice. Patient-facing, intelligent, EHR-based information tools could challenge physician dominance of the medical interaction, even as they improve patient participation in and compliance with physicians' recommendations. Such data products may also support virtual care through telemedicine applications and a variety of home-based care innovations. The impact of the digital revolution in health care on medical practice will likely dwarf any effects of the ACA. Watch this space.

The Biomedical Revolution

Another profound influence on medical practice that has only the most indirect relationship to the ACA is the accelerating biomedical revolution that represents the culmination of 70 years of intensive US investment in biomedical research, including the mapping of the human genome. This research is now yielding therapies that are dramatically improving the health of patients suffering from age-old scourges, in some cases curing them outright.

Patients with previously fatal cancers are now experiencing prolonged, apparently disease-free remissions. We can cure hepatitis C. Genetically derived therapies have changed the course of cystic fibrosis and may eliminate sickle cell disease and hemophilia.

These developments are good news for practicing physicians who encounter such patients, but they also pose stark dilemmas because of their costs. Physicians will soon be grappling at the frontlines with a huge societal dilemma. Protected by complex intellectual property laws, the pharmaceutical companies manufacturing these new therapies are charging prices that, collectively, are likely to prove unaffordable for the nation. Physicians will be dealing personally with the consequences of price-based rationing—knowing they have tools that could cure patients but unable to dispense them because of their cost. This challenge is not without precedent. The US health care system has always rationed access to health care, to some extent, on the basis of patients' financial resources. But the numbers of patients who may be excluded from life-saving care and the financial hurdles that must be overcome will be unprecedented.

Conclusion

Throughout recorded history the medical profession has been in continuous evolution. The pace of that change in medical practice now seems to be accelerating, like the pace of change affecting all aspects of modern society. The ACA should be seen as one of a panoply of forces contributing to this rapid evolution of medical practice.

Correspondingly, the ACA may best be regarded as representing and continuing trends that preexisted the legislation and will likely persist long after the ACA recedes as the potent political and policy topic that it has been over the last 10 years. The nation continues to struggle with the reform of a health system for which the word "dysfunctional" hardly seems adequate. The ACA made a number of attempts to correct manifest flaws in that system that are traceable to medical practice—through increasing the supply of primary care and through promoting financial and organizational experiments intended to increase physicians' accountability for cost and quality and, thereby, improve systemic performance. In the process the ACA has affected medical practice, though it has done so in ways that are hard to document with precision. The practice of medicine is central to health system performance, and physicians need help to participate effectively and usefully in global health system reform. Providing that help remains an open policy agenda.

Part V

THE FUTURE

CHAPTER 17

THE IMPACT OF THE ACA ON THE DEBATE OVER DRUG PRICING REGULATION

Rachel E. Sachs and Steven D. Pearson

One primary aim of the Affordable Care Act (ACA) was to expand insurance coverage and provide all Americans with quality, affordable health care. Although substantial debate during the ACA's development focused on how to ensure affordability for individual patients, employers, and public and private insurers, the ACA steered clear of proposing major changes to how drugs are priced or covered. Ten years later, drug prices and costs to patients and the health system have risen to become the single greatest health care concern of the American public.

Nothing in the ACA explicitly caused drug costs to rise faster than other components of health spending. The ACA did not create high-deductible insurance plan designs that leave individual patients at risk for significant financial burdens. The ACA did not construct the drug development and delivery chain that allowed Martin Shkreli to massively increase the price of an older, inexpensive drug or that encouraged the drug company Mylan to increase the price for the EpiPen or that led the many makers of insulin to raise list prices year after year while pharmacy benefit managers (PBMs) pocketed substantial rebates. The ACA is not responsible for these features of the byzantine,

Rachel E. Sachs, JD, MPH, is an associate professor of law at Washington University in St. Louis.

Steven D. Pearson, MD, MSc, is the founder and president of the Institute for Clinical and Economic Review (ICER).

dysfunctional drug market in the United States, although it also did not address these problems. Today, however, as policymakers sift through the lessons of the first decade of the ACA and contemplate the next phase of health care reform, drug pricing sits at the center of their challenge to make sustainable the vision of expanded insurance coverage that can reconcile access with affordability.

In this chapter we consider several essential themes that policymakers must tackle when moving forward in this space. Part 1 describes the relatively few provisions that made it into the final ACA that addressed drug pricing and coverage, against the political background of the negotiations over the ACA between the White House, Congress, and the pharmaceutical industry. Part 2 considers how the landscape has changed a decade after the ACA's passage and how drug affordability has become far more salient to American patients than it was in 2010. Part 3 considers potential pathways for future drug-pricing reform. Given both the complexity of the problem and the range of options available to policymakers, we offer general themes and values that ought to be considered moving forward and explain how several policy proposals fit within those paradigms.

The Limited Effects of the ACA on Drug Pricing

The ACA included pay cuts to hospitals and insurers to both control costs and to help pay for broad expansions of insurance coverage. One key industry escaped largely unscathed: the pharmaceutical industry. Reporting has explained this outcome by framing it as the bargain that the White House and Congress struck with drug makers to gain their support for the bill.[1] PhRMA, the drug industry lobbying group led by former Louisiana Republican representative Billy Tauzin, negotiated an agreement whereby drug companies agreed to help fund the law's insurance expansion by paying approximately $90 billion over 10 years through larger Medicaid discounts and a new Branded Prescription Drug Fee. Industry's support came as part of an understanding that none of the major structural changes to drug pricing being proposed in Congress at the time would move forward as part of the ACA: no reimportation of medicines from countries like Canada, where they are sold at a fraction of what Americans pay, and no government negotiations of drug prices. PhRMA ultimately spent a mere $150 million in advertising to support the ACA's passage[2]—and received tens of millions of new customers with insurance coverage in return.

Although the ACA did not include the major structural changes to drug pricing that some advocates had called for, it did contain several provisions that have influenced access to drugs and elements of the drug market. Most importantly, the large coverage expansions made possible by the ACA, both in the individual market and through Medicaid expansion, have so far provided nearly 20 million Americans with access to health insurance.[3] This insurance has enabled many patients to obtain and afford the prescription drugs they need, perhaps for the first time. In addition, the ACA included a requirement that all individual and small-group plans include prescription drug coverage as one of 10 essential health benefits they must provide,[4] ensuring that drug coverage could no longer be excluded in the private market.

The ACA also closed Medicare Part D's donut hole, enabling the tens of millions of seniors in that program to more easily afford the prescriptions they need. The donut hole, a strange feature of Part D's original 2003 legislation meant to help the law fit within a budget target, required beneficiaries to pay the entire cost of their prescription drugs once their spending reached a certain level, with coverage only kicking back in after beneficiaries reached a much higher, catastrophic spending level. For instance, in 2010 Part D beneficiaries paid 25% of the cost of their drugs (after an initial deductible of $310) until the total plan spend on their drugs reached $2,830. Then beneficiaries were 100% responsible for the next $3,610 of medications, at which point they would enter the catastrophic phase of their benefits and would pay just 5% of drug costs.[5] The ACA included provisions to close the donut hole gradually by 2020, and a more recent budget deal accelerated that closure to 2019.[6] Now, with no donut hole, patients pay 25% of the cost of their drugs until they reach the catastrophic phase, at which point their responsibility drops to 5%.

Three other provisions of the ACA had major implications for pharmaceutical pricing and payment. First, the ACA increased the mandatory minimum Medicaid rebates for both branded and generic drugs. Medicaid has historically required pharmaceutical companies to remit to Medicaid a rebate per unit when selling pharmaceuticals for program beneficiaries. Before the ACA, companies making branded prescription drug products were obligated by federal statute to remit either 15.1% of a drug's average manufacturer price (AMP) or the difference between the AMP and the best price provided to a subset of other payers for the drug, whichever was larger, while companies making generic products were obligated to remit 11% of the AMP per unit. The ACA increased these minimum rebate obligations to 23.1% and 13%, respectively, requiring pharmaceutical companies to provide larger baseline discounts to the program than they had previously.[7] State Medicaid programs are also empowered to seek supplemental rebates beyond these statutory minimums.

Second, the ACA expanded the range of entities eligible to participate in the 340B program, which was developed to permit certain types of health care facilities to purchase drugs for their patients at prices at or below the rates available to Medicaid. Those facilities are then able to charge insurers full price when administering these drugs, allowing them to use this spread between the full and discounted price to subsidize other aspects of care for vulnerable populations. Before the ACA, the set of facilities eligible to purchase drugs through the 340B program was limited to 12 categories, including federally qualified health centers, Ryan White facilities, and disproportionate share hospitals. The ACA expanded the range of covered entities further to include children's hospitals, freestanding cancer hospitals, critical access hospitals, and rural referral centers.[8] These additions have significantly expanded the program's scope. From 2011 to 2016 there was a 60% increase in the number of hospitals participating in the program, largely attributable to growth in hospital types that were newly eligible after the ACA.[9]

And third, the ACA created a new path to approval for biosimilar drugs in the hopes of improving competition in that growing market. The Biologics Price Competition and Innovation Act (BPCIA) provided innovator biologic drugs—cell-based therapies that are more complicated to manufacture than are traditional small-molecule drugs like cholesterol-lowering statins—with 12 years of data exclusivity protections.[10] Twelve years of exclusivity was viewed as a victory for drug makers, as it far exceeds the 5 years that small-molecule drugs typically receive, resulting in a much longer time period during which drug makers can often set monopoly prices.

The ACA envisioned that at the end of the exclusivity period biologics would face significant competition from biosimilar versions of the original biologics. To make this possible, the ACA created a new regulatory pathway for biosimilar approval by specifying the process through which these products could rely on the data submitted by the innovator biologic in their initial approval process. Essentially, the BPCIA sought to do for biologics what the Hatch-Waxman Act did for generic small-molecule drugs, although there are additional considerations involving the more complex science behind biologics.[11]

The BPCIA was intended to promote the development of competing biosimilars and, thereby, lower the price of many of the most expensive pharmaceuticals being sold in 2010. Unfortunately, the vision of a robust biosimilar market in the United States has not come to pass. The US Food and Drug Administration (FDA) still lacks a clear path for biosimilars to be labeled as interchangeable with the original version, while even those that are approved face byzantine patent thickets curated by originator companies that keep most approved biosimilars from the market.[12] While Europe has seen significant progress and financial benefits from biosimilars, 10 years after the ACA the biosimilar market in the United States remains stuck in neutral, far from what the ACA's authors would have hoped.

However, there were important missed opportunities where the Act's drafters could have more significantly impacted drug pricing and coverage in the longer term. None of the ACA's provisions significantly altered the fundamental market dynamics of the pharmaceutical pricing and payment system. Pharmaceutical companies today remain free to amass large patent portfolios and receive lengthy exclusivity periods on new drugs. Medicare and Medicaid remain legally obligated to cover most and, in many cases, *all* branded drugs. And there is no process for the federal government or a private-sector partner to evaluate the evidence used to approve a new drug and deploy that evidence in negotiations over pricing or coverage. As had occurred with earlier health insurance coverage expansion efforts in Massachusetts, coverage expansion was the ACA's primary focus, and many of the cost drivers that would go on to make insurance affordability a growing problem were not directly addressed.

One important missed opportunity was the creation of the Patient-Centered Outcomes Research Institute (PCORI). The ACA established PCORI as an independent nonprofit organization to fund the generation and dissemination of comparative clinical effectiveness research (CER) on different health care treatment options. As the ACA was under development, multiple advocacy groups and policy experts touted CER as an important mechanism for reducing unnecessary variation and overuse of medical treatments. The hope was that PCORI's work could lead to lower costs through the creation and use of better evidence by patients, clinicians, and insurers.[13]

Existing programs of CER evidence review in other countries strongly influenced the establishment of this new national CER program. These programs, such as the Pharmaceutical Benefits Advisory Committee in Australia and the National Institute for Health and Clinical Excellence in England, had for many years reviewed the clinical and cost effectiveness of new drugs and were integral parts of the coverage decision-making process within their respective national health systems.[14] In a small minority of cases over the years these agencies had denied coverage for approved, effective medicines when the clinical benefit in relation to the cost was viewed as providing insufficient value, given other priorities in a resource-constrained health care system. This ability to deny coverage enabled their national health systems to obtain far lower prices on prescription drugs than in the United States.

Given these precedents, it was a short conceptual leap for some in the United States to surmise an analogous role for the new federal CER program under discussion. If this was the intended path, it looked to many that the outcome would be explicit governmental rationing of expensive treatments, as opposed to the existing implicit rationing through access to insurance. In the midst of a rising chorus of warnings about the dangers of expanded federal powers, commentators argued that a national CER institute would serve as an "assault against seniors" and would "necessitate rationing."[15] This claim galvanized opposition, was amplified by PhRMA and aligned interests, and rattled Democrats framing the legislation. Some commentators, policymakers, and physician groups continued to argue that evidence on cost and cost effectiveness should be integral components of CER and part of PCORI's mandate.[16] They believed that it was disingenuous to pretend that cost was not an important consideration and that added rigor and transparency could be brought to discussions if evidence on clinical effectiveness and cost were included as part of CER reviews.

Nevertheless, concerns about the political consequences of cost-effectiveness research ultimately led to ACA language labeling PCORI's task as "comparative *clinical* effectiveness research" and prohibiting its funding of research that would use the traditional metric of cost effectiveness—the cost per additional quality-adjusted life year (QALY) gained—to set thresholds that might serve as a basis for recommending pricing or payment within Medicare.[17]

In the eyes of many, PCORI was "hamstrung" from the beginning by these restrictions on its research and its ability to make recommendations.[18] But there was no blanket exclusion of cost or value measures, and when PCORI released the first draft definition of patient-centered outcomes research in 2011, it did include a goal of assessing health care value. When drug companies and providers raised strong concerns that use of the word "value" might signal that cost analyses would be part of future PCORI studies, PCORI's executive director made a point of saying in public, "You can take it to the bank that PCORI will never do a cost-effectiveness analysis."[19] The contrast with some of the most prominent national health technology agencies in other countries was unmistakable.

In addition to steering away from cost considerations, the early years of PCORI's allocation of research funding also showed a marked lack of interest in comparing the clinical effectiveness of drugs, despite widespread acknowledgment that head-to-head trials of drugs were sorely needed. In the end, partly through design but also through implementation, PCORI would not be the vehicle through which the United States would tackle hard questions about the value of pharmaceuticals and whether prices aligned with patient benefits. One of the fundamental cost drivers of the health care system was placed off limits. Coverage expansion would not be twinned with strong mechanisms for cost control. Much work was left to be done.

The Increasing Public Salience of Pharmaceutical Prices

A decade after the ACA's passage, the issue of prescription-drug affordability has rapidly increased in its salience for both patients and the system as a whole, and the need for another step in the health care reform process now appears more urgent. Patients—particularly those on Medicare with no out-of-pocket limit—are increasingly exposed to high out-of-pocket costs for their prescription drugs, and those costs have continued to rise. At the same time, those costs impose ever-increasing burdens on the overall system, which lacks sufficient tools to respond.

In short, drug prices are not only high; they are also rising faster than any other segment of health care. Drug companies have strong incentives to regularly raise the list prices of their products. Similarly, the launch prices of many new drugs continue to rise, even when other drugs already exist in the same class. Although some of these new products are highly effective, others command a premium even if they have limited efficacy. Often this is because payers are compelled by law to cover these products and are limited in their legal authority to negotiate lower prices for them.[20]

These factors create challenges for patients. The large increase in drug costs over the past decade means that overall patient spending on drugs has increased, and many patients bear large financial burdens. This problem has been driven by 2 factors: (1) an increasing number of patients with chronic conditions such as arthritis and multiple sclerosis are now being treated with very expensive specialty medications, and (2) employers and other plan sponsors have shifted their health-benefit offerings toward plans that require increased deductibles and co-insurance in place of lower co-payments. In 2010, 35% of patients' cost sharing was in the form of deductibles, the rest coming through co-payments and co-insurance. But by 2016 deductible spending had risen to 52% of cost sharing, and overall patient out-of-pocket spending increased accordingly.[21] Importantly, when patients are in this deductible phase or are responsible for co-insurance rather than a co-payment, their out-of-pocket responsibility is typically based on the ever-increasing list price of the drug in question, not the (often, though not always much lower) net price their insurer has negotiated for the product.[22]

Many patients have difficulty with these high out-of-pocket costs, with 1 in 4 Americans reporting that they have difficulty affording their prescriptions.[23] Patients may skip doses, take less medication per dose, or delay filling the prescription entirely.[24] Patients who must make these choices may suffer adverse health consequences as a result, whether that is a worsening of their symptoms, hospitalization,[25] or even death.[26] Although the debate over health care reform remains politically polarized, there is broader agreement around pharmaceutical pricing, with bipartisan support for at least some reforms and a full 80% of survey respondents agreeing that prescription drug prices are "unreasonable."[27]

These factors also pose challenges for our health care system as a whole. System-wide spending is rising, perhaps particularly for public payers. Between 2007 and 2016 Medicare Part D spending more than doubled, from $46.2 billion[28] to $99.5 billion.[29] Medicare Part B spending on prescription drugs may be increasing even more quickly, nearly doubling from $15.4 billion in 2009 to $29.1 billion in 2016.[30] More than half of this Part B total comes from anticancer medications.[31] In 2015 overall national prescription drug spending totaled about $457 billion, or 16.7% of overall personal health care services.[32] At the current rates of increase, over time even larger shares of total health spending will be spent on prescription drugs.[33]

The aforementioned requirements that public payers cover many or all of these products exacerbate these challenges. Medicare Part B has no ability to decline to cover FDA-approved drugs whose prices continue to rise year after year or who enter at unsustainable or unjustified prices. Similarly, Part D plans must cover at least 2 FDA-approved drugs per therapeutic class, and in 6 therapeutic classes, plans must cover essentially all drugs. On top of these coverage requirements, the Medicare program itself is legally prohibited from negotiating for the prices of prescription drugs and, therefore, cannot leverage the full size of the program in negotiations. These legal requirements provide manufacturers with significant bargaining power in their negotiations with Medicare-plan sponsors. If plans cannot walk away from the coverage negotiation process if they do not like a branded company's offer and must negotiate on behalf of smaller pools of beneficiaries, that limits their ability to obtain lower prices on these drugs.

Policymakers, recognizing not only that patients are being harmed but also that these long-term trends are not sustainable for our system as a whole, have begun to address these issues. However, several institutional actors—particularly the states and the executive branch—are limited in their ability to effect change. States are limited in what actions they can take by the separation of powers between them and the federal government. The executive branch, primarily the Department of Health and Human Services, on its own can have a more meaningful impact on Medicare and Medicaid than it can for patients with private insurance, but its authority is limited even within those government programs. As with the ACA, federal legislation will be needed to more fully address the drivers of these problems and their impact on American patients.

Potential Paths Forward

Importantly, there are multiple ways to lower drug prices. Many different countries have adopted different strategies to restructure their pharmaceutical markets, each of which has tradeoffs and each of which may be a particular fit for the country adopting it. In our view, though, policymakers should consider strategies that would serve 3 main goals: (1) lowering patients' out-of-pocket costs, (2) addressing misaligned incentives in the payment system, and (3) reducing overall health care spending. Because there are many different ways to pursue each of these goals, each of which has its own advantages and disadvantages, we highlight options within each category and note the potential tradeoffs between and among them.

Lowering Patients' Out-of-Pocket Costs

The ACA's focus on patients' out-of-pocket costs in general can be applied more specifically to patients' out-of-pocket costs for drugs. Confronting this problem would not only relieve the financial pressures facing many patients but also address the health consequences that can come with those financial pressures. Several stakeholders have suggested strategies that would limit or cap patients' out-of-pocket costs, particularly in Medicare. These strategies provide policymakers with many options to consider, as they may differ by the drugs they apply to, the patients who would benefit, how far they would cap costs, and a range of other dimensions.

Three different proposals help illustrate the range of possibilities. First, policymakers are considering capping overall out-of-pocket costs in Medicare Part D above the catastrophic threshold,[34] where patients currently remain responsible for 5% of the costs of their medication without limit. This would assist the more than a million Medicare beneficiaries who must pay many thousands of dollars out of pocket for their medications each year.[35] Second and relatedly, one Democratic-sponsored bill would have capped out-of-pocket costs per month in ACA-regulated plans at $250 per person, enabling patients to both lower and smooth their expenses over the year.[36] Third, the Trump administration had considered (though it then rejected) reforms to the Part D rebate system that would pass along plan-negotiated discounts to patients at the point of sale, lowering out-of-pocket costs for seniors who take medications with high negotiated rebates.[37]

Proposals like these would benefit patients who have difficulty affording their medications due to high out-of-pocket costs and would follow in the spirit of the ACA's focus on sharing risk broadly across larger pools of patients. However, lowering out-of-pocket costs for this group alone is likely to increase costs for other patients and the system as a whole. This is because lowering costs for these patients has the positive effect of enabling them to more easily afford the medications they need, meaning that there is increased utilization and, therefore, increased costs for the system as a whole. These increased costs result in higher premiums for other beneficiaries as well. As a result, it is important to pair solutions to this problem with other reforms that would have the ability to lower prices more directly.

Addressing Misaligned Incentives

Throughout our system of prescription drug reimbursement, there are many misaligned incentives that drive prices up, rather than down, over time and that disincentivize robust competition. Academics and policymakers have often focused on PBMs. In the traditional PBM business model, PBMs were paid a percentage of the rebates (discounts) they were able to negotiate off the list price of drugs on behalf of their clients, plan sponsors, and insurance companies. When choosing between 2 similar drugs for preferential formulary placement, this model gave PBMs an incentive to favor the drug that had a higher list price—and a correspondingly higher rebate—over the drug with a lower list price, even if the drug with a lower list price would have been less expensive for the plan sponsor or insurer. This incentive encourages pharmaceutical companies to raise their list prices over time but then provide larger rebates. Although recent scrutiny has led many employers and other plan sponsors to change their contracts with PBMs to avoid this perverse incentive, its influence persists, and it is still possible to find Part D plans offering more favorable formulary placement to branded drugs than to lower-priced generics,[38] let alone competitors. Policymakers have also focused on incentives for physicians in Medicare Part B to prescribe more expensive drugs than would otherwise be therapeutically justified because they are reimbursed more for prescribing more expensive drugs.[39]

Proposals to address these incentives would follow in the model of the ACA's efforts on delivery-system reform. The ACA identified similar distortions in the system for providing health care services and aimed to address them through innovative models such as accountable care organizations (ACOs), medical homes, and bundled payments. To address perverse incentives for PBMs and others in the drug delivery chain that have encouraged list price increases, options include eliminating rebates or returning rebates to plan sponsors and sharing them with patients. For Medicare Part B the essential need is to move away from paying providers based on a percentage of the drug's price. Importantly, although these proposals would help remedy distortions in our current system, they would not fundamentally address the underlying problem of high drug prices.

Reducing Overall Health Care Spending

Just as other countries have adopted different strategies for providing universal health care, they have also adopted different strategies for reducing overall health care spending.[40] One theme policymakers commonly consider is how to align drug prices with their clinical value. Health technology assessment groups around the world evaluate the comparative clinical effectiveness and cost effectiveness of new drugs, using that information to make reimbursement decisions.[41] Using these strategies, other countries are able to negotiate far lower prices for prescription drugs than are US payers. For example, in the UK the National Institute for Health and Care Excellence evaluates the clinical and economic evidence for a new drug, asking whether it represents a good value for the health care system at the price offered by the manufacturer. Only if the drug's cost per QALY gained meets a certain threshold will it be recommended for insurance coverage through the NHS.

Germany's approach is quite different. There, the health technology assessment process is focused on analyzing comparative clinical effectiveness. If a new drug demonstrates no added benefit relative to other drugs (perhaps in the same therapeutic class), it is then subject to reference pricing based on the lowest price charged within the class. For drugs with added clinical benefit, a confidential negotiation phase seeks a mutually agreeable price, with comparisons to prices in other countries playing a significant role. If industry and government negotiators fail to reach a deal, arbitration serves as the final step in setting a reimbursement rate.

When the pharmaceutical industry is faced with the possibility of actions that would lower drug prices, it typically argues that innovation will be reduced as a result, meaning that patients may lack new treatments in the future. However, it is critical to keep in mind not only the amount of innovation we receive but also the kind. The goal of proposals like these is to align drug prices with the value we receive from those drugs. Choosing to pay more for drugs that provide better clinical value and less or not at all for drugs that provide no benefit over existing treatments may lead pharmaceutical companies to invest in a different set of research projects, but that set of projects is likely to be more beneficial for society.[42] Even now pharmaceutical companies are discouraged from developing certain kinds of pharmaceuticals, such as those that would treat early-stage cancers, even if they would be highly socially valuable. Keeping not just innovation but also the social value of that innovation at the forefront of policy discussions will be relevant for decisionmakers.

Conclusion

The ACA's primary focus on coverage expansion allowed its drafters to ignore many of the fundamental cost drivers of the system, including drug pricing and spending. The next phase of health care reform must grapple with these issues. Such reform is undoubtedly difficult, but it is one that other developed nations have tackled successfully. This next phase will consider the difficult social and ethical challenges of how to manage limited resources and must particularly aim to lower patients' out-of-pocket costs, address misaligned incentives, and reduce overall spending.

CHAPTER 18

TOWARD EQUALITY AND THE RIGHT TO HEALTH CARE

Sara Rosenbaum

Introduction

Examined through the lens of health equality, the Affordable Care Act (ACA) represents the most significant advance in more than a half century. In truth, the law's coverage reforms in their entirety represent an effort to mitigate health inequality. But the ACA also amends earlier laws that themselves stand as legal landmarks in health equity, and these amendments merit closer attention. Of particular interest in this regard are Medicaid, the community health centers program, and civil rights laws aimed at ending discrimination in federally funded health programs.

Were this essay to fully address the ACA's health equality provisions, it would discuss many of its private insurance reforms: its prohibition against preexisting condition exclusions and discriminatory insurance pricing, its guaranteed access and renewal protections, and its premium tax credit and cost-sharing reduction provisions. It would also discuss the law's essential health benefit coverage rules for individual and small-group plans that take aim at certain longstanding discriminatory coverage practices such as exclusion of maternity care, exclusion of habilitative services for people with developmental disabilities, and discriminatory benefit designs and coverage determination procedures that historically have barred coverage for patients with significant

Sara Rosenbaum, JD, is the Harold and Jane Hirsh Professor of Health Law and Policy, Milken Institute School of Public Health, George Washington University.

disabilities who need care for health maintenance rather than recovery reasons.

Medicaid, civil rights, and community health centers warrant special focus. Each has played a historic role in the fight for greater health equality, and each became part of the legal foundation on which the ACA rests, with new responsibilities. The Medicaid amendments were conceived as fundamental to the law's near-universal coverage framework—an insurance pathway for the poorest Americans. Community health centers were tasked—as they have so often been before—with translating coverage into health care access for medically underserved communities and populations. A preexisting body of civil rights law was redesigned to follow the contours of a modern health care system that integrates financing and care and to better reflect evolving health, social, and cultural norms regarding the types of people and health needs meriting special legal protections against discrimination and exclusion.

Taken as a whole, the ACA constitutes a seminal advance in law. But it is more than just a law: as Professor Abbe R. Gluck has suggested, the ACA is a "superstatute," a special law whose power is such that it has transformed social expectations regarding government's role in health care.[1] The health equality provisions play a major role in this transformation. Public support for Medicaid is high, with 74% of Americans viewing the program favorably,[2] and for decades there has been bipartisan consensus for expanding community health centers. Furthermore, Americans overwhelmingly reject prejudice by health care providers, even for religious reasons.[3]

Of course, the picture is not entirely rosy; in important ways the law's health equality achievements fall short. There still is no pathway to affordable coverage for unauthorized US residents. The private insurance affordability reforms offer inadequate protection against high costs; pointedly, its "family glitch"[4] excludes financial help altogether for workers who can afford their own employer-sponsored coverage but not coverage for their spouses and children. Above all, a solution is urgently needed to remedy the damage done to the Medicaid expansion by the Supreme Court's decision in *National Federation of Independent Businesses v. Sebelius*,[5] which effectively made expansion optional for states and created an entirely unforeseen coverage crisis for the poor.

Normally, as has been the case previously, legislative shortcomings would have been addressed through incremental amendments. This, after all, is the story of Medicare and Medicaid, which have steadily evolved over more than 5 decades. But the bitter politics of health reform have defeated any semblance of evolutionary normalcy; instead, the law has endured unprecedented attack—in Congress, by state officials, by the Trump administration, and in court.

Despite its failings, the ACA has achieved dramatic, measurable gains in health equality, opening greater access for previously uninsured Americans who, after all, were disproportionately low income and underserved. Ten years after the ACA's passage Medicaid now covers an additional 15 million people.[6] Community health center funding has more than doubled, and capacity has grown by nearly 50%, from 19.5 million patients in 2010[7] to over 28 million served in 2018.[8] Civil rights laws have been reconfigured and modernized. Although this reconfiguration will take time to be felt, especially given the legal backlash the reforms generated, early signs point to its long-term impact, particularly with respect to patients who have experienced exclusion based on gender identity.[9] In short, even if the nation has a ways to go, it is on the right path.

Transformation and Achievement

Medicaid

In an amendment of fewer than 100 words, the ACA transformed Medicaid policy. Previously, federal law limited coverage to certain categories of low-income and medically vulnerable people—children and pregnant women, exceptionally poor parents of minor children, the elderly, and persons with severe disabilities. The ACA created what was to be a new, mandatory eligibility group consisting of working-age adults not enrolled in Medicare who are citizens or long-term US residents and whose household incomes do not exceed 138% of the federal poverty level ($28,676 for a family of 3 in 2018). As a legislative drafting matter, the amendment was modest. But its policy impact was profound—a victory over 4 centuries of social welfare discrimination against able-bodied adults dating to the original English Poor Law.[10]

From a legal perspective the Medicaid expansion was simply the latest step in the program's constant evolution over a half century.[11] This evolution reflects Medicaid's ability, as the nation's largest public health investment in health care, to change with relative speed in the face of enormous needs that confront any national health care financing system grounded in market principles and dependent for its survival on predictable risks and the presence of strict controls against adverse selection. Unconstrained by features essential to standard insurance norms such as a healthy risk pool, prospective enrollment, and tightly controlled benefits,[12] Medicaid has grown into the nation's largest public-health first responder. Its accessibility in time of need, broad benefits, nominal cost sharing, and relatively low per-capita costs compared to private insurance made it the logical coverage pathway for the poor. Indeed, numerous states had already expanded Medicaid on an experimental basis.[13] To ease adoption, Congress also provided generous federal funding: 100% of the cost of medical assistance for the expansion population between 2014 and 2016, slowly declining to 90% in 2020 and beyond.

By effectively making expansion optional, *NFIB* deeply scarred the law, which (logically) had made no alternative provision in the event of expansion's failure. Not only did the decision legally foreclose nationwide implementation as a basic condition of state Medicaid participation, but in framing the expansion as an unconstitutional overreach by Congress, the ruling essentially became instrumental in triggering a resurgence of prejudice against the poor. In seeking a justification for his decision, Chief Justice John Roberts took a broad swipe at the very concept of Medicaid expansion, characterizing it not as simply a natural outgrowth of a 50-year evolution but instead as a "shift in kind, not merely degree"[14]—by implication not merely a legal overreach but a policy one as well.

The chief justice's framing has had enormous consequences. The most visible victims have been 2.5 million working-age adults living in 14 states who fall into a coverage gap—too poor for marketplace subsidies that become available once household income reaches the federal poverty threshold ($21,330 for a family of 3 in 2019) but ineligible for Medicaid in their nonexpansion state. Most of the gap's victims reside in the historic South, where poverty and a lack of insurance coverage are highest; 4 states alone (Texas, Florida, North Carolina, and Georgia) account for over ⅔ of the coverage-gap population.[15] But the Court's framing of the underlying policy helped pave the way for ramped-up attacks on expansion—by opponents determined to thwart state adoption,[16] by federal opponents determined to eliminate the expansion as part of their 2017 repeal-and-replace effort,[17] and by the Trump administration, which not only has continued to support legislative action to eliminate expansion funding and redesign Medicaid as a block grant but also has pursued 2 administrative strategies whose impact is to eliminate coverage.

The first such administrative strategy has involved the use of special demonstration powers found in Section 1115 of the Social Security Act to encourage states to pursue experiments designed to significantly reduce the size of their expansion populations. This strategy began with a March 2017 letter from senior administration officials to governors that characterized the expansion as "a clear departure from the core, historical mission of the program"[18] while offering states experimental permission to impose a range of restrictions, including work mandates, premium obligations, complex reporting rules, restricted benefits, high cost sharing, and exclusionary periods (known as lock-outs) for failure to comply.[19] Thus, whereas the Obama administration had used Section 1115 to encourage states to adopt expanded eligibility under somewhat more restrictive terms than otherwise would apply (and had refused to allow mandatory work experiments), the Trump administration repurposed 1115 to achieve coverage reduction goals.

In relatively rapid order, federal courts have issued opinions[20] halting work experiments on the ground that the administration intentionally failed to acknowledge their adverse impact on coverage, but not before Arkansas actually had launched its demonstration. Within 6 months of launch nearly 17,000 had lost coverage; a major evaluation of the Arkansas demonstration (not conducted by the government, as required under law, but instead with foundation funding) documented a 12-percentage-point decline in Medicaid enrollment, with no gains in either employment or private insurance. This research further documented that over 95% of those losing coverage either met the work requirements or qualified for an exemption.[21] The administration has appealed the court rulings.

The Trump administration's second strategy has been regulations that dramatically expand the circumstances under which Medicaid enrollment by eligible legal immigrants can trigger a public charge determination that, in turn, would make them ineligible for permanent residency (green card) status.[22] Experts predict that the rule will lead to a Medicaid enrollment decline of between 1.0 and 3.1 million people, as immigrants and their families flee the program (along with food and housing benefits) out of fear of legal repercussions.[23] Multiple federal courts declared the rule illegal and preliminarily enjoined the rule from taking effect, citing its impact on health and health care as a major harm that would follow if an unlawful regulation was permitted to stand.[24] As of fall 2019, the Trump administration has appealed these decisions.

Despite the blow landed by *NFIB* and the attacks on Medicaid mounted under the Trump presidency, the expansion has achieved major gains by 2019: 37 states have embraced it (in some cases, in lesser form under 1115 authority), with enormous coverage gains as a result. Furthermore, the attacks on the program and the ensuing struggle to gain nationwide acceptance arguably have reinforced the fact of Medicaid's irreplaceable structural brilliance and its importance to people and health care.

Indeed, the logic of Medicaid expansion remains as firm today as it was a decade ago. Expansion has had an enormous, positive impact. As of July 2018 Medicaid and its small companion, the Children's Health Insurance Program (CHIP), enrolled over 73 million people—15.6 million more than in 2013 and a 27.5% growth over Medicaid's national 2013 enrollment baseline.[25] Medicaid expansion accounts for most of the ACA's remarkable coverage gains and the concomitant decline in the proportion of Americans without insurance: the largest declines have come in expansion states, which experienced a nearly 20-percentage-point drop in the number of uninsured residents, compared to a 10-percentage-point drop in nonexpansion states.[26] Extensive research[27] has documented Medicaid's impact on access to care, uncompensated care, and positive labor market effects, along with positive effects on physical and mental health[28] and, indeed, on mortality itself.[29]

Community Health Centers

To ensure that coverage would translate into health care access for communities with a high concentration of poverty and a shortage of primary care, the ACA established a fund to underwrite a major expansion of the community health centers program; the fund subsequently has been extended twice, in 2015 and again in 2017,[30] and a further extension is expected by the end of 2019.

The fund has yielded enormous results where health equity is concerned, along with Medicaid fueling major growth. This growth has been integral to the success of the Medicaid expansion, enabling coverage gains to translate into health care itself. Furthermore, as they always have, health centers have continued to serve as access points for those left out of the coverage reforms—in particular, the millions left out of the Medicaid expansion and immigrants who remain without a pathway to coverage. Indeed, nearly 1 in 4 patients remains uninsured,[31] a figure nearly 3 times higher than the national average,[32] and it is far higher in the Medicaid nonexpansion states, where in 2018 the uninsured patient figure stood at 35%, compared to 18% in expansion states.[33]

Like the decision to build on Medicaid, investing in health centers in order to bridge coverage and care for the medically underserved was a matter of basic logic. The first health centers—an experimental outgrowth of the War on Poverty and civil rights reform—opened their doors in Boston, Massachusetts, and Mound Bayou, Mississippi.[34] Over the decades the program has undergone exponential growth but has continued to hew closely to its roots—comprehensive primary health care, community governance, charges adjusted by income, and location in medically underserved urban and rural communities. Health centers have remained true to their roots, providing not only primary care but also services and supports aimed at addressing the underlying social conditions that threaten both patient and community health.

Today's health centers increasingly operate as integrated primary-care networks serving patients of all ages, with full participation in a heavily modernized Medicaid system of managed-care plans and accountable care organizations (ACOs), along with active network participation in marketplace plan provider networks, given the relatively low income that characterizes so many marketplace enrollees. Furthermore, in keeping with the original vision,[35] health centers also remain entry points into a wide array of health, educational, nutrition, and social services. For this reason, the program also has become a principal means of addressing the needs of patients with complex and chronic health conditions requiring enhanced primary care and links to more specialized services.

Even in the bitterness of the ACA's postenactment period, health centers held on to bipartisan support, along with the National Health Service Corps, which supplies many of the health professionals working at health centers as well as the teaching health centers program, established under the ACA and designed to better utilize health centers as primary care training sites.[36] As health centers would be the first to admit, their special status as a public health intervention that enjoys bipartisan support carries a certain irony, given the communities they serve and the fact that their sustainability is intertwined with their patients' access to insurance.

Transforming Civil Rights and Health Care

The battle to desegregate health care represents one of the most important chapters in the nation's civil rights history.[37] Health care desegregation played a major role in the design of the 1964 Civil Rights Act, in particular Title VI, which bars discrimination by federally assisted health programs based on race, color, or national origin. The use of federal funding to advance civil rights ultimately served as the model for other important civil rights laws that followed: Section 504 of the Rehabilitation Act of 1973 (barring discrimination on the basis of handicap—later incorporated into the Americans with Disabilities Act), the Age Discrimination Act of 1975, and the Title IX Education Amendments of 1972 (barring discrimination by federally assisted educational entities).

Building on these legal precedents, the ACA enhanced and restructured preexisting civil rights laws, shaping them into a new law, codified at Section 1557 of the Act. Section 1557 accomplishes several things, 2 of which are especially notable. First, it broadens the range of protected classes, for the first time addressing discrimination by federally assisted health programs on the basis of sex, just as the 1972 Education Amendments were designed to do in an education context. Second, in a historic move, Section 1557 explicitly defines health programs to include contracts of insurance, which would include health plans purchased with Medicare, Medicaid, CHIP, or premium tax credit funding. Under longstanding civil rights law principles that apply civil rights obligations entity-wide, this extension of the term "federal financial assistance" to include health insurance public subsidies means that insurers that sell publicly financed insurance are now expected to comply with civil rights laws across *all* of their products, including insured or administered employer-sponsored plans not receiving direct federal funding.

Implementing federal enforcement regulations issued by the Obama administration in 2016[38] hewed to this entity-wide principle while also adopting a definition of discrimination on the basis of sex that includes gender identity and sexual orientation. The 2016 rule also expanded the language-access obligations of covered entities, reflecting a modernization of earlier language-access standards established in policies from 2000. At the same time—and consistent with law—the 2016 rule preserved a longstanding religious-conscience exception for health care workers in cases involving abortion and sterilization, thereby permitting health professionals involved in direct care to refuse to provide abortions. By simultaneously expanding civil rights law to include sex discrimination and adopting an expanded definition of sex (as the regulations do) and extending civil rights obligations to all forms of health insurance (not just plans purchased with direct federal subsidies such as Medicaid or premium tax credits), Section 1557 sought to ensure that care can no longer be withheld from transgender patients and that no insurance plan—whether directly purchased or provided through an employer—can exclude coverage of necessary medical and surgical treatment.

Threats and Challenges Going Forward

The ACA's health equality provisions have resulted in major gains in coverage and health care access, and the extension of civil rights protections under Section 1557 already have produced measurable early gains in expanding access to coverage and care. But the ACA's health equality provisions also face challenges. Some arise from the limits of the original law, others attributable to the Court's 2012 decision and the lack of a nationwide pathway forward, and others are attributable to congressional opponents or Trump administration policies. The 2019 health insurance report from the US Census Bureau[39] shows the cumulative effect of these problems—uninsurance levels in nonexpansion states among the poor double the national average, and widespread Medicaid coverage losses among children and adults, with startling declines among children who are legal immigrants or naturalized citizens. This suggests that widespread fear of green card consequences had begun even before final rules were issued in the summer of 2019.

Harmful administrative policies can be reversed. But the blow landed by *NFIB* demands more—potentially significant political and programmatic tradeoffs along with new spending. Even relatively moderate proposals aimed at rectifying remaining coverage gaps or creating new access points for underserved communities and populations require new financial investment. The question is whether the will exists to overcome political hurdles and commit new funding.

Coverage

Without a doubt, overcoming *NFIB*'s downstream consequences for Medicaid represents the single largest threat not only in states that remain in the nonexpansion column but also in expansion states that could freely change their minds and roll back.

The question is what to do about this problem. One option is to continue the kinder, gentler approach of the Obama administration—that is, continue to encourage more limited expansion via Section 1115, without going as far as the Trump administration has sought to do. But this approach has had only a modest impact in encouraging expansion; only a handful of states have done so on a demonstration basis. If, as the chief justice correctly observed in *NFIB*, the ACA as written transformed Medicaid "into a program to meet the health care needs of the entire nonelderly population with income below 138% of the poverty level,"[40] then in the wake of the impact of *NFIB* on that promise, the nation needs a better solution.

One approach might be to expand legislative pot-sweeteners in order to make expansion even more attractive. Options might be fully federally funding the expansion population on a permanent basis, allowing states to expand only to 100% of the federal poverty level (i.e., partial expansion), and in these partial-expansion states, leaving people at 100% of poverty or higher in marketplace plans. These enhancements could be joined with additional federal funds for expansion states that would help support broader and deeper health system transformation efforts aimed at improving the quality and efficiency of health care itself while giving states the means to increase funding for social services. Finally, federal funding could be enhanced to help expansion states meet the heightened needs of traditional populations with serious disabilities, who represent the costliest Medicaid population.

But anyone who has been through the state Medicaid expansion wars will say that if money were the issue, we would be at full expansion now. The ACA offered incredibly generous terms, with permanent funding set at 90% of medical assistance expenditures for the expansion populations, a federal contribution level never offered previously for any new eligibility group. What the nation is dealing with is ideology. One need only look at a state such as Utah, whose lawmakers literally refused to move forward with an expansion that had been overwhelmingly approved by a voter referendum, insisting instead on substituting a far more constrained and punitive model containing a host of eligibility restrictions. Or consider Texas, where the issue cannot even get traction, even as its rural hospitals collapse. These examples underscore that even "blandishments," as the chief justice in *NFIB* termed the special Medicaid financial incentives, may do no good.

So the deeper question is what are more fundamental structural changes that can be suggested in the name of health equity. One option might be to fully federalize Medicaid coverage for adults and children, including pregnant women, whose eligibility is based on low income. This would enable a single national eligibility standard. But beyond the politics of a federalization carve-out, there are 2 problems. The first is the historic importance of the federal-state partnership where innovation in health care delivery is concerned; the fact of the matter is that states have been the active partners in trying to develop more effective care approaches, particularly delivery approaches aimed at bridging health, educational, employment, and social services. Second, one need only watch the process of state health system reforms to know that states have proven more nimble at rapidly changing coverage policies in response to public health threats such as local spikes in infant mortality. At the federal level local crises are more likely to simply wash out.

Another, more plausible option may be to utilize the same federalism model on which the ACA's private insurance regulatory reforms and insurance exchanges are based. This model gives states the option of expanding Medicaid or electing to default to a federal system, which in this case could be zero premium coverage through a marketplace plan, with high cost-sharing subsidies. We know that, unlike the Medicaid approach of mandatory conditions of participation, this model would pass constitutional muster because it is used with relative frequency in both health care and non–health care laws. This fallback could be coupled with additional Medicaid investments in expansion states to incentivize them to maintain their expansions. No one can predict with any real certainty how many states would roll back coverage. But from a policy and ethical perspective, there is little question that the harm to millions of people left out of coverage entirely in the nonexpansion states outweighs the downside of additional funding that would be required to establish a federal default system that can better ensure coverage equality.

Access to Care and Civil Rights Protections

Where the expansion of community health centers is concerned, the threat, as noted, is to sustainability, and the answer to this threat is to insure the poor. Congress has repeatedly shown itself to be all in on the program; the question is whether lawmakers recognize that the program is only as strong and durable as the financial base on which health centers rest. Once, grant funding was synonymous with the health center business model. Today, grants represent less than 20% of health centers' annual operating revenue. If health centers are to perform as envisioned, their patients must be insured—the Medicaid expansion battle has taught us that.

The fate of the civil rights reforms is more complicated. It is fair to say that all major civil rights advances—whether achieved through the legislature or the courts—have faced enormous resistance. At a time when tensions over deregulation, culture, and religion have never been greater, it is no surprise that enormous tensions would surround a civil rights law spanning virtually the entire system of health care financing in the United States and designed to modernize the meaning of discrimination on the basis of sex.

The Obama administration interpreted the ACA's new civil rights protections relatively robustly. The Trump administration, in contrast, has sought to dramatically broaden the reach of religious-conscience protections while downgrading the civil rights protections themselves. In the case of religious-conscience protections, soon after the Obama administration issued its rule expanding the concept of sex discrimination and barring discrimination against women with reproductive health–related conditions, a federal court in Texas enjoined its application to religious entities.[41] But in May 2019, following the Trump administration's own expanded religious-conscience rule, numerous states and cities, threatened with the loss of federal funding for noncompliance, immediately challenged that rule. This challenge led to a decision by the administration to delay the rule's effective date to November 2019 while litigation ensued.[42] By November 2019, the rule had been enjoined nationally, as had the administration's expanded religious- and moral-exemption rule, protecting employers that object to covering contraceptives.[43] Thus, by September 2019 the administration's contraceptive employer exemption rules, along with religious-conscience protection rules covering both coverage and care, either had been blocked by the courts or delayed.

Still pending as of fall 2019 is an additional rule that would fundamentally roll back the key elements of the Section 1557 rule itself. The proposed rule would eliminate the expansive definition of discrimination based on sex so as to exclude transgender status and limit the scope of 1557 to insurance plans only when purchased with public program funding (tax credits would not be considered public funding), thereby eliminating the entity-wide rule and allowing insurers to continue discriminating through products that do not receive direct federal subsidies. The rule would also eliminate enhanced language-access protections for people whose primary language is not English while also eroding access protections for persons with disabilities.[44] When published in final form, this rule will likely face multiple legal challenges as well.

Ultimately, all of these cases will make their way through the judicial system. Indeed, during its 2019–2020 term, the Supreme Court is expected to decide major cases focused on the meaning of sex discrimination under different federal civil rights laws applicable to employment. Although these cases arise under civil rights laws separate from Section 1557, they are expected to have a major impact on how the term "on the basis of sex" is interpreted in health care settings. And, of course, the contraceptive cases go on and on, with dueling nationwide injunctions in place preventing employers from taking advantage of a broad exemption but creating an enormous lack of clarity as to where matters ultimately will end up. Such turmoil is not particularly unusual with respect to breakthrough laws that attempt to do no less than define the legal contours of social relationships and culture. But it has caused disruption and uncertainty, to say the least.

Concluding Thoughts

For more than half a century this nation has been on a slow—much of the time painfully slow—journey toward greater health care equality. But the successes also have been enormous, none more so than the ACA. Despite its limits—and even considering the damage done by the Court—the law has created new rights and legal expectations while also setting a framework for future action.

By now, however, the nation should have accomplished more— near-universal coverage, an even stronger expansion of access to care, and a civil rights framework capable of guiding the system. Backsliding, stalling, and retrenchment have been painful to experience; more importantly, as demonstrated by research into coverage and mortality, the price paid has been measurable in human terms. But as noted at the outset of this essay, by moving decisively toward the goal of an affordable health insurance coverage pathway for all citizens and legal residents, the ACA has in turn fundamentally affected social attitudes regarding the relationship between people and health care in a national health system that so decisively depends on health insurance as the means for gaining access to care. Public support means that its gains are here to stay; it is time to resume forward movement.

CHAPTER 19

THE ACA'S LESSONS FOR FUTURE HEALTH CARE REFORMS

Rahm Emanuel

When I think about rating the Affordable Care Act (ACA), my overarching view is that the statute has been extraordinary. The ACA gets an A for meeting its goal of expanding health care coverage. It gets a B for controlling costs. It probably gets a C for innovation in the health care system. And, if I am being totally honest, in politics I would say it gets a C+.

Looking Back:
The Politics of Taking on Health Care Reform

In assessing the ACA, one needs to be cognizant of the fact that health care reform is inherently tough politics. I have seen and studied many health care fights. Here is one rule that governs them all: nobody starts a health care reform fight and ends the fight a political winner.

Take the passage of Medicare and Medicaid in 1965 and then the Democratic Party's disappointing performance in the 1966 midterm election. The Democrats did retain their majority, but they suffered big losses: 47 in the House and 3 in the Senate. The Clinton health care reform offers another example. In 1994 the Democrats lost 54 seats in

Rahm Emanuel, MA, was senior adviser to President Clinton (1993–1998), a congressman from Chicago's 5th District (2003–2009), chief of staff to President Obama (2009–2010), and most recently mayor of Chicago (2011–2019). This chapter is based on a keynote address delivered at the "Affordable Care Act at 10: History, Legacy, Challenges" conference on September 26, 2019, at Yale Law School.

the House and 8 seats in the Senate. In both chambers the Democrats lost the majority and Republicans took control. To be sure, there are other factors that affected both the 1966 and 1994 elections—and of course Johnson won with Medicare and Medicaid while Clinton failed to enact his reform—but a primary rule of health care reform is that nobody starts a health care fight with high popularity and ends higher than where they started. It does not happen. Health care reform produces short-term political losses. The credit—when it comes—comes later, which is true also for the ACA, Medicare, Medicaid, and CHIP.

A second rule about health care reform in the United States is that we are adept at universalizing care for segments of the population but have had much less success achieving universal coverage for the entire population. Before the ACA was enacted we had already achieved universal coverage for different segments of the population: seniors with Medicare; the poor, disabled, pregnant women, and mothers with dependent children under Medicaid (some states were more generous and included additional populations); veterans with the Veterans Health Administration System; and low-income children with CHIP.

My own recommendation to President Obama was to follow this tested path: he could push for universal coverage but in the drawer keep a plan to universalize some segments of the population. My vote was to expand coverage to all families and small businesses. Both groups are appealing constituents like seniors, veterans, and children. And they vote. Expanding coverage to them would be good politics and good policy.

A third rule of health reform is about the relationship between the president and Congress. I wrote a memo early on for President Obama about lessons from President Clinton's experience. Among the lessons was for the president to lay out principles rather than an entire piece of legislation. A president should not introduce a bill—that is the work of Congress. The president should enunciate the principles and goals that guide the legislation, but the actual drafting should be left to Congress. Let Congress do the work and get the credit as well. Another lesson from 1993 to 1994 was to take the major medical interest groups— hospitals, insurance companies, physicians, drug companies—off the political field entirely. Neutralize them. Those groups cannot actively work against health care reform or else it will die—it is much easier to scare people when it comes to health reform than it is to persuade people. But the medical interest groups cannot lobby too intensely *for* it either, or else it will be perceived as something that is not "real" reform. In addition, the bill needs to be flexible enough to accommodate a wide range of interests: it needs to be broad enough that those who want to hear about costs hear cost control and those who want to hear about expanding coverage hear about expanding coverage and so on. As a former ballet dancer, I can personally attest to the benefits of that kind of flexibility.

There is a fourth rule: timing. The ACA's timing was less than ideal. We were in the midst of the Great Recession. Congress had spent $800 billion rescuing the banks and the financial sector, and the Obama administration enacted the Recovery Act, spending an additional $800 billion. Average Americans were losing their houses, their jobs, and their life savings, while Washington was spending $1.5 trillion in the blink of an eye—and asking taxpayers to foot the bill for this bailout— so the bankers and auto executives would not need to take a pay cut. That is a bad political cocktail, and there were strong feelings that the corporate sector should be held accountable for their failures.

My argument at the time was, therefore, to push for banking reform before health reform—I advocated "Old Testament Justice" for those who created the worst recession since the Great Depression. In addition, the financial industry would oppose financial reform. This is exactly the political fight one wanted. Holding the titans of the financial industry accountable and battling against them was good politics. With a robust financial reform package, there would be a catharsis in the body politic that could at least begin to address the middle-class anger and frustration. That, in turn, would make for a much better moment for health reform to follow.

There was another consideration that many people forget. We had a very crammed legislative agenda. In 2009 we were not just doing health care reform; we were also revising our Afghanistan policy. And the president wanted to get climate change (cap and trade) done. Everybody in the Afghan room was against health care. Everybody in the health care room was against Afghanistan. As chief of staff, I had to keep both of those on track without having them running into each other and blowing the place up.

With these rules about health reform in mind, I advised the president that he should start with financial reform—what became the Dodd-Frank Wall Street Reform and Consumer Protection Act. After that, he could move on to expansion of universal coverage, focusing first on families and small businesses.

As the historical record reveals, he rejected my advice on the sequencing of financial and health care reform. The good news is that he wanted and welcomed a healthy debate.

A Bridge to a Bipartisan Bill

The Republican stance on health care was another critical consideration. In reality there were only 3 or 4 Republican senators who mattered during the period of the ACA's enactment. The same held true for the Recovery Act. I was locked in Senator Majority Leader Harry Reid's room for 48 hours with the 3 Republicans who ultimately voted for the Recovery Act: Olympia Snowe (R-ME), Susan Collins (R-ME), and Arlen Specter (R-PA) (wavering Ben Nelson (D-NE) was also in the room). By the time we were voting on the ACA, at the end of 2009, Specter had become a Democrat and we were really just focusing on Snowe and Collins. (Incidentally, 6 months after the ACA it was the same few—Collins and Snowe from Maine, plus Scott Brown from Massachusetts—who voted with the Democrats for Dodd-Frank.)

Getting those 2 Republican votes on health care reform became harder as time passed. Despite Senator Max Baucus's optimism for a broader bipartisan coalition for the ACA as he negotiated the bill from his perch as the chair of the Senate Finance Committee, in my view we were never going to get Senators Chuck Grassley or Mike Enzi or any other member of the so-called Gang of 8 or Gang of 6 moderates. Between the vote on the Recovery Act and the vote on the ACA, we saw the rise of a concentrated force of middle-class dissatisfaction that became known as the Tea Party. Tea Party activists were angry about Cash for Clunkers and about the mortgage bailout, but they were especially angry about health care. In August 2009, just when Congress was home for recess, members from across the country really felt the physical force of that rage, and it unnerved everybody pushing for health care reform. A very effective expression of this were the signs that read, "Keep your government hands off my Medicare."

The Democrats' goal should have been to give the few Republican senators in play a bridge away from the Republicans. And remember: the Republican side was fighting us with all they had. We were able to help the 3 Republicans resist that pressure when it came to the Recovery Act—a vote that, in my view, saved the American economy from a depression.

But for the ACA we should have understood better what bridge these few senators wanted to walk on. Not the bridge we wanted them to walk on—rather, what bridge they would feel comfortable on to go with the Democrats. That is a very lonely walk. To get Olympia Snowe to leave the Republican comfort zone, the Democratic side needs to be extremely receptive to her. Despite the many compromises the ACA did make to conservative policy ideas, ultimately there wasn't enough offered for her to feel that comfort. From the Finance Committee, where she was working with Senator Baucus, to the Senate floor, where she was working with Republicans, the bridge just fell short.

The ACA did pass without the Republicans. That was a major loss, even as the ACA passed. Looking at the history of major social welfare legislation, for legitimacy and long-term viability, it is always better to enact with bipartisan support. Whether Social Security, Medicare, Medicaid, or the Civil Rights Act, early bipartisan support enhanced the legislation's legitimacy and the ability to build off of and expand it in subsequent years. The ACA's story is very different: 10 years in, we are still dealing with charges about its legitimacy because we did not get a single Republican vote.

The political arc of the ACA did turn back toward the Democrats. Many people claim the ACA was instrumental in the Democrats' victory in 2018. I worry, however, about overselling the political potency of health care in this way. In my view the most important aspect of the ACA to the 2018 elections was just one provision in particular—the ban on exclusions from coverage for preexisting conditions. That provision has turned out to be enormously popular—and I think that provision and maybe that provision alone is what won in 2018. To otherwise oversell the ACA's success for the party will lead us to mistakes. The other advantage in 2018 is Trump did not reform or improve the

ACA—he wanted to repeal the ACA. That helped make the ACA even more politically potent and valuable.

Looking Ahead: Medicare for All and the Politics of Health Care Reform 2020

That brings us to 2020. Democrats have a massive political advantage on health care going into the election. Among voters, they are up by about 22 percentage points on health care. But—and this is very important—the Democrats do not have a huge political advantage on any one specific policy; rather, the polling numbers reflect the voters' feeling that they can trust the Democrats more on this issue. Therefore, depending on what Democrats offer, health care can be a really big advantage or a big liability.

This polling advantage goes away with Medicare for All. Medicare for All may be good policy, but I think it is a real political liability for the Democrats. First, 160 million people—people in the private insurance system—lose what they have. I have never seen an electoral strategy that wins when the politician says, "I'll take this away from you. Trust me, I've got something better for you." I think that approach is a mistake.

Second, there is no legislative path to Medicare for All. Democrats barely passed the ACA with 58 votes in the Senate and 257 votes in the House. What makes progressive Democrats think Medicare for All with 49 or 51 votes in the Senate is a winner? If anyone can produce the 9 Republicans who are going to vote for Medicare for All, I will publicly declare New York pizza better than Chicago pizza.

Third, running on Medicare for All and not delivering it would be a political disaster for the Democrats. Progressives believe in the government as an affirmative force. The worst thing to do to voters is to say, "I'm going to enact this policy," then get elected and say, "Well, I can't do it." That will further undermine the faith and belief those voters have in government and in Democrats. And all the other things the Democrats are trying to get done in addition to health care will be imperiled.

So what is my proposal for Democrats in 2020 and beyond? Go back to the salami slice. Democrats should expand coverage for a particular population. And in my view in 2020 that population should be early retirees. Remember Clinton's impeachment: 7 days after the Monica Lewinsky affair was revealed, Clinton gave his 1998 State of the Union Address. His number-one policy proposal? Allowing early retirees to buy into Medicare. It is good politics. It is also good policy: early retirees are the fastest growing uninsured population today.

Beyond allowing early retirees to buy into Medicare, we should create a public option—not around Medicare but around the Federal Employee Health Benefit Program. Every cabinet secretary and every cabinet secretary's family, every senator and every congressman, and the president of the United States all get their health insurance through the Federal Employee Health Benefit Program. It is basically an insurance exchange not unlike the ACA's own. And the government negotiates on behalf of the consumer on matters from premiums to co-pays to drug formularies. This is exactly what a public option would do, and the sales pitch to the public would be very appealing: "You have been paying for the best health care in America. It is your elected representatives who happen to get it. Now, we are going to give you access to the same insurance that your senator and congressman have." That is a political winner.

What should the Democrats *not* do besides Medicare for All? They should not rush to give health care to immigrants crossing the borders. In the first Democratic presidential debate for the 2020 primaries there was a moment when everybody on the stage raised their hands in favor of giving health care immediately to people crossing the border. That was not smart or right. Democrats cannot tell 160 million people who are content with their current insurance that they are going to take their health care away to introduce a brand-new program and then also promise something entirely new to immigrants who are not here legally. Forget the moral argument—this is political malpractice. To quote Bill Clinton, that dog just don't hunt.

Democrats have an advantage in health care. It is a winner only if they are smart about it. But they could squander it by emphasizing Medicare for All or health care for undocumented immigrants. Democrats need to move in steps, and they need to be the right steps. Democrats need to be good on policy and good on politics.

Finally, the other major hot-button issue—and one Democrats should take on—is drug prices. Both through the National Institutes of Health (NIH) and high drug pricing, America subsidizes the rest of the world on pharmaceuticals. That cannot continue indefinitely, and I do think in the next 5 years it will end. Democrats can make this happen if they adopt the right strategy.

Most importantly, Democrats should not put up just one bill on drug pricing; instead, they should put on the table separate bills about negotiated drug prices, reimportation, and transparency of pricing—including transparency across all federal and state agencies. The reason for separate bills as a political strategy is that it would have the pharmaceutical industry spending its political capital fighting at least 3 different fights—that will be hard to do at once. But Democrats should force that fight across the entire waterfront and make the companies choose which policies they want to battle on. What they do not battle on, Congress can pass. If the Democrats take the Senate in 2020, they will probably enact drug price negotiations, which is the harder lift. If the Democrats do not take the Senate, the bill may be about reimportation.

Are the Republicans ready to come on board for more health care legislation? It depends on what the Democrats decide to do. In 2008 George Bush vetoed the reauthorization of the Children's Health Insurance Program (CHIP). Barack Obama, once in office, tried to reauthorize and expand CHIP up to 12 million children. That bill passed with 45 Republican votes in the House and bipartisan Senate support. So the question is: What is the health policy the Democrats want passed? If they are trying to enact universal coverage, there are likely no Republican votes for that in either Chamber. But if they try to achieve other aspects of health reform, like prescription drug price control or expanding coverage to vulnerable parts of society such as early retirees, small business owners, and recent college graduates, there probably are a small but significant number of Republicans—10 or so, and potentially shrinking every day—who could be convinced to walk across that bridge. Every step is an important one.

CHAPTER 20

FROM THE ACA TO MEDICARE FOR ALL?

Jacob S. Hacker

On September 13, 2017, a packed audience gathered to watch the unveiling of a hotly anticipated new product. They were not, however, in Silicon Valley, where the newest iPhone had been announced the day before. They were in Washington, DC, where a new Medicare for All bill was being launched by Independent senator Bernie Sanders of Vermont.

New bills typically receive little notice. In 2013, when Sanders first introduced a Medicare for All bill, there was not a single cosponsor. By 2017 Sanders's proposal had 16 cosponsors, a third of the Senate Democratic caucus. They included 5 of the top contenders for the Democratic nomination: Cory Booker of New Jersey, Kristen Gillibrand of New York, Kamala Harris of California, Elizabeth Warren of Massachusetts, and of course Sanders himself.[1] Though Sanders had lost the nomination in 2016, he seemed to be defining the Democratic Party's health care vision for 2020.

Progressive elements of the party have celebrated this shift. For most of 2017 the left and center-left joined forces to fight a fierce—and ultimately successful—battle to block Republicans from repealing and replacing the Affordable Care Act (ACA). But the left wing of this alliance has always demanded much more than the ACA. When Senate Majority Leader Mitch McConnell (R-KY) said he was giving up on the GOP repeal efforts in late 2017, progressive ground troops happily

---

Jacob S. Hacker, PhD, is Stanley Resor Professor of Political Science and director of the Institution for Social and Policy Studies at Yale University.

turned from the legislative trenches to the campaign battlefield, making support for Medicare for All a litmus test for 2020 Democratic presidential contenders.

Along with the defeat of the 2017 Republican drive for retrenchment, the newly intense push for Medicare for All has transformed the character of Washington's perennial health care debate. Although Republicans continue to pursue regulatory and legal strategies to gut the ACA, Democrats are beginning to see a path to universal health care that builds on Medicare rather than expanding private insurance. In a way that was not true during the last fight—indeed, *because* of the last fight and its legacies—a growing share of those on the left are making the case that the United States is finally ready for Medicare for All.[2] Is it? And if not, is there another way to achieve the goal it embodies: affordable, high-quality health care for all?

The Perils of "Path Dependence"

To tackle these questions, we need to start with another: How did we get here? Why does the United States have a patchwork quilt of health coverage that costs roughly twice as much per person as most other rich nations', all while leaving tens of millions of Americans without insurance?

The basic story can be told in a single sentence: for much of the twentieth century, America's fragmented political institutions, the powerful medical and business lobbies, and the receptivity of the public to antigovernment fearmongering all conspired to kill big expansions of public insurance. Even at the height of the Great Depression, with overwhelming Democratic majorities in Congress, President Franklin D. Roosevelt decided not to include health insurance in the Social Security Act of 1935. His personal physician had warned him about doctors' intense opposition, and he feared their lobbying would kill the whole deal, including Social Security.[3]

FDR's decision turned out to be fateful. With America's entry into World War II, the nation's agenda shifted away from domestic affairs. Unions, corporations, and private insurers stepped into the breach—thanks in part to favorable tax laws and federal support for collective bargaining—and by the 1950s the majority of working-age Americans received health benefits via work. Although Harry Truman briefly picked up the banner of national health insurance in the late 1940s, the opposition of the American Medical Association (AMA)—along with Republicans and most southern Democrats—doomed the effort. By the time advocates of government insurance finally had another bite at the apple after Lyndon B. Johnson's landslide election in 1964, they had strategically retreated to the goal of covering those left out of the employment-based system: the elderly and the poor. The result was Medicare and Medicaid—the biggest steps toward universal health care until the passage of the ACA in 2010.[4]

The system that resulted was neither universal nor efficient. But as reform-minded leaders discovered in the 1970s and then again in 1993, it was also near impossible to restructure. Resistance not only came from a hugely expensive medical-industrial complex; it also came from ordinary citizens who had good benefits at work or through Medicare or Medicaid and could be scared into thinking that even commonsense reforms might make them worse off. To add to the difficulties, most of these well-insured Americans had no idea how much their benefits really cost because the expense was hidden in their pay packages or spread across all taxpayers.

It would be hard to design a less-welcoming context for Medicare for All. Enacting a universal program means taking on a lobbying juggernaut to impose taxes on people generally suspicious of government, most of whom were insulated from the true costs of their care. Reformers found again and again that the system's deep-pocketed defenders could transform initially positive public opinion into fear and hostility.

This problem has a social-scientific name: path dependence. This is the notion that past developments can heavily constrain and channel the scope of feasible institutional or policy change. When policies involve major shifts in public and private resources and social structures, they can give rise to strong vested interests, widespread expectations, and entrenched institutions that constrain the options confronting policymakers.[5] These so-called policy feedback effects can make comprehensive reform nearly impossible even when the resulting policy configurations are widely considered to be ineffective. The American health care system is Exhibit A for such ineffective policy mixes, and many policy changes would make it better. The challenge is figuring out how to achieve those changes politically, given path dependence and the increasing polarization of American politics.

The Difference a Decade Makes

The ACA was very much a response to the lessons of the past. It not only built on employment-based insurance; it also contained relatively limited measures to control costs. Prior chapters have described in detail what the law contains. Here I want to talk about what it does not contain: a public option modeled after Medicare.

The public option was designed to move the nation toward a broader Medicare program while accommodating the path-dependent history of American health insurance. In brief, the plan would have let Americans who did not have coverage through work or existing public programs buy into a Medicare-like national health program. Thanks to the work of advocacy organizations, such as the progressive group Health Care for America Now!, the public option eventually made its way into the reform plans of all the leading Democratic candidates for president in 2008, including Barack Obama.

The idea of the public option was to give people who were covered through the state-based marketplaces, where the uninsured could buy private coverage, a public plan that used Medicare's payment rates to hold down prices. Doing so, advocates argued, would guarantee good backup insurance in the many parts of the nation—such as rural areas—where there are not many competing insurers as well as put pressure on health insurance companies to bring down their own costs.

Needless to say, those insurance companies were not fans of the idea, and they hammered the public option relentlessly. Critics on the right described it as a backdoor route to Medicare for All, despite the fact that it would be available only to uninsured Americans who were buying coverage through the marketplaces. In the end the public option died a death of a thousand cuts. A pared-back version passed through the House but was eventually stripped from the final bill in the Senate.[6] It was a reminder of just how difficult it is to expand federal health insurance, even when one party controls all 3 branches.

Many progressives rallied to the public option in 2009 and 2010. Yet they are now setting their sights much higher. The movement toward Medicare for All has occurred quickly, and it has caught many in the party's establishment by surprise. But it is not a passing enthusiasm. Its roots go back to the very first bills for universal coverage, such as the Wagner-Murray-Dingell bills of the 1940s. And its resurgence reflects major shifts in the politics of health care since the fights of the Obama presidency.[7]

The main source of these shifts is the ACA itself. The law has had profound effects. Yet it has also further polarized the politics of health care. Although based on a bipartisan model, the ACA has faced scorched-earth GOP opposition from day one. By contrast, Democrats at first proved timid defenders of the law. Trump's election changed that: the threat posed by unified Republican control galvanized Democrats, especially the party's most progressive voters. Having preserved the ACA—at least for now—virtually all parts of the Democratic coalition are returning to the health care fight with full awareness of the futility of bipartisan outreach in the near term.

Yet the increasing boldness of the Democratic left reflects more than political calculations; it also reflects serious shortcomings of the Massachusetts-inspired approach. The marketplaces in particular have failed to live up to expectations. Of course, their travails reflect in part the ceaseless GOP attacks on them. But that is yet another reason Democrats are gravitating away from them. Many were not that enthusiastic about the Massachusetts model to begin with. They saw it as a second-best route to expanded coverage and political accommodation—one that had a chance of winning some Republican support, if not at the outset then at least down the road.[8] But if the expansion is lackluster and the political accommodation nonexistent, why cling to second best?

According to Gallup, more than ⅔ of Democratic voters now support a "government-run health care system"—up significantly from just a few years ago.[9] (Even Republican voters' support for the idea has gone up, but it is still well short of a majority.[10]) Even as most Democrats tell pollsters they want to preserve and improve the ACA, when those supportive Democrats are given the choice, roughly ¾ said they would rather replace it "with a federally funded health care program providing insurance to all Americans."[11]

In sum, the case for Medicare for All is much stronger than it was during the straitjacketed debate of 2009. Will that case be strong enough, and if not, what might be able to deliver on Medicare for All's promise?

Medicare for All: What and Why?

What is the case for Medicare for All? Although the label has recently come into vogue, American progressives have advocated for a national insurance plan since at least the 1940s. Truman and his allies called their goal "national health insurance." After the defeat of reform plans in the 1970s, however, many on the left began speaking of "single payer"—a reference to the unified payment systems found in universal systems abroad.

In fact, most major countries on earth do not have single payer; they have multiple payers, but all the payers pay the same negotiated health care prices and play by the same strict rules to ensure more or less equal treatment of all subscribers. Even Medicare is not really a single payer: a component of Medicare called Medicare Advantage allows beneficiaries to enroll in private insurance plans that meet strict standards, and roughly a third of Medicare beneficiaries are in such plans.[12]

The defining feature of the systems found in other rich democracies is not the way payments are channeled; it is who is covered, what is covered, and how medical prices are set. First, these systems are universal. The government guarantees all citizens coverage and then figures out how to pay for it. Second, these systems have a single, uniform benefits package. Finally, they use government's bargaining power to restrain costs. In recent years a consensus has formed among health care experts that the major reason US health care spending is so high is because we pay such high health care *prices*. When a nation's leaders commit themselves to providing insurance to everyone, they become much more worried about what health care costs. They also discover that government has a unique capacity to do something about it: set prices.

Medicare does not cover the entire population, but it has evolved in the same direction. At first it paid whatever health care providers

demanded, and costs then soared. Since the 1980s, however, it has gradually improved its ways of paying for care, and costs have risen significantly more slowly than in the private sector. The prices Medicare
pays are much lower than those paid by private insurers. They also vary
much less across providers. And the gap between Medicare and private insurance has been growing, as doctors and hospitals increasingly
consolidate into large medical systems demanding premium prices. In
recent years Medicare's overall tab has risen as the baby boomer generation has been retiring. Yet its spending per enrollee has been essentially
flat, rising less quickly than either economic growth or inflation.[13]

As a blueprint, then, Medicare for All is grounded in evidence about
what works both here and abroad. Yet for its backers, the political logic
is just as important as the policy rationale. The political message of
Medicare for All enthusiasts is that the days of technocracy and tri-
angulation are over. Stop offering Rube Goldberg contraptions that
Americans will barely understand and activists will not rally behind.
Stop trying to fill the gaps in a flawed system and smuggle in cost-control through the backdoor. Just say everyone is covered by Medicare,
period. Republicans are certain to call *anything* the Democrats try to
do a "government takeover"—so why not embrace the epithet and offer voters a takeover they seem to like? Medicare.

Another Road to Nowhere?

Yet the path to Medicare for All is far more daunting than many em-
barking on it may understand. The biggest challenges are political: employer-sponsored health plans cover more than 160 million Americans.
These plans have become less common, more expensive, and more
restrictive. Still, every reasonably well-insured group—whether union
workers or well-paid white-collar employees—is inherently distrustful
of change. Remember: the extremely modest dislocations caused by
the ACA, affecting at most 2 million enrollees, precipitated a bipartisan scramble to ensure people could keep their current plans, however
ill-designed or inadequate.

Financing the transition to Medicare for All would also be a formidable challenge—again, mostly for political reasons. We do not know

exactly how much a universal Medicare program would cost, but independent analysts who have looked at Sanders's proposal estimate it would require new federal spending on the order of $2 to $3 trillion per year.[14] Whatever the exact number, we are talking about a historic tax increase: $2 trillion represents roughly 10% of our economy. By way of comparison, the 1942 tax hike to fund World War II amounted to 5% of GDP. The 1993 tax hike under President Bill Clinton that Republicans (falsely) claimed was the "largest in history" equaled just over half a percent of the GDP.[15]

Now, it is important to note that these taxes would replace private sources of financing. As Sanders put it in an interview after his plan was released: "My Republican friends say, 'Well, Bernie wants to raise your taxes.' They [conveniently] forget to . . . mention that Bernie wants to do away with the private insurance premiums that you're now paying."[16]

The rub is that most well-insured Americans have no idea how much they are now paying. What they see is their portion of the premium and their out-of-pocket spending. What they are *actually* paying is much greater. It includes the lower wages they receive because they get health benefits instead of cash as well as the higher taxes they pay on everything else because the federal government does not tax health benefits as pay.

Our system is almost perfectly designed to hide the true costs of health care; indeed, it would be hard for a system with such outrageous costs to survive if this were not so. Much of what makes American health care so complicated reflects the preferences of those who benefit from a lack of transparency: drug companies, highly paid specialists, medical device manufacturers, commercial insurers, and so on. Yet the cure offered by Medicare for All—immediately bringing all these costs into the open—could very well kill the patient. Those with good coverage would suddenly face a steep tax bill for something they mistakenly believed they were getting on the cheap.

To be sure, Medicare for All could generate big savings. Supporters tout the fact that Medicare's current administrative costs are a fraction of commercial plans', and it does not need to earn profits or pay CEO salaries. The largest and most fundamental source of savings under Medicare for All, however, would be the federal government's proven ability to set prices below what doctors and hospitals charge private insurers.

Technically, such price restraint is doable. Politically, it is dicier. Quickly ratcheting down prices system-wide will encounter fierce industry resistance. The familiar adage that every dollar of health spending is someone's income is *literally* true when it comes to physicians, who make much more than doctors in most other rich nations (especially specialists). But it is essentially true for every part of our medical-industrial complex: drug companies, hospitals, medical device manufacturers, and on and on. Only insurers, perhaps, do not have a lot at stake if prices come down. By proposing to basically do away with insurers, however, Medicare for All would give them plenty of reason to fight too.

Moreover, extending Medicare to the whole population would involve new spending as well as new savings—not only to cover those currently uninsured but also to raise payment levels for the 70+ million Americans covered by Medicaid, a notorious under-payer. And single-payer advocates not only want to expand Medicare; they also want to upgrade its benefits. Sanders's new bill offers extremely broad services, including dental and vision benefits, without cost sharing. That is much more than what Medicare now offers—or than does almost any country, for that matter—and would likely raise spending substantially. It would also mean enormous changes for an extremely large range of stakeholders, from health care providers to pharmaceutical manufacturers to employers.

Here it is worth emphasizing another perverse feature of our system: it enriches a whole set of deep-pocketed stakeholders willing to spend whatever it takes to block changes that threaten them. All the political liabilities of a plan will be found and ruthlessly exploited. That has been the story of every health care debate our nation has had, including the failure of the Clinton health plan back in 1994.[17] When President Clinton described his plan before a joint session of Congress, it actually commanded majority support among voters. But after a few months of GOP and industry attacks, its poll numbers were in the basement. By the time Democrats gave up on trying to pass it, a majority in favor of congressional action had turned into a majority afraid of it.[18]

Medicare for All has political advantages over complex public-private partnerships of the sort envisioned by the Clinton plan: among other things, it is easy to understand and builds on a popular program.[19] But it still has vulnerabilities that opponents will ruthlessly exploit. In polls, support for single payer declines substantially when these vulnerabilities—higher taxes, a greater government role—are mentioned even innocuously. Figure 20.1, based on the work of the Kaiser Family Foundation, shows just how significant this falloff is.

The longtime reform advocate Richard Kirsch, who headed Health Care for America Now! during the struggle to pass the ACA, puts it this way: "The solution is the problem."[20] When public attention shifts from problems to solutions, every bit of rhetorical ammunition will be used to demonize the solution. And overcoming this initial impression can be close to impossible. In politics, opponents do not have to offer an alternative—they can just destroy yours.

In sum, Medicare for All has a great deal going for it, but it also poses serious political risks. Thus, its advocates—and all those sympathetic with its goals—must ask: Is there a path to universal, affordable coverage based on Medicare that is less risky?

Medicare for All, or Medicare for More?

The case for building on Medicare is powerful. Medicare provides valuable and valued coverage through a simple enrollment and financing system, and it has proven much more capable of controlling costs than the private sector. Perhaps most important, Medicare is not just effective; it is also overwhelmingly popular. Republican and Democratic voters alike embrace the program, and everyone knows what it is and roughly how it works. This helps explain why a range of proposals that create a new system quite different from the current Medicare system use the label "Medicare for All."[21]

Yet Medicare for All is not the only way to build on Medicare. In fact, a wide range of Medicare-based plans are on the table, with more, it seems, arriving daily. They range, in rough order of ambition, from plans to augment the ACA with a public option based on Medicare, to proposals to expand Medicare to specific populations (e.g., people

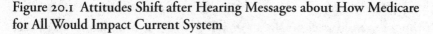

Figure 20.1 Attitudes Shift after Hearing Messages about How Medicare for All Would Impact Current System

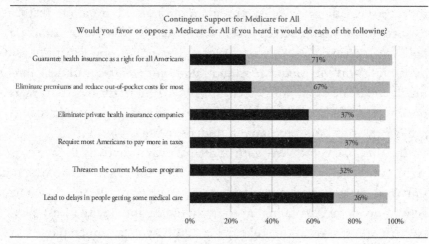

Source: Kaiser Family Foundation Health Tracking Poll (January 9–14, 2019).

aged 55 to 65), to proposals that would guarantee all Americans either Medicare or comparable coverage through regulated private plans.

Many of these plans, however, have a different problem from Medicare for All: they are not designed to match the international standard of performance. They have a better chance of getting enacted, but they are not likely to get us to universality and effective cost control.

In particular, proposals that would simply create a Medicare buy-in option or add Medicare to the ACA's marketplaces do not seem well poised to create sufficient expansionary pressures. The main problem is scale: the public plan envisioned in these proposals just would not cover a lot of people. Small scale is a policy liability, increasing the chances that the plan would end up attracting enrollees with disproportionately high costs and decreasing its leverage over the system. It is also a political liability because these problems and the lack of a strong constituency or serious stakeholder investment could quell opportunities for expanding the public plan to a substantial share of Americans.

Proposals for categorical expansion raise similar difficulties, though; depending on their design, they could cover a much larger group. The case for expanding Medicare to Americans nearing retirement—what Paul Starr calls "mid-life Medicare"—is strong: this is a group facing increasing vulnerability in the labor market that has paid into Medicare for a good chunk of time.[22] Yet there is also a serious risk that such proposals could peel off the most sympathetic groups just as Medicare did, creating a bigger Medicare program but not a clear path to further expansions. We only need to look to Medicare's history to see how a policy can create a robust constituency but not strong expansionary dynamics. Mid-life Medicare would build on the current understanding of Medicare as an entitlement for older Americans based on years of contributions. Partly for this reason, it might make it even harder to achieve reforms built on different understandings.

In sum, a big problem with most partway proposals is that they seem poorly suited to create strong momentum to go all the way to universal coverage and systemwide price regulation. Indeed, they may actively work against going all the way by leaving out the least sympathetic groups—working-age single adults who are unemployed or whose employer does not offer insurance. One important implication, I have come to believe, is that all Medicare expansion plans should contain the foundations for universal, automatic enrollment. Without such provisions, proposals are basically designed to give up before the game begins. With them, they are better poised to ramp up the size of the public plan and build a big support coalition quickly. They are also better fortified against the inevitable efforts to undermine a Medicare expansion once it passes.

How might universality be hardwired into Medicare expansion? Two changes are crucial. The first is to transform the ACA's "play-or-penalty" approach into a true "play-or-pay" system; that is, employers would still need to provide insurance ("play") or make a payment to the federal government. But these payments would be considered *contributions* rather than penalties, with workers and their families then enrolled in Medicare. Thus, all Americans with direct or family ties to the workforce would be covered automatically. Independent contractors could pay the contribution directly, and those without any tie to the workforce could be signed up through other public programs or when they sought care without insurance.

Once someone was enrolled under this system, moreover, they should remain enrolled, without action on their part and with any premiums automatically deducted. These 2 basic features—a play-or-pay requirement and continuous coverage provisions—would quickly reach the vast majority of Americans. More important, they would quickly defuse the most effective attack on universal health care: that reformers want to help "them" at the expense of "us." Instead of focusing expansions of Medicare just on those without insurance, the goal would be to make Medicare a potential source of health security for *all* Americans, regardless of age and income.

At the same time, any Medicare expansion of this sort needs to offer something tangible to 2 crucial constituencies: current Medicare beneficiaries and workers whose employers continued to provide insurance. If the fight over the ACA carries any lesson, it is that current beneficiaries need assurances that their coverage is secure and improving. It should not take 3 elections for them to find out that their benefits are better and the threat of death panels a bogeyman. Medicare needs to be improved as it is expanded.

A similar imperative applies to workers who remain in private employment-based plans—plans that still leave tens of millions of Americans vulnerable to high medical bills and unexpected insurance gaps. The simplest way to ensure that a Medicare expansion delivers for those in employment-based coverage would be to make the benefits offered by Medicare the new standard for private insurance. Initially, this might not affect a large number of plans—though, remember, the Medicare benefits package would be improved for existing beneficiaries, making it more comparable to employment-based insurance in generosity and scope. But over time, as Medicare was improved and expanded to reach more Americans, the Medicare benefits standard would ensure a rising floor of protection for all Americans who remain in private plans, tangibly linking the fates of those within Medicare and those covered by private insurance.

The Road to Somewhere?

Make no mistake: even a partial Medicare expansion will face fierce resistance. Providers, drug manufacturers, and private insurers will vigorously fight any plan that threatens their profits, and concessions will need to be made to overcome their resistance. No country has gotten to universal health insurance without propitiating industry stakeholders.

(Asked how he overcame doctors' resistance, the architect of the British National Health Service replied that he "stuffed their mouths with gold."[23]) But every step toward a bigger Medicare program will increase government's capacity to resist such special pleading in the future.

The approach I have advocated would take that step while taming some of Medicare for All's most serious political liabilities. First, it would reduce disruption to employment-based plans. That is because a large share of employers that now provide benefits would likely continue to do so. After all, the penalty in the ACA is modest, but most larger employers still offer health insurance. Some might feel less compunction about paying the fee if it were a contribution rather than a penalty. Some might not want to upgrade their plans to match an improved Medicare program, either initially or as the Medicare benefits package improved over time. But most employers now providing coverage would likely feel they still had a reason to sponsor insurance, at least in the medium term.

Second, the employer contribution would not only create a system in which high-quality private insurance could continue but would also ensure a steady source of financing. Additional sources would be needed, of course. For example, enrollees should be asked to pay a premium based on income (similar in concept to the "employee" share of private premiums or the Medicare Part B premium). Still, the new revenues required—on top of current investments in the ACA—would be modest compared with that required by Medicare for All.

In short, opening up Medicare to everyone as I have described would deliver much of what is most inspiring about Medicare for All. But it would not require ending employment-based health insurance in one fell swoop or replacing all the hidden sources of private financing with federal taxes overnight.

A final virtue of this approach is that, if the barriers still looked too formidable, its core components could be pursued through a series of self-reinforcing steps. I call this "sequencing," to distinguish it from the planned roll-out or "staging" of a new law. Staging is when a bill implements specific provisions over time. Medicare for All bills, for example, often include some initial moves toward that goal. But these early provisions are staged, not sequenced, and opponents will inevitably focus on the final stage. Senator Kamala Harris's recent campaign proposal for Medicare for All, for example, envisions a 10-year window in which a system much like the one I have outlined is put in place, followed by the establishment of Medicare for All. In the best case, staging gives advocates time to get things right and foster political support. In the worst, it gives opponents time to undermine or reverse the policy.

Sequencing, by contrast, involves multiple rounds of policymaking in which each policy ideally creates momentum for the next. It is the kind of process that the architects of the ACA hoped to spark but has proved much harder to achieve than they envisioned. Part of the problem with the ACA is that it lacks a central focal point, such as Medicare. And part of the problem is that it is very complex—a reflection, in part, of the restricted political window through which it passed.

By contrast, Medicare expansion would focus people on a familiar program in which most had a stake. It would also give employers incentives to see Medicare as a means of insuring their workers. In the past, business opposition to social programs withered once employers realized they were a good deal. Such dynamics will surely be more muted today. Nonetheless, employers who pay the contribution are likely to become more supportive, and more employers are likely to take advantage of the option over time.

Consider the following sequence. First Medicare benefits could be upgraded and employers given the option of enrolling their workers in the upgraded program. At the same time, the standards for employment-based plans could be raised. Then, the ACA penalty could be transformed into a contribution requirement—first for larger employers, then for all employers. Each of these steps would be popular, do much good, and create momentum for further action.

The test with any sequenced approach is whether each step will increase the pressure for more. I have argued that adding Medicare to the ACA marketplaces or expanding Medicare to new groups might not meet that test. I have also argued that the approach I have presented has a better chance of achieving that goal—that it is more likely to get us to guaranteed universal coverage through a self-reinforcing process.

The passion of those who resist partial measures is essential. And there are indeed partial measures that should be resisted. But passion should not blind us to political risks. The test of seriousness should not be whether candidates say "I support Medicare for All" or raise their hands when asked if they would eliminate private insurance. It is whether they are willing to support policies that will truly deliver quality health care to all Americans at a cost our nation can afford.

ACKNOWLEDGMENTS

This book could not have come to fruition without the tireless and brilliant contributions of Eugene Rusyn, the senior fellow at the Solomon Center for Health Law and Policy at Yale Law School. Eugene helped lead this project from conception through completion. He played an integral role in shaping all of its content and attending to every detail—making sure it actually was delivered with every "i" dotted and "t" crossed. Our gratitude to and admiration for him are boundless.

We are also grateful for the support we received from our respective institutions. The Solomon Center for Health Law and Policy at Yale Law School has been at the forefront of national scholarship and legal practice related to the Affordable Care Act, and we have benefited enormously from the years of academic and legal collaborations around the ACA it has facilitated. We thank Yale Law School Deans Robert Post and Heather Gerken, the Solomon family, Yale School of Medicine Dean Robert Alpern, Solomon Center executive staff Katherine Kraschel and Kathryn Mammel, and Senior Administrative Assistant Lise Cavallaro for their support of our work. We are also grateful to Penn's Healthcare Transformation Institute. The Institute is dedicated to taking the ACA framework and reducing health care costs through physician behavior change. It has provided a generative intellectual home for thinking about how to improve upon the ACA.

This book also received generous support from the Commonwealth Fund, the Milbank Memorial Fund, and the Robert Wood Johnson Foundation. We also owe appreciation to the National Academy of Social Insurance and the Oscar M. Ruebhausen Fund at Yale Law School for cosponsoring the conference supporting the book.

We thank Clive Priddle and the fantastic team at PublicAffairs for recognizing the value of a comprehensive assessment of the ACA at 10 years and for being able to expedite the book's publication to ensure both timeliness and inclusion of the latest facts in an ever-changing environment.

Finally, we thank our all-star list of contributors for their insights and commitment to the project as well as all the work they have put in over the past decade in service of governance, law, and better health care.

GLOSSARY

ACA—Affordable Care Act
ACOs—accountable care organizations
Advanced APM—Advanced Alternative Payment Model
AHCA—American Health Care Act
AIA—Anti-Injunction Act
AMA—American Medical Association
AMP—average manufacturer price
APIs—application programming interfaces
APNs—advanced practice nurses
AQC—Alternative Quality Contract
PGP—Medicare Physician Group Practice
BCRA—Better Care Reconciliation Act
BCRA—Bipartisan Campaign Reform Act
BPCIA—Biologics Price Competition and Innovation Act
BPCI—Bundled Payments for Care Improvement
CBO—Congressional Budget Office
CER—clinical effectiveness research
CHF—congestive heart failure
CHIP—Children's Health Insurance Program
CLASS Act—Community Living Assistance Services and Supports
   Act
CMMI—Center for Medicare and Medicaid Innovation
CMS—Centers for Medicaid and Medicare Services
COPAs—Certificates of Public Advantage
CPC—Comprehensive Primary Care
CPC+—CPC Plus
CSR—cost-sharing reduction
DOJ—Department of Justice
DSRs—delivery-system reforms
E&E—eligibility and enrollment
EDE—enhanced direct enrollment
ED—emergency department

EHRs—electronic health records

ERISA—Employee Retirement Income Security Act

ESI—employer-sponsored insurance

FFE—federally facilitated exchange

FFS—fee-for-service

FPL—federal poverty level

FQHCs—federally qualified health centers

FTC—Federal Trade Commission

GDP—gross domestic product

HCERA—Health Care and Education Reconciliation Act

HHI—Herfindahl-Hirschman Index

HHS—Health and Human Services

HIMs—health insurance marketplaces

HIPAA—Health Insurance Portability and Accountability Act

HIT—Health Information Technology

HITECH Act—Health Information Technology for Economic and Clinical Health Act

HRRP—Hospital Readmissions Reduction Program

HSAs—Health Savings Accounts

IPAB—Independent Payment Advisory Board

LEJR—lower-extremity joint replacement

MACRA—Medicare Access and CHIP Reauthorization Act

MA—Medicare Advantage

MCOs—managed care organizations

MedPAC—Medicare Payment Advisory Commission

MIPS—Merit-Based Incentive Payment System

MMA—Medicare Modernization Act

MSSP—Medicare Shared Savings Program

NAIC—National Association of Insurance Commissioners

NFIB—*National Federation of Independent Business v. Sebelius*

NHE—national health expenditures

NHSC—National Health Service Corps

NIH—National Institutes of Health

OCM—Oncology Care Model

OECD—Organisation for Economic Co-operation and Development

OHIE—Office of Health Insurance Exchanges

ONC—Office of the National Coordinator for Health Information Technology

PAs—physician assistants

PBMs—pharmacy benefit managers

PCORI—Patient-Centered Outcomes Research Institute

PCPs—primary care physicians

PPACA—Patient Protection and Affordable Care Act

QALY—quality-adjusted life year

QHP—qualified health plan

SBE-FP—SBEs on the federal platform

SBEs—state-based exchanges

SNAP—Supplemental Nutrition Assistance Program

SNFs—skilled nursing facilities

ABOUT THE CONTRIBUTORS

Melinda K. Abrams, MS, is a senior vice president at the Commonwealth Fund and oversees the Delivery System Reform and International Health Policy programs. She has served on many national committees and boards and was the recipient of the Research Leadership Award from the Primary Care Collaborative and the Champion Award from the Primary Care Development Corporation. Ms. Abrams holds a BA in history from Cornell University and an MS in health policy and management from the Harvard School of Public Health.

Joseph Antos, PhD, is the Wilson H. Taylor Resident Scholar in Health Care and Retirement Policy at the American Enterprise Institute (AEI). He is also an adjunct associate professor of emergency medicine at the George Washington University and vice chair of the Maryland Health Services Cost Review Commission. Prior to AEI, he held senior positions at the Congressional Budget Office, the US Department of Health and Human Services, and other federal agencies.

Joel Ario, MDiv, JD, has 30 years of experience shaping and implementing health policy at the state and federal levels. He has provided strategic consulting and policy analysis to state governments, foundations, health plans, and other stakeholders as a managing director at Manatt Health since 2012. Previously he was the first director of the US Department of Health and Human Services' Office of Health Insurance Exchanges (2010–2011) and also served as insurance commissioner in Pennsylvania (2007–2010) and Oregon (2000–2007). He is a graduate of St. Olaf College, Harvard Divinity School, and Harvard Law School.

Nicholas Bagley, JD, is a law professor at the University of Michigan. From 2007 to 2010 he served as an attorney in the Civil Division at the US Department of Justice. Before that, he was a clerk to Justice John Paul Stevens of the US Supreme Court and Judge David Tatel of the US Court of Appeals for the DC Circuit. He writes extensively about health care and, in particular, the implementation of the Affordable Care Act.

Katherine Baicker, PhD, is a health economist and is dean of the University of Chicago's Harris School of Public Policy. She has served as a member of the President's Council of Economic Advisers from 2005 to 2007, on the Medicare Payment Advisory Commission from 2010 to 2016, as chair of the Massachusetts Group Insurance Commission from 2014 to 2017, and on the CBO Panel of Health Advisors from 2009 to the present. She is one of the leaders of the Oregon Health Insurance Experiment assessing the multifaceted effects of Medicaid expansion.

David Blumenthal, MD, MPP, is president of the Commonwealth Fund. Previously he served as chief health information and innovation officer at Partners Health System in Boston and was Samuel O. Thier Professor of Medicine and Professor of Health Care Policy at Massachusetts General Hospital/Harvard Medical School. From 2009 to 2011 Dr. Blumenthal served as the national coordinator for Health Information Technology under President Barack Obama and was charged with building an interoperable, private, and secure nationwide health information system and supporting the widespread, meaningful use of health IT.

Sylvia Mathews Burwell is the 15th president of American University in Washington, DC. From 2014 to 2017 she served as the 22nd secretary of the US Department of Health and Human Services, and from 2013 to 2014 she served as director of the Office of Management and Budget under President Barack Obama. She has also served as president of the Global Development Program, chief operating officer at the Bill & Melinda Gates Foundation, and president of the Walmart Foundation.

Eric Cantor, JD, is the vice chairman and a managing director at Moelis & Company, an independent, global investment bank. Previously Mr. Cantor served as a US representative from Virginia from 2001 to 2014. He served as House majority leader from 2010 to 2014, during which time he led the public policy agenda for the US House. Mr. Cantor holds a BA from the George Washington University, a JD from the College of William and Mary, and an MA from Columbia University.

James C. Capretta, MA, is a resident fellow at the American Enterprise Institute. As an associate director in the White House Office of Management and Budget from 2001 to 2004, he helped the Bush administration craft and pass the Medicare Modernization Act of 2003. He serves as a senior adviser to the Bipartisan Policy Center and on the Advisory Board of the National Institute for Health Care Management.

Paul Clement, JD, is a partner at Kirkland & Ellis and a distinguished lecturer in law at the Georgetown University Law Center. He served as the 43rd solicitor general of the United States from 2004 to 2008. He has argued over 95 cases before the US Supreme Court, including 4 cases involving the Affordable Care Act. Paul is a graduate of Georgetown University, Cambridge University, the Harvard Law School, and the public schools of Cedarburg, Wisconsin. He clerked for Judge Laurence H. Silberman and for Associate Justice Antonin Scalia.

Jonathan Cohn is senior national correspondent at *HuffPost* and the author of *Sick: The Untold Story of America's Health Care Crisis—and the People Who Pay the Price*. He has also written for such publications as the *Atlantic* and *New York Times* as well as the *New Republic* and *American Prospect*, where he was a senior editor. Jonathan has won awards from the Sidney Hillman Foundation, World Hunger Year, the National Women's Political Caucus, and the Association of Health Care Journalists.

Carrie H. Colla, PhD, is a health economist focusing on provider payment, health insurance markets, and insurance benefit design. Her work is aimed at improving the quality, accessibility, and cost of health care. Dr. Colla's research is dedicated to examining health system performance and the effectiveness of payment and delivery-system reforms, including accountable care organizations. Colla received her undergraduate degree from Dartmouth College and her MA in economics and PhD in health policy from the University of California, Berkeley.

Leemore S. Dafny, PhD, is the Bruce V. Rauner Professor of Business Administration at the Harvard Business School and a member of the faculties of the John F. Kennedy School of Government and the interdisciplinary Program in Health Policy. From 2012 to 2013 Dafny was deputy director for health care and antitrust in the FTC's Bureau of Economics.

Nancy-Ann DeParle, JD, is a partner and cofounder of Consonance Capital Partners, a health care–focused private equity firm, and a director of CVS Health and HCA Healthcare. From 2011 to January 2013 she was assistant to the president and deputy chief of staff for policy in the Obama

White House and counselor to the president and director of the White House Office of Health Reform from 2009 to 2011.

Ezekiel J. Emanuel, MD, PhD, is the vice provost for Global Initiatives, Diane and Robert Levy University Professor, and codirector of the Healthcare Transformation Institute at the University of Pennsylvania. From 2009 to 2011 he was a special assistant in the Office of Management and Budget in the Obama administration. He has written *Reinventing American Health Care* and *Prescription for the Future* and in June 2020 will publish *Which Country Has the World's Best Health Care?* One component of his research focuses on designing and evaluating alternative payment models, especially bundled payment and capitation models.

Rahm Emanuel, MA, was senior advisor to President Bill Clinton from 1993 to 1998. After leaving the White House he became an investment banker with Wasserstein Perella and served on the board of Freddie Mac. In 2003 he became congressman from Chicago's 5th District, serving in the US House of Representatives until 2009. He served as President Obama's chief of staff from January 2009 to October 2010. From 2011 to 2019 he served as mayor of Chicago. He is author of *The Nation City: Why Mayors Are Now Running the World.*

Abbe R. Gluck, JD, is professor of law and founding faculty director of the Solomon Center for Health Law and Policy at Yale Law School and professor of internal medicine at Yale Medical School. She has written extensively on the political and legal challenges to the ACA and coauthored US Supreme Court briefs in both major cases. She is a former law clerk to US Supreme Court Justice Ruth Bader Ginsburg and currently chairs the Uniform Law Commission's Health Care Committee and is an elected member of the leadership body of the American Law Institute.

Jacob S. Hacker, PhD, is Stanley Resor Professor of Political Science and director of the Institution for Social and Policy Studies at Yale University. A regular policy advisor and expert commentator, he is the author or coauthor of 5 books, numerous journal articles, and a wide range of popular writings on American politics and public policy. His recent honors include a fellowship at the Radcliffe Institute for Advanced Study and induction into the American Academy of Arts and Sciences.

Nicole Huberfeld, JD, is professor of health law, ethics, and human rights as well as professor of law at Boston University. Her scholarship explores health law and constitutional law, often addressing health reform (especially Medicaid), federalism, and the spending power. She is author of 2 health law casebooks and many book chapters and articles, including "What Is Federalism in Healthcare For?" (*Stanford Law Review*, 2018, with Abbe R. Gluck) and "Federalizing Medicaid," cited in the first Supreme Court decision on the ACA.

Timothy Stoltzfus Jost, JD, is an emeritus professor at the Washington and Lee University School of Law. He is a coauthor of a casebook, *Health Law*, used widely throughout the United States and now in its 8th edition. He has written numerous monographs on legal issues in health care reform for national organizations and until 2018 blogged regularly for *Health Affairs*, where he is a contributing editor. He is a member of the National Academy of Medicine.

Corinne Lewis, MSW, is the senior research associate at the Commonwealth Fund's Delivery System Reform Program. Before joining the Fund, she held research positions at Mathematica Policy Research, Inc. and the Laboratory for Youth Mental Health at Harvard University. Ms. Lewis holds a BA in psychology from Boston University and an MS in social policy from Columbia University's School of Social Work.

John E. McDonough, DrPH, MPA, is a professor of practice at the Harvard TH Chan School of Public Health. Between 2008 and 2010 he served as a senior advisor on National Health Reform to the US Senate HELP Committee, where he worked on passage of the ACA. Between 2003 and 2008 he was executive director of Health Care for All, Massachusetts's consumer advocacy organization, where he played a leading role in the passage of the 2006 Massachusetts health reform law. From 1985 to 1997 he was a member of the Massachusetts House of Representatives, where he cochaired the Joint Committee on Health Care.

Amol S. Navathe, MD, PhD, is a physician and health economist at the University of Pennsylvania. He is a leading scholar on payment-model design and evaluation and serves on the Medicare Payment Advisory Commission. His scholarship is unique because of its bidirectional translation between basic scientific discovery and real-world practice. He is founding coeditor-in-chief of *Health Care: The Journal of Delivery Science and Innovation*, and from 2009 to 2011 he led the nation's Comparative Effectiveness Research strategy in the Obama administration.

Peter R. Orszag, PhD, is CEO of Financial Advisory at Lazard Freres & Co. LLC, leading the firm's advisory businesses that serve companies and governments across the globe. In the Obama administration he served as the director of the Office of Management and Budget from 2009 to 2010 and before that as the director of the Congressional Budget Office from 2007 to 2008. He graduated summa cum laude in economics from Princeton University and obtained a PhD in economics from the London School of Economics, which he attended as a Marshall Scholar. Dr. Orszag is married to Bianna Golodryga of CNN.

Steven D. Pearson, MD, MSc, is the founder and president of the Institute for Clinical and Economic Review (ICER). Dr. Pearson is also a lecturer in the Department of Population Medicine at Harvard Medical School. Previously he has served as a visiting scientist in the Department of Bioethics at the NIH, and special advisor on Technology and Coverage Policy at the Center for Medicare and Medicaid Services. His publications include the book *No Margin, No Mission: Health Care Organizations and the Quest for Ethical Excellence*.

Rahul Rekhi, MSc, is a vice president in financial advisory at Lazard Freres & Co. LLC. Prior to that, he was a staff economist on the Council of Economic Advisers in the Obama White House from 2015 to 2017. Rahul attended Oxford and the London School of Economics as a Marshall Scholar and was previously named a Truman Scholar, a World Economic Forum Global Shaper, and a member of the Forbes "30 under 30." His writings have appeared in the *Guardian*, the *Los Angeles Times*, and *Health Affairs*, among others.

Sara Rosenbaum, JD, is Harold and Jane Hirsh Professor of Health Law and Policy and founding chair of the Department of Health Policy at George Washington University's Milken Institute School of Public Health. She has devoted her career to health justice for medically underserved populations. A member of the National Academies of Sciences,

Engineering, and Medicine, Professor Rosenbaum has worked with successive presidential administrations and Congresses. She served as an original commissioner on Congress's Medicaid and CHIP Payment and Access Commission (MACPAC) and chaired MACPAC from January 2016 through April 2017. She worked on the ACA with both the Obama administration and Congress.

Rachel E. Sachs, JD, MPH is an associate professor of law at Washington University in St. Louis. Her research explores the interaction of intellectual property law, food and drug regulation, and health law. Her scholarship has appeared in journals, including the *Harvard Law Review*, the *Michigan Law Review*, the *New England Journal of Medicine*, and the *Journal of the American Medical Association*. Sachs was previously an academic fellow at the Petrie-Flom Center for Health Law Policy, Biotechnology, and Bioethics and a lecturer in law at Harvard Law School.

Kathleen Sebelius, MPA, has been engaged in health policy for decades in the public and private sectors. She served in President Obama's cabinet as the 21st secretary of the US Department of Health and Human Services from 2009 to 2014 and was elected statewide 4 times in Kansas as governor (2003–2009) and insurance commissioner (1995–2003). Sebelius is the CEO of Sebelius Resources LLC. She serves as a director for Dermira, Devoted Health, Exact Sciences, Myovant Sciences, and several private health-sector interests. She coleads the Health Strategy Group for the Aspen Institute.

Shanoor Seervai, MPP, is a senior research associate and communications associate at the Commonwealth Fund. Ms. Seervai holds a BA in international relations from Brown University and a master's in public policy from the Harvard Kennedy School. Before joining the Fund, she worked as a reporter for the *Wall Street Journal's* South Asia Bureau.

Jonathan Skinner, PhD, is the James O. Freedman Presidential Professor in Economics at Dartmouth College and a professor at the Geisel School of Medicine's Institute for Health Policy and Clinical Practice. Skinner's research interests include the economics of government transfer programs, technology growth and disparities in health care, and the savings behavior of aging baby boomers. He is currently director of the Aging Program at the National Bureau of Economic Research (NBER) and a member of the National Academy of Medicine. Skinner received a PhD in economics from UCLA and a BA in economics and political science from the University of Rochester.

Benjamin D. Sommers, MD, PhD, is a professor of health policy and economics at the Harvard School of Public Health and associate professor of medicine at Harvard Medical School. He is a health economist and primary care physician whose main research interests are health policy for vulnerable populations and the health care safety net. From 2011 to 2012 he served as a senior adviser in the US Department of Health and Human Services. His research has received numerous awards, and he was elected to the National Academy of Medicine in 2019.

Donald B. Verrilli, Jr., JD, is a partner in the law firm of Munger, Tolles & Olson and founded the firm's Washington, DC, office. Before joining the firm, he served as solicitor general of the United States from 2011 to 2016. As solicitor general, Verrilli successfully defended the Affordable Care Act in 2 landmark cases, *National Federation of Independent Businesses v. Sebelius* and *King v. Burwell*. He also represented the United States before the Supreme Court in many other cases, including *Obergefell v. Hodges* (marriage equality) and *United States v. Arizona* (immigration).

NOTES

Preface

1. Heidi L. Allen et al., "Can Medicaid Expansion Prevent Housing Evictions?" *Health Affairs* 38, no. 9 (2019): 1451–1457, https://doi.org/10.1377/hlthaff.2018.05071.

2. Sara R. Collins et al., "How the Affordable Care Act Has Improved Americans' Ability to Buy Health Insurance on Their Own: Findings from the Commonwealth Fund Biennial Health Insurance Survey, 2016," Commonwealth Fund, February 2017, 1–16, https://www.commonwealthfund.org/sites/default/files/documents/___media_files_publications_issue_brief_2017_feb_1931_collins_biennial_survey_2016_ib.pdf.

3. Larisa Antonisse et al., "The Effects of Medicaid Expansion Under the ACA: Updated Findings from a Literature Review," Medicaid, Kaiser Family Foundation, August 15, 2019, https://www.kff.org/medicaid/issue-brief/the-effects-of-medicaid-expansion-under-the-aca-updated-findings-from-a-literature-review-march-2018/; and Sarah Miller et al., "Medicaid and Mortality: New Evidence from Linked Survey and Administrative Data," NBER Working Paper No. 26081, National Bureau of Economic Research, Cambridge, MA, August 2019, https://doi.org/10.3386/w26081.

4. Kenneth Brevoort, Daniel Grodzicki, and Martin B. Hackman, "Medicaid and Financial Health," NBER Working Paper No. 24002, National Bureau of Economic Research, Cambridge, MA, November 2017, https://doi.org/10.3386/w24002.pdf.

5. Ryan M. McKenna et al., "The Affordable Care Act Attenuates Financial Strain According to Poverty Level," *INQUIRY: A Journal of Medical Care Organization, Provision and Financing* 55 (2018): 1–14, https://doi.org/10.1177/0046958018790164.

6. "Reforming the Health Care System," in *Economic Report of the President* (Washington, DC: 2017), 195–298, https://obamawhitehouse.archives.gov/sites/default/files/docs/chapter_4-reforming_health_care_system_2017.pdf.

7. Wikipedia, s.v. "Ronald Reagan Speaks Out Against Socialized Medicine," last modified June 28, 2019, https://en.wikipedia.org/wiki/Ronald_Reagan_Speaks_Out_Against_Socialized_Medicine.

8. "The Reagan Presidency," https://web.archive.org/web/20080517013218/http://www.reagan.utexas.edu/archives/reference/presssketch.html.

9. Sarah Kliff, "Under Trump, the Number of Uninsured Americans Has Gone Up by 7 Million," *Vox*, January 23, 2019, https://www.vox.com/2019/1/23/18194228/trump-uninsured-rate-obamacare-medicaid.

10. "KFF Health Tracking Poll: The Public's Views on the ACA," Health Reform, Kaiser Family Foundation, last modified October 15, 2019, https://www.kff.org/interactive/kff-health-tracking-poll-the-publics-views-on-the-aca/#?response=Favorable--Unfavorable&aRange=twoYear.

11. MaryBeth Musumeci, "Explaining Texas v. U.S.: A Guide to the 5th Circuit Appeal in the Case Challenging the ACA," Health Reform, Kaiser Family Foundation, July 3, 2019, https://www.kff.org/health-reform/issue-brief/explaining-texas-v-u-s-a-guide-to-the-5th-circuit-appeal-in-the-case-challenging-the-aca/.

Introduction

1. On March 30 President Obama signed a second bill, the Health Care and Education Reconciliation Act of 2010, which made a few important changes to the ACA, including raising the amount of the insurance subsidies, improving Medicare's pharmaceutical benefit, and delaying the implementation on taxing high-cost, so-called Cadillac health-care plans until 2018.

Chapter 1. The Path to the Affordable Care Act

1. Max Baucus, "Call to Action: Health Reform 2009," US Senate Committee on Finance, Washington, DC, November 2008, https://www.finance.senate.gov/imo/media/doc/finalwhitepaper1.pdf.

2. Whitney Blair Wyckoff, "Number of Americans with Health Insurance Fell in 2009," NPR, September 16, 2010, https://www.npr.org/sections/health-shots/2010/09/16/129908672/number-of-insured-americans-dropped-in-2009.

3. Max Fisher, "Here's a Map of the Countries that Provide Universal Health Care (America's Still Not on It)," *The Atlantic*, June 28, 2012, https://www.theatlantic.com/international/archive/2012/06/heres-a-map-of-the-countries-that-provide-universal-health-care-americas-still-not-on-it/259153/.

4. "Coverage at Work: The Share of Nonelderly Americans with Employer-Based Insurance Rose Modestly in Recent Years, but Has Declined Markedly over the Long Term," Kaiser Family Foundation, last modified February 1, 2019, https://www.kff.org/health-reform/press-release/coverage-at-work-the-share-of-nonelderly-americans-with-employer-based-insurance-rose-modestly-in-recent-years-but-has-declined-markedly-over-the-long-term/.

5. Elisa Gould, "A Decade of Decline in Employer-Sponsored Health Insurance Coverage," Economic Policy Institute, February 23, 2012, https://www.epi.org/publication/bp337-employer-sponsored-health-insurance/.

6. Len Burman, Surachai Khitatrakun, and Sarah Goodell, "Tax Subsidies for Private Health Insurance: Who Benefits and at What Cost?," The Synthesis Project, The Robert Wood Johnson Foundation, Princeton, NJ, July 2009, https://www.taxpolicycenter.org/sites/default/files/alfresco/publication-pdfs/1001297-Tax-subsidies-for-private-health-insurance-Who-benefits-and-at-what-cost-.pdf.

7. "Health at a Glance 2011—OECD Indicators," Organization of Economic Cooperation and Development, November 23, 2011, https://www.oecd.org/els/health-systems/49084488.pdf.

8. Rabah Kamal and Cynthia Cox, "How Has U.S. Spending on Healthcare Changed over Time?," Peterson-Kaiser Health System Tracker, December 10, 2018, https://www.healthsystemtracker.org/chart-collection/u-s-spending-healthcare-changed-time/#item-start.

9. "National Health Expenditures 2010: Sponsor Highlights," Centers for Medicare and Medicaid Services, 2011, https://www.cms.gov/Research-Statistics-Data-and-Systems/Statistics-Trends-and-Reports/NationalHealthExpendData/downloads/sponsors.pdf.

10. Michelle Long et al., "Trends in Employer-Sponsored Insurance Offer and Coverage Rates, 1999–2014," Kaiser Family Foundation, March 21, 2016, https://www.kff.org/private-insurance/issue-brief/trends-in-employer-sponsored-insurance-offer-and-coverage-rates-1999-2014/.

11. Glenn A. Melnick and Katya Fonkych, "Hospital Pricing and the Uninsured: Do the Uninsured Pay Higher Prices?" *Health Affairs* 27, Supplement 1 (2008): w116–122, https://doi.org/10.1377/hlthaff.27.2.w116.

12. Committee on the Quality of Health Care in America, *Crossing the Quality Chasm: A New Health System for the 21st Century* (Washington, DC: National Academy Press, 2001), 1.

13. Nicole Carafella Lallemand, "Reducing Waste in Health Care," Brief, Health Affairs, December 13, 2012, https://www.healthaffairs.org/do/10.1377/hpb20121213.959735/full/.

14. Perry Beider and Stuart Hagen, "Limiting Tort Liability for Medical Malpractice," CBO Economic and Budget Issue Brief, Washington, DC, January 2004, https://www.cbo.gov/sites/default/files/108th-congress-2003-2004/reports/01-08-medicalmalpractice.pdf, 4.

15. See, for example, Stuart Altman and David Shactman, *Power, Politics and Universal Health Care: The Inside Story of a Century-Long Battle* (Amherst, NY: Prometheus Books, 2011), and John E. McDonough, *Inside National Health Reform* (Berkeley: University of California Press; New York: Milbank Memorial Fund, 2011), Chapters 1–4.

16. "Rep. Wilson Shouts, 'You Lie' to Obama During Speech," Politics, CNN, last modified September 10, 2009, https://www.cnn.com/2009/POLITICS/09/09/joe.wilson/.

17. Douglas W. Elmendorf, Director of the US Congressional Budget Office to Speaker Nancy Pelosi, Washington, DC, March 20, 2010, https://www.cbo.gov/sites/default/files/111th-congress-2009-2010/costestimate/amendreconprop.pdf. In fact, the Affordable Care Act was projected to lower the national deficit by $124 billion over 10 years.

18. Title IX of the Affordable Care Act raises taxes on high-income households, insurance companies, medical device makers, pharmaceutical companies, and more. Patient Protection and Affordable Care Act, 42 U.S.C. § 9001–23.

19. Maximum-rate ratios control discrepancies in price contributions between distinct groups in the risk pool. For example, older persons can pay a maximum of 3 times the price young people are asked to pay. Pre-ACA, no control on pricing existed, and cost discrepancies varied widely.

20. National Federation of Independent Business v. Sebelius, 567 U.S. 519 (2012).

21. See C. Stephen Redhead et al., "Discretionary Spending Under the Affordable Care Act (ACA)," prepared by the Congressional Research Service (Washington, DC, February 2017), https://fas.org/sgp/crs/misc/R41390.pdf; see also C. Stephen Redhead, "Appropriations and Fund Transfers in the Affordable Care Act (ACA)," prepared by the Congressional Research Service (Washington, DC, February 2017), https://fas.org/sgp/crs/misc/R41301.pdf.

22. "Open Payments," Centers for Medicare and Medicaid Services, last modified June 28, 2019, https://www.cms.gov/openpayments/.

23. Elmendorf to Pelosi, Washington, DC, March 20, 2010.

24. Sara R. Collins et al., "The Comprehensive Congressional Health Reform Bills of 2009: A Look at Health Insurance, Delivery System, and Financing Provisions," Commonwealth Fund, last modified January 7, 2010, https://affordablecareactlitigation.files.wordpress.com/2018/09/1333_collins_comprehensive_congressional_hlt_reform_bills_2009_revised_172010_v2.pdf.

25. Discussed in Abbe R. Gluck and Nicole Huberfeld's article in this same volume.

26. Joanne Spetz et al., "Scope-of-Practice Laws for Nurse Practitioners Limit Cost Savings That Can Be Achieved in Retail Clinics," *Health Affairs* 32, no. 11 (November 2013): 1977–1984, https://doi.org/10.1377/hlthaff.2013.0544.

Chapter 2. Policy Design: Tensions and Tradeoffs

1. Office of Management and Budget, *A New Era of Responsibility: Renewing America's Promise* (Washington, DC: US Government Printing Office,

2009), 27. All further quotations in this paragraph are from this document, which can be consulted at https://www.govinfo.gov/content/pkg/BUDGET -2010-BUD/pdf/BUDGET-2010-BUD.pdf.

2. Carmen DeNavas-Walt, Bernadette D. Proctor, and Jessica C. Smith, "Income, Poverty, and Health Insurance Coverage in the United States: 2008," Census Bureau, Washington, DC, September 2009, https://www.census.gov /prod/2009pubs/p60-236.pdf, and Peter R. Orszag, "Counting the Un- insured: 46 Million or 'More than 30 Million'?," blog, Office of Manage- ment and Budget, last modified September 10, 2009, https://web.archive.org /web/20100305220333/https://www.whitehouse.gov/omb/blog/09/09/10 /CountingtheUninsured46MillionorMorethan30Million/.

3. These include premiums linked to health status that priced many Amer- icans out of coverage, preexisting conditions exclusions and other forms of coverage denial (e.g., retroactive cancellations of coverage), and unstandard- ized plans that were difficult for consumers to understand and compare.

4. Lydia Saad, "Americans Rate National and Personal Healthcare Dif- ferently," Gallup, last modified December 4, 2008, https://news.gallup.com /poll/112813/americans-rate-national-personal-healthcare-differently.aspx, and "Covering the Uninsured: Options for Reform," Kaiser Family Foundation, September 16, 2008, https://www.kff.org/health-reform/issue-brief/covering -the-uninsured-options-for-reform/.

5. This estimate includes those directly employed by health and medical insurance carriers as well as estimates of employment in insurance agencies, brokerages, and related services. It does not include employment within pro- vider organizations or other entities linked to private insurance administra- tion (e.g., revenue cycle).

6. There is some evidence that the impact of the health insurance–wage offset could differ across types of workers (e.g., part-time vs. full-time work- ers), Katherine Baicker and Amitabh Chandra, "The Labor Market Effects of Rising Health Insurance Premiums," *Journal of Labor Economics* 24, no. 3 (2006): 609–634, https://doi.org/10.1086/505049) and older vs. younger workers (Mark V. Pauly and Bradley Herring, *Pooling Health Insurance Risks* [Washington, DC: AEI Press, 1999]).

7. Both the ACA and the Massachusetts health reform efforts also con- tained a range of additional coverage reform provisions, such as the individual and employer mandates and the extension of dependent coverage eligibility through the age of 26. Ian Duncan and Ryung Suh, "Massachusetts Health Insurance Reform: Impact on Insurance Markets, Pricing, and Profitability," Society of Actuaries, August 2016, https://www.soa.org/globalassets/assets /Files/Research/Projects/research-2016-ma-health-insurance-reform.pdf.

8. Jacob Wallace and Zirui Song, "Traditional Medicare versus Private In- surance: How Spending, Volume, and Price Change at Age Sixty-Five," *Health Affairs* 35, no. 5 (2016), 864–872, https://doi.org/10.1377/hlthaff.2015.1195,

and Daria Pelech, "An Analysis of Private-Sector Prices for Physicians' Services," working paper, Congressional Budget Office, Washington, DC, January 2018, https://www.cbo.gov/publication/53441.

9. Laura Wheaton, Victoria Lynch, and Martha C. Johnson, "The Overlap in SNAP and Medicaid/CHIP Eligibility, 20013," Urban Institute, January 9, 2017, https://www.urban.org/research/publication/overlap-snap-and-medicaidchip-eligibility-2013.

10. For example, Medicaid coverage of behavioral health services, rehabilitative services, and personal care services is usually more comprehensive than the coverage that has been offered by exchange plans (Ken Cannon, Jenna Burton, and MaryBeth Musumeci, "Adult Behavioral Health Benefits in Medicaid and the Marketplace," Medicaid, Kaiser Family Foundation, June 11, 2015, https://www.kff.org/medicaid/report/adult-behavioral-health-benefits-in-medicaid-and-the-marketplace/).

11. Benjamin D. Sommers et al., "Reasons for the Wide Variation in Medicaid Participation Rates Among States Hold Lessons for Coverage Expansion in 2014," *Health Affairs* 31, no. 5 (2012): 909–919, https://doi.org/10.1377/hlthaff.2011.0977; Arik Levinson and Sjamsu Rahardja, "Medicaid Stigma," working paper, Department of Economics, Georgetown University, Washington, DC, April 2004, http://units.georgetown.edu/economics/pdf/406.pdf; and Jennifer P. Stuber et al., "Beyond Stigma: What Barriers Actually Affect the Decisions of Low-Income Families to Enroll in Medicaid?," Health Policy and Management Issue Briefs, Himmelfarb Health Sciences Library, George Washington University, Washington, DC, July 2000, https://hsrc.himmelfarb.gwu.edu/cgi/viewcontent.cgi?article=1052&context=sphhs_policy_briefs.

12. By contrast, covering the uninsured (for whom health care often went uncompensated) with public insurance would provide a net financial benefit for care providers.

13. 567 U.S. 519 (2012).

14. Matthew Buettgens, "The Implications of Medicaid Expansion in the Remaining States: 2018 Update," Research, Urban Institute, May 17, 2018, https://www.urban.org/research/publication/implications-medicaid-expansion-remaining-states-2018-update.

15. Whereas eligibility for exchange subsidies in Medicaid expansion states begins at a household income of 138% of the FPL, in nonexpansion states this threshold falls to 100%. In effect, the exchanges provided a vehicle for partially inoculating beneficiaries from unforeseen state decisions to forgo Medicaid expansion.

16. Based on subsidized nongroup enrollment data for households earning up to 400% of the FPL in nonexpansion states per Buettgens, "The Implications of Medicaid Expansion."

17. See Chapters 4 and 5 in this volume.

18. Daniel W. Sacks et al., "How Do Insurance Firms Respond to Financial Risk Sharing Regulations? Evidence from the Affordable Care Act," NBER Working Paper No. 24129, National Bureau of Economic Research, Cambridge, MA, December 2017, https://doi.org/10.3386/w24129.

19. In part because of the resultant actuarial volatility (and due to higher-than-expected offer rates of ESI), exchange enrollment has lagged behind initial projections, particularly among those receiving few or no subsidies; insurer participation in the exchanges is lower than in the early years of ACA implementation (Rachel Fehr, Cynthia Cox, and Larry Levitt, "Individual Insurance Market Performance in Early 2019," Private Insurance, Kaiser Family Foundation, June 27, 2019, https://www.kff.org/private-insurance/issue-brief/individual-insurance-market-performance-in-early-2019/), and premium growth in the exchanges since 2017 has outpaced earlier projections that did not incorporate the effects of these shocks.

20. Aditi P. Sen and Thomas Deleire, "The Effect of Medicaid Expansion on Marketplace Premiums," Office of the Assistant Secretary for Planning and Evaluation, US Department of Health and Human Services, August 2016, https://aspe.hhs.gov/pdf-report/effect-medicaid-expansion-marketplace-premiums.

21. Anita Cardwell, "Revisiting Churn: An Early Understanding of State-Level Health Coverage Transitions under the ACA," National Academy for State Health Policy, last modified August 8, 2016, https://nashp.org/revisiting-churn-an-early-understanding-of-state-level-health-coverage-transitions-under-the-aca/, and Benjamin D. Sommers et al., "Insurance Churning Rates for Low-Income Adults Under Health Reform: Lower Than Expected but Still Harmful for Many," *Health Affairs* 35, no. 10 (2016): 1816–1824, https://doi.org/10.1377/hlthaff.2016.0455.

22. This in addition to a number of narrower dimensions (e.g., increasing exchange plan standardization). This figure does not include undocumented immigrants.

23. Matthew Fiedler et al., "Building on the ACA to Achieve Universal Coverage," *New England Journal of Medicine* 380, no. 18 (2019): 1685–1688, https://doi.org/10.1056/NEJMp1901532.

24. Aviva Aron-Dine, "Data: Silver Loading Is Boosting Insurance Coverage," *Health Affairs Blog*, September 17, 2019, https://www.healthaffairs.org/do/10.1377/hblog20190913.296052/full/.

25. Amy Finkelstein, Nathaniel Hendren, and Mark Shepard, "Subsidizing Health Insurance for Low-Income Adults: Evidence from Massachusetts," *American Economic Review* 109, no. 4 (2019): 1530–1567, https://doi.org/10.1257/aer.20171455.

26. Though reinsurance partially offsets overall subsidy levels due to the ACA's premium-linked tax credit structure, on balance it makes coverage more

affordable for the unsubsidized and the comparatively undersubsidized. Chris Sloan, Neil Rosacker, and Elizabeth Carpenter, "State-Run Reinsurance Programs Reduce ACA Premiums by 19.9% on Average," Press Releases, Avalere, March 13, 2019, https://avalere.com/press-releases/state-run-reinsurance -programs-reduce-aca-premiums-by-19-9-on-average.

27. Alan J. Auerbach, William G. Gale, and Aaron Krupkin, "If Not Now, When? New Estimates of the Federal Budget Outlook," Brookings, February 11, 2019, https://www.brookings.edu/research/if-not-now-when-new -estimates-of-the-federal-budget-outlook/.

28. Rachel Fehr, Cynthia Cox, and Larry Levitt, "Insurance Participation on ACA Marketplaces, 2014–2019," Health Reform, Kaiser Family Foundation, November 14, 2018, https://www.kff.org/health-reform/issue-brief /insurer-participation-on-aca-marketplaces-2014-2019.

29. To illustrate, in 2018 Medicaid carriers participated in the nongroup exchanges in about 1 in 4 counties nationwide and, in competitive markets, sold the lowest-cost silver plan about 70% of the time; Katherine Hempstead and Joanna Seirup, "Medicaid MCOs in the Individual Market: Past, Present . . . and Future?," *Health Affairs Blog*, August 30, 2018, https://www.health affairs.org/do/10.1377/hblog20180823.490433/full/. In effect, these coverage options resemble conventional public option proposals but, all else equal, with lower premiums, more active care management, and narrower networks.

30. John E. Wennberg et al., "Improving Quality and Curbing Health Care Spending: Opportunities for the Congress and the Obama Administration," The Dartmouth Institute for Health Policy and Clinical Practice Center for Health Policy Research, Dartmouth Medical School, Lebanon, NH, 2008, http://archive.dartmouthatlas.org/downloads/reports/agenda_for_change.pdf.

31. Based on National Health Expenditures data. By comparison, net costs of private health insurance, consisting of insurance-side administrative costs and profit, represents less than 7% of overall spending.

32. Based on CBO projections at the time, this rapid cost growth in health care would ultimately provide a drag on both the federal budget (via increased expenditures on Medicare and Medicaid and reduced tax revenues) and the economy as a whole—for instance, with Medicare spending net of premiums expected to rise from 5% of GDP in 2009 to over twice that by 2040.

33. Amy N. Finkelstein et al., "Effect of Medicaid Coverage on ED Use—Further Evidence from Oregon's Experiment," *New England Journal of Medicine* 375, no. 16 (2016): 1505–1507, https://academic.oup.com/qje/article-abstract/131/4/1681/2468872?redirectedFrom=fulltext.

34. William Patrick Luan et al., "Using Compulsory Relocation to Understand Drivers of Geographic Variation in the U.S. Military," paper presented at the 2018 Academy Health Annual Research Meeting, Seattle, WA, June 2018, https://academyhealth.confex.com/academyhealth/2018arm/mediafile /Handout/Paper22234/AcademyHealth_poster_luan_variations.pdf.

35. Keith D. Moore and Dean C. Coddington, "The Work Ahead: Activities and Costs to Develop an Accountable Care Organization," American Hospital Association, Washington, DC, April 2011, https://www.aha.org/system /files/content/11/aco-white-paper-cost-dev-aco.pdf.

36. Excludes spending associated with Veterans Affairs facilities.

37. See, for example, Jeffrey Clemens and Joshua D. Gottlieb, "In the Shadow of a Giant: Medicare's Influence on Private Physician Payments," *Journal of Political Economy* 125, no. 1 (2017): 1–39, https://doi.org/10.1086/689772.

38. To illustrate, broad bipartisan consensus around the imperative of delivery-system reform in the wake of the ACA led to significant incentives for payment-model uptake by providers via the enactment of MACRA in 2015.

39. "Measuring Progress: Adoption of Alternative Payment Models in Commercial, Medicaid, Medicare Advantage, and Fee-for-Service Medicare Programs," Health Care Payment Learning and Action Network, October 2018, https://hcp-lan.org/2018-apm-measurement/.

40. David M. Cutler et al., "Explaining the Slowdown in Medical Spending Growth Among the Elderly, 1999–2012," *Health Affairs* 38, no. 2 (2019): 222–229, https://doi.org/10.1377/hlthaff.2018.05372.

41. Joseph P. Newhouse et al., *Variation in Health Care Spending: Target Decision Making, Not Geography* (Washington, DC: The National Academies Press, 2013).

42. Michael L. Barnett et al., "Two-Year Evaluation of Mandatory Bundled Payments for Joint Replacement," *New England Journal of Medicine* 380, no. 3 (2018): 252–262, https://doi.org/10.1056/NEJMsa1809010.

43. Bill Frack, Andrew Garibaldi, and Andrew Kadar, "Why Medicare Advantage Is Marching Toward 70% Penetration of U.S. Healthcare Market," *L.E.K. Consulting's Executive Insights* 19, no. 69 (2017), https://www.lek.com /sites/default/files/insights/pdf-attachments/1969_Medicare_AdvantageLEK _Executive_Insights_1.pdf.

44. Peter J. Huckfeldt et al., "Less Intense Postacute Care, Better Outcomes for Enrollees in Medicare Advantage Than Those in Fee-for-Service," *Health Affairs* 36, no. 1 (2017): 91–100, https://doi.org/10.1377/hlthaff.2016.1027.

45. Peter R. Orszag and Rahul Rekhi, "The Economic Case for Vertical Integration in Health Care," *NEJM Catalyst: Innovations in Care Delivery* (forthcoming).

46. Karen Stockley, "How Do Changes in Medical Malpractice Liability Laws Affect Health Care Spending and the Federal Budget?," Working Paper Series 2019.03, Congressional Budget Office, Washington, DC, April 2019, https:// www.cbo.gov/system/files/2019-04/55104-Medical%20Malpractice_WP.pdf.

47. Michael Frakes and Anupam B. Jena, "Does Medical Malpractice Law Improve Health Care Quality?," *Journal of Public Economics* 143 (2016): 142–158, https://doi.org/10.1016/j.jpubeco.2016.09.002. Such safe harbors likely require implementation at the state level.

48. Gerard F. Anderson et al., "It's the Prices, Stupid: Why the United States Is So Different from Other Countries," *Health Affairs* 22, no. 3 (2003): 89–105, https://doi.org/10.1377/hlthaff.22.3.89.

49. Zack Cooper et al., "The Price Ain't Right? Hospital Prices and Health Spending on the Privately Insured," *Quarterly Journal of Economics* 134, no. 1 (2019): 51–107, https://doi.org/10.1093/qje/qjy020.

50. Irene Papanicolas, Liana R. Woskie, and Ashish K. Jha, "Health Care Spending in the United States and Other High-Income Countries," *JAMA* 319, no. 10 (2018): 1024–1039, https://doi.org/10.1001/jama.2018.1150.

51. Cooper et al., "The Price Ain't Right?"

Chapter 3. The Road Not Taken

1. James C. Robinson, Timothy T. Brown, and Christopher Whaley, "Reference Pricing Changes the 'Choice Architecture' of Health Care for Consumers," *Health Affairs* 36, no. 3 (2017): 524–530, https://doi.org/10.1377/hlthaff.2016.1256.

2. Lisa Clemans-Pope and Nathaniel Anderson, "How Many Non-Group Policies Were Canceled? Estimates from December 2013," *Health Affairs Blog*, March 3, 2014, https://www.healthaffairs.org/do/10.1377/hblog20140303.037517/full/.

3. The 2019 FPL is $12,490 for an individual, with $4,420 added for each additional family member. See "HHS Poverty Guidelines for 2019," Office of the Assistant Secretary for Planning and Evaluation, US Department of Health and Human Services, last modified January 11, 2019, https://aspe.hhs.gov/poverty-guidelines.

4. 567 U.S. 519 (2012).

5. Discussed in Chapter 10 of this volume.

6. See Chapter 14 of this volume.

7. Robert Mechanic and Clifton Gaus, "Medicare Shared Savings Program Produces Substantial Savings: New Policies Should Promote ACO Growth," *Health Affairs Blog*, September 11, 2018, https://www.healthaffairs.org/do/10.1377/hblog20180906.711463/full/.

8. Government Accountability Office, "CMS Innovation Center: Model Implementation and Center Performance," March 2018, https://www.gao.gov/assets/700/690875.pdf.

9. Douglas W. Elmendorf, Director of the Congressional Budget Office, to Speaker Nancy Pelosi, March 20, 2010, "Estimates of Spending and Revenue Effects of H.R. 4872, Reconciliation Act of 2010 (Final Health Care Legislation)," https://www.cbo.gov/publication/21351.

10. This paragraph is excerpted from Joseph R. Antos et al., "Improving Health and Health Care: An Agenda for Reform," *Health Affairs Blog*, Decem-

ber 9, 2015, https://www.healthaffairs.org/do/10.1377/hblog20151209.052181
/full/.

11. For a detailed description of a reform plan consistent with this perspective, see Joseph Antos et al., "Improving Health and Health Care: An Agenda for
Reform," American Enterprise Institute, December 2015, https://www.aei.org
/wp-content/uploads/2015/12/Improving-Health-and-Health-Care-online.pdf.

12. Rachael Bade, Josh Dawsey, and Jennifer Haberkorn, "How a Secret
Freedom Caucus Pact Brought Down Obamacare Repeal," *Politico*, March
26, 2017, https://www.politico.com/story/2017/03/trump-freedom-caucus
-obamacare-repeal-replace-secret-pact-236507.

13. Timothy Jost, "House Passes AHCA: How It Happened, What It
Would Do, and Its Uncertain Senate Future," *Health Affairs Blog*, May 4,
2017, https://www.healthaffairs.org/do/10.1377/hblog20170504.059967/full/,
and "Summary of the American Health Care Act," Kaiser Family Foundation, May 2017, http://files.kff.org/attachment/Proposals-to-Replace-the
-Affordable-Care-Act-Summary-of-the-American-Health-Care-Act.

14. "Cost Estimate: H.R. 1628, American Health Care Act of 2017," Congressional Budget Office, Washington, DC, May 24, 2017, https://www.cbo
.gov/publication/52752.

15. Ibid.

16. Vernon K. Smith, "Can States Survive the Per Capita Medicaid Caps
in the AHCA?," *Health Affairs Blog*, May 17, 2017, https://www.healthaffairs
.org/do/10.1377/hblog20170517.060155/full/.

17. Timothy Jost, "Republican ACA Replacement Effort Collapses; States
Defend *House v. Price* Intervention Request," *Health Affairs Blog*, July 18,
2017, https://www.healthaffairs.org/do/10.1377/hblog20170718.061095/full/.

18. Erin Kelly and Eliza Collins, "Where We Are Now on the Senate Health
Care Bill: Clean Repeal Dead as GOP Plods Through Debate," *USA Today*,
July 26, 2017, https://www.usatoday.com/story/news/politics/2017/07/26
/senate-health-care-bill-whats-happening-now/511889001/.

19. "Compare Proposals to Replace the Affordable Care Act," Health Reform, Kaiser Family Foundation, undated, https://www.kff.org/interactive
/proposals-to-replace-the-affordable-care-act/.

20. Timothy Jost, "ACA Round-Up: A Double-Threat Presidential Tweet,
Cassidy-Graham-Heller, Bipartisan Market Stabilization Ideas, and Good
News from Ohio," *Health Affairs Blog*, July 31, 2017, https://www.health
affairs.org/do/10.1377/hblog20170801.061345/full/.

21. Gabrielle Levy, "GOP Leaders Signal Graham-Cassidy Support,"
U.S. News and World Report, September 19, 2017, https://www.usnews.com
/news/politics/articles/2017-09-19/gop-leaders-signal-graham-cassidy-support
-as-negotiations-to-stabilize-obamacare-stall.

22. "Public Opinion on Single-Payer, National Health Plans, and Expanding Access to Medicare Coverage," Kaiser Family Foundation, last modified

October 15, 2019, https://www.kff.org/slideshow/public-opinion-on-single-payer-national-health-plans-and-expanding-access-to-medicare-coverage/.

23. Stan Dorn, "Maryland's Easy Enrollment Health Insurance Program: An Innovative Approach to Covering the Eligible Uninsured," *Health Affairs Blog*, May 13, 2019, https://www.healthaffairs.org/do/10.1377/hblog20190510.993788/full/.

24. Joseph Antos, "Capping the Tax Exclusion Will Not Destroy Employer Health Insurance," *Forbes*, April 26, 2016, http://www.forbes.com/sites/realspin/2016/04/26/capping-the-tax-exclusion-will-not-destroy-employer-health-insurance/#5791e0005647.

25. For a more detailed examination of price transparency, see James C. Capretta, "Toward Meaningful Price Transparency in Health Care," American Enterprise Institute, June 2019, https://www.aei.org/wp-content/uploads/2019/06/Toward-meaningful-price-transparency-in-health-care.pdf.

26. We do not recommend adding Part D when combining Part A and Part B. Unlike Part B, which is optional but enrolls nearly all beneficiaries, about 30% of Medicare beneficiaries are not enrolled in Part D. See Juliette Cubanski, Anthony Damico, and Tricia Neuman, "10 Things to Know About Medicare Part D Coverage and Costs in 2019," Medicare, Kaiser Family Foundation, June 4, 2018, www.kff.org/medicare/issue-brief/10-things-to-know-about-medicare-part-d-coverage-and-costs-in-2019/.

27. Rachel Garfield, Kendal Orgera, and Anthony Damico, "The Coverage Gap: Uninsured Poor Adults in States That Do Not Expand Medicaid," Medicaid, Kaiser Family Foundation, March 21, 2019, https://www.kff.org/medicaid/issue-brief/the-coverage-gap-uninsured-poor-adults-in-states-that-do-not-expand-medicaid/.

Chapter 4. Present at the Creation

1. Kathleen Sebelius served as secretary of the Department of Health and Human Services from April 2009 through April 2014, and Nancy-Ann DeParle was counselor to the president and director of the White House Office of Health Reform from March 2009 to January 2011 and assistant to the president and deputy chief of staff for policy from February 2011 to January 2013. The authors wish to acknowledge the significant contributions—both to this chapter and to the passage and implementation of the ACA—of their friend and former colleague Phil Schiliro; he served as director of the White House Office of Legislative Affairs from 2009 to 2010, special adviser to President Obama in 2011, and President Obama's White House adviser for the ACA and health policy from 2013 to 2014.

2. "14 States Sue to Block Health Care Law," CNN, March 23, 2010, http://www.cnn.com/2010/CRIME/03/23/health.care.lawsuit/index.html.

3. This Office of Consumer Information and Insurance Oversight, which reported directly to the HHS secretary, became the Center for Consumer Information and Insurance Oversight within the Centers for Medicare and Medicaid Services in late 2010 because Congress refused to allow the secretary to create and fund a new operating division to run the ACA. Ironically, we had set out to create the separate operating division because we thought it would be more acceptable to the ACA's detractors in Congress, who had said they did not want it to be a public program like Medicare and Medicaid.

4. "Obama: 'If You Like Your Health Care Plan, You'll Be Able to Keep Your Health Care Plan,'" Politifact, https://www.politifact.com/obama-like -health-care-keep/.

5. Mike Rogers, interview by David Gregory, *Meet the Press*, NBC, December 1, 2013, http://www.nbcnews.com/id/53707062/ns/meet_the_press -transcripts/t/dec-mike-rogers-chris-van-hollen-timothy-dolan-ezekiel -emanuel-david-brooks-stephanie-rawlings-blake-andrea-mitchell-chuck -todd-harry-smith/#.XbCWBuhKiUk.

6. National Federation of Independent Business v. Sebelius, 567 U.S. 519 (2012).

7. Mitch McConnell, interview by Major Garrett, "Top GOP Priority: Make Obama a One-Term President," *National Journal*, October 23, 2010, https://www.nationaljournal.com/member/magazine/top-gop-priority-make -obama-a-one-term-president-20101023/.

8. Maine Community Health Options v. United States, which was argued before the Supreme Court on December 10, 2019. The case was consolidated with Moda Health Plan Inc. v. United States and Land of Lincoln Mutual Health Insurance Co. v. United States.

9. By the time it was settled, the case was known as US House of Representatives v. Hargan and Mnuchin. The case can be found here: https:// images.law.com/contrib/content/uploads/documents/398/6808/16-5202 _Documents.pdf.

10. Patient Protection and Affordable Care Act, 42 U.S.C. §2713.

11. Kimberly Daniels, William D. Mosher, and Jo Jones, "Contraceptive Methods Women Have Ever Used: United States, 1982–2010," *National Health Statistics Reports* 62 (February 2013), https://www.cdc.gov/nchs/data /nhsr/nhsr062.pdf.

12. "Survey: Nearly Three in Four Voters in America Support Fully Covering Prescription Birth Control," Planned Parenthood, last modified January 30, 2014, https://www.plannedparenthood.org/about-us/newsroom/press -releases/survey-nearly-three-four-voters-america-support-fully-covering -prescription-birth-control.

13. Unitarian Universalist Women's Federation, "UU Women Speak Out for Contraception and Freedom of Conscience," https://www.uuwf.org/actions /uu-women-speak-out-for-contraception-and-freedom-of-conscience/.

14. Jamila Taylor and Nikita Mhatre, "Contraceptive Coverage Under the Affordable Care Act," Center for American Progress, October 6, 2017, https://www.americanprogress.org/issues/women/news/2017/10/06/440492 /contraceptive-coverage-affordable-care-act/.

15. "U.S. Rates of Pregnancy, Birth and Abortion among Adolescents and Young Adults Continue to Decline," Guttmacher Institute, September 7, 2017, https://www.guttmacher.org/news-release/2017/us-rates-pregnancy -birth-and-abortion-among-adolescents-and-young-adults-continue.

16. Burwell v. Hobby Lobby, 537 U.S. (2014).

17. Little Sisters of the Poor Home for the Aged v. Burwell, 578 U.S. (2016).

18. 567 U.S. 519 (2012).

19. Representative Mark Meadows to Speaker John Boehner and House Majority Leader Eric Cantor, Washington, DC, August 21, 2013, https://web .archive.org/web/20131006003805/http://meadows.house.gov/uploads /Meadows_DefundLetter.pdf.

20. Quoted in Karen Tumulty, "Government Shutdown or Not, Obamacare Moves Forward," *Washington Post*, October 1, 2013, https://www.washington post.com/politics/government-shutdown-or-not-obamacare-moves-forward /2013/09/30/788e99f4-29ed-11e3-b139-029811dbb57f_story.html.

21. "National Scorecard on Rates of Hospital-Acquired Conditions 2010 to 2015: Interim Data from National Efforts to Make Health Care Safer," Agency for Healthcare Research and Quality, Rockville, MD, last modified December 2016, https://www.ahrq.gov/hai/pfp/2015-interim.html, and Accreditation Insider, "CMS: Hospital Readmission Rate Drop Nationwide," Accreditation and Quality Compliance Center, September 20, 2016, https:// www.accreditationqualitycenter.com/articles/cms-hospital-readmission -rate-drop-nationwide.

Chapter 5. Implementing the Insurance Exchanges

1. This article generally uses the term "exchange team" to identify the Office of Health Insurance Exchanges (OHIE) and other parts of the Obama administration charged with initial responsibility for the ACA exchanges. Whereas OHIE was responsible for day-to-day work on the exchanges, the exchange team was multilayered and typically included a much larger group of Health and Human Services (HHS) staff and for significant decisions often included White House personnel as well. Indeed, by late 2011 OHIE had been reorganized, with many functions reassigned to other offices.

2. Minnesota subsequently applied for and received a planning grant when Mark Dayton was elected governor in November 2010. Alaska failed

to execute on its grant, leaving the final tally at 49 states (though some states drew down little or none of their allotted funds).

3. Abbe R. Gluck and Nicole Huberfeld, "What Is Federalism in Health-care For?," *Stanford Law Review* 70, no. 6 (2018): 1689–1803, https://review .law.stanford.edu/wp-content/uploads/sites/3/2018/06/70-Stan.-L.-Rev .-1689.pdf.

4. The ACA referred to "exchanges," while more recent regulations replace "exchange" with "marketplace." The use of the terms "federally facilitated exchange" and "state-based exchange" reflect the original language.

5. Pennsylvania Cons. Stat. 40 § 9301 (2019), and New Jersey Rev. Stat. § 17B:27A-58 (2019).

6. See Chapter 10 in this volume.

7. Blue Cross Blue Shield Association, "BCBS Companies and Licensees," Blue Cross Blue Shield, https://www.bcbs.com/bcbs-companies-and -licensees.

8. Medicare actually includes 3 insurer-based products: Medicare Supplement policies to offset high cost sharing in Medicare fee-for-service (Social Security Act § 1882, and 42 U.S.C. § 1395ss[p]), prescription drug plans (PDPs) (Social Security Act § 1860D-1, and 42 U.S.C. §1395w-101), and Medicare Advantage plans, which typically rely on narrow networks to offer products that combine all Medicare coverages (Social Security Act § 1851, and 42 U.S.C. §1395w-21).

9. Chapin White and Christopher Whaley, *Prices Paid to Hospitals by Private Health Plans Are High Relative to Medicare and Vary Widely: Findings from an Employer-Led Transparency Initiative* (Santa Monica, CA: RAND Corporation, 2019), https://doi.org/10.7249/RR3033.

10. Patient Protection and Affordable Care Act, 42 U.S.C § 1311(c)(1).

11. Ibid., § 1413(a).

Chapter 6. The ACA, Repeal, and the Politics of Backlash

1. Hendrik Hertzberg, "Electoral Dissonance," *New Yorker*, November 7, 2010, https://www.newyorker.com/magazine/2010/11/15/electoral-dissonance.

2. John B. Judis, "A Lost Generation," *The New Republic*, November 3, 2010, https://newrepublic.com/article/78890/a-lost-generation, and Gary Langer, "2010 Elections Exit Poll Analysis: The Political Price of Economic Pain," ABC News, November 3, 2010, https://abcnews.go.com/Politics/2010 -midterms-political-price-economic-pain/story?id=12041739.

3. "KFF Health Tracking Poll: The Public's Views on the ACA," Health Reform, Kaiser Family Foundation, last modified October 15, 2019, https:// www.kff.org/interactive/kff-health-tracking-poll-the-publics-views-on-the

-aca/#?response=Favorable--Unfavorable&aRange=all, and "Public Approval of Health Care Law," Polls, RealClear Politics, https://www.realclearpolitics.com/epolls/other/obama_and_democrats_health_care_plan-1130.html.

4. Nate Cohn, "What Democrats' Losses in 2010 Can Tell Us About G.O.P.'s Chances in 2018," *New York Times*, May 5, 2017, https://www.nytimes.com/2017/05/05/upshot/what-democrats-losses-in-2010-can-tell-us-about-gops-chances-in-2018.html.

5. See also Brendan Nyhan et al., "One Vote Out of Step? The Effects of Salient Roll Call Votes in the 2010 Election," *American Politics Research* 40, no. 5 (2012): 844–879, https://doi.org/10.1177/1532673X11433768.

6. Tara Golshen, "Why Wasn't the Blue Wave Bigger?" *Vox*, November 7, 2018, https://www.vox.com/2018/11/7/18041006/midterm-election-results-democrat-win-house-gerrymander.

7. Harry Enten, "Latest House Results Confirm 2018 Wasn't a Blue Wave. It Was a Blue Tsunami," Politics, CNN, December 6, 2018, https://www.cnn.com/2018/12/06/politics/latest-house-vote-blue-wave/index.html.

8. Hannah Fingerhut, "Support for 2010 Health Care Law Reaches New High," FactTank, Pew Research Center, February 23, 2017, https://www.pewresearch.org/fact-tank/2017/02/23/support-for-2010-health-care-law-reaches-new-high/.

9. Ashley Kirzinger et al., "KFF Election Tracking Poll: Health Care in the 2018 Midterms," Polling, Kaiser Family Foundation, last modified October 18, 2018, https://www.kff.org/health-reform/poll-finding/kff-election-tracking-poll-health-care-in-the-2018-midterms/.

10. "2018: The Health Care Election," Wesleyan Media Project, last modified October 18, 2018, http://mediaproject.wesleyan.edu/101818-tv/.

11. Among the Republican candidates making these claims were Senate candidates Martha McSally (AZ) and Josh Hawley (MO) and House candidates Mike Bishop (MI) and John Faso (NY). See Jonathan Cohn and Kevin Robillard, "GOP Senate Candidates Are Scrambling to Rewrite Their Record on Pre-Existing Conditions," *HuffPost*, September 2, 2018, https://www.huffpost.com/entry/republicans-lying-pre-existing-conditions_n_5b8964a2e4b0162f4722ab9d, and Jonathan Cohn, "Republicans Are Using Their Families to Defend Their Records on Health Care," *HuffPost*, October 9, 2018, https://www.huffpost.com/entry/pre-existing-conditions-obamacare-bishop-slotkin_n_5bbbad09e4b01470d0540f38.

12. Emily Badger, "How the Rural-Urban Divide Became America's Political Fault Line," *New York Times*, May 21, 2019, https://www.nytimes.com/2019/05/21/upshot/america-political-divide-urban-rural.html, and Dave Wasserman, "The Congressional Map Has a Record-Setting Bias Against Democrats," FiveThirtyEight, August 7, 2017, https://fivethirtyeight.com/features/the-congressional-map-is-historically-biased-toward-the-gop/.

13. Jacob Hacker and Paul Pierson, *Winner-Take-All Politics: How Washington Made the Rich Richer—and Turned Its Back on the Middle Class* (New York: Simon & Schuster, 2010).

14. Eric Levitz, "The Democrats' Irrational Love of the Filibuster Could Doom Their Agenda," *New York Magazine*, February 1, 2019, https://nymag .com/intelligencer/2019/02/dems-irrational-love-of-filibusters-could-doom -their-agenda.html, and Thomas E. Mann and Norman Ornstein, *It's Even Worse Than It Looks* (New York: Basic Books, 2012), 84–100.

15. Atul Gawande, "Getting There from Here," *New Yorker*, January 18, 2009, https://www.newyorker.com/magazine/2009/01/26/getting-there-from -here.

16. For background on the history of the ACA's enactment, see Steven Brill, *America's Bitter Pill: Money, Politics, Backroom Deals, and the Fight to Fix Our Broken Healthcare System* (New York: Random House, 2015); John McDonough, *Inside National Health Reform* (Berkeley: University of California Press, 2011); and Paul Starr, *Remedy and Reaction: The Peculiar American Struggle over Health Care Reform* (New Haven, CT: Yale University Press, 2011). See also Jonathan Cohn, "How They Did It," *New Republic*, May 20, 2010, https://newrepublic.com/article/75077/how-they-did-it.

17. Tessa Berenson, "Reminder: The House Voted to Repeal Obamacare More Than 50 Times," *Time*, March 24, 2017, https://time.com/4712725/ahca -house-repeal-votes-obamacare/.

18. As discussed in Chapter 8 of this volume.

19. Rachel Garfield, Kendal Orgera, and Anthony Damico, "The Coverage Gap: Uninsured Poor Adults in States That Do Not Expand Medicaid," Medicaid, Kaiser Family Foundation, March 21, 2019, https://www.kff.org /medicaid/issue-brief/the-coverage-gap-uninsured-poor-adults-in-states-that -do-not-expand-medicaid/.

20. Texas v. U.S., also discussed in Chapters 8 and 9.

21. James A. Morone, "Partisanship, Dysfunction, and Racial Fears: The New Normal in Health Care Policy?," *Journal of Health Politics, Policy, and Law* 41, no. 4 (2016): 827–846, https://doi.org/10.1215/03616878-3620965; Jonathan Oberlander, "Implementing the Affordable Care Act: The Promise and Limits of Health Care Reform," *Journal of Health Politics, Policy, and Law* 41, no. 4 (2016): 803–826, https://doi.org/10.1215/03616878-3620953; and Michael Grunwald, "The Victory of 'No'," *Politico*, December 4, 2016, https:// www.politico.com/magazine/story/2016/12/republican-party-obstructionism -victory-trump-214498.

22. Robert Pear, "Marco Rubio Quietly Undermines Affordable Care Act," *New York Times*, December 9, 2015, https://www.nytimes.com/2015/12/10/us /politics/marco-rubio-obamacare-affordable-care-act.html.

23. Op. cit. note 3.

24. Benjamin D. Sommers, "Insurance Cancellations in Context: Stability of Coverage in the Nongroup Market prior to Health Reform," *Health Affairs* 33 no. 5 (2014): 887–894, https://doi.org/10.1377/hlthaff.2014.0005, and Lisa Clemans-Cope and Nathaniel Anderson, "How Many Nongroup Policies Were Canceled? Estimates from December 2013," *Health Affairs Blog*, March 3, 2014, https://www.healthaffairs.org/do/10.1377/hblog20140303.037517/full/.

25. Nancy Cook, "Democratic Rift Spurs Questions About Obamacare's Future," *Politico*, January 19, 2016, https://www.politico.com/story/2016/01/obamacare-bernie-sanders-hillary-clinton-218001, and Paul Demko, "Obama Defends Obamacare, Acknowledges Problems with the Law," *Politico*, October 20, 2016, https://www.politico.com/story/2016/10/barack-obama-obamacare-defends-problems-230110.

26. For more on the institutional and structural reasons for the ACA's political weakness, see Jacob Hacker and Paul Pierson, "The Dog That Almost Barked: What the ACA Repeal Fight Says About the Resilience of the American Welfare State," *Journal of Health Politics, Policy, and Law* 43, no. 4 (2018): 551–577, https://doi.org/10.1215/03616878-6527935.

27. Ryan Koronowski, "68 Times Trump Promised to Repeal Obamacare," ThinkProgress, March 24, 2017, https://thinkprogress.org/trump-promised-to-repeal-obamacare-many-times-ab9500dad31e/.

28. Robert Costa and Amy Goldstein, "Trump Vows 'Insurance for Everybody' in Obamacare Replacement Plan," *Washington Post*, January 15, 2017, https://www.washingtonpost.com/politics/trump-vows-insurance-for-every body-in-obamacare-replacement-plan/2017/01/15/5f2b1e18-db5d-11e6-ad42-f3375f271c9c_story.html, and Donald J. Trump, "Trump Gets Down to Business on 60 Minutes," interviewed by Scott Pelley, CBS News, September 27, 2015, https://www.cbsnews.com/news/donald-trump-60-minutes-scott-pelley/.

29. Craig Gilbert, "Ryan: Obamacare Phaseout Will Leave 'No One Worse Off,'" *Milwaukee Journal-Sentinel*, December 5, 2016, https://www.jsonline.com/story/news/politics/elections/2016/12/05/ryan-obamacare-phaseout-leave-no-one-worse-off/94998966/.

30. Larry Levitt, "JAMA Forum: What Might an ACA Replacement Plan Look Like?," News@JAMA, January 24, 2017, https://newsatjama.jama.com/2017/01/24/jama-forum-what-might-an-aca-replacement-plan-look-like/, and Jeffrey Young, "There Is No GOP Obamacare Replacement and There Never Has Been," *HuffPost*, March 27, 2019, https://www.huffpost.com/entry/no-gop-obamacare-replacement_n_5c9bcff1e4b07c88662fd2d3.

31. For an example of such analysis, see "H.R. 1628, Obamacare Repeal Reconciliation Act of 2017," Congressional Budget Office Cost Estimate, Washington, DC, July 19, 2017, https://www.cbo.gov/publication/52939.

32. Robert J. Blendon and John M. Benson, "Public Opinion About the Future of the Affordable Care Act," *New England Journal of Medicine* 377, no.

e12 (2017), https://doi.org/10.1056/NEJMsr1710032, and Dylan Scott and Sarah Kliff, "Why Obamacare Repeal Failed," *Vox*, July 31, 2017, https://www.vox .com/policy-and-politics/2017/7/31/16055960/why-obamacare-repeal-failed.

33. Kristen Bailik and A. W. Geiger, "Republicans, Democrats Find Common Ground on Many Provisions of Health Care Law," FactTank, Pew Research Center, December 8, 2016, https://www.pewresearch.org/fact-tank/2016/12/08 /partisans-on-affordable-care-act-provisions/, and Liz Hamel, Jamie Firth, and Mollyann Brodie, "Kaiser Health Tracking Poll: March 2014," Health Reform, Kaiser Family Foundation, March 26, 2014, https://www.kff.org/health -reform/poll-finding/kaiser-health-tracking-poll-march-2014/.

34. Kendal Orgera and Jennifer Tolbert, "The Opioid Epidemic and Medicaid's Role in Facilitating Access to Treatment," Medicaid, Kaiser Family Foundation, last modified May 24, 2019, https://www.kff.org/medicaid /issue-brief/the-opioid-epidemic-and-medicaids-role-in-facilitating-access -to-treatment/, and Brendan Saloner et al., "The Affordable Care Act in the Heart of the Opioid Crisis: Evidence from West Virginia," *Health Affairs* 38, no. 4 (2019): 633–642, https://doi.org/10.1377/hlthaff.2018.05049.

35. "Sabotage Watch: Tracking Efforts to Undermine the ACA," Center on Budget and Policy Priorities, last modified October 9, 2019, https://www .cbpp.org/sabotage-watch-tracking-efforts-to-undermine-the-aca.

36. Jeffrey Young, "Trump Says He Should Let Obamacare 'Collapse.' That's Cruel and Irresponsible," *HuffPost*, March 24, 2017, last modified July 18, 2017, https://www.huffpost.com/entry/trump-says-he-should-let-obamacare -collapse-thats-cruel-and-irresponsible_n_58d59c8ee4b03787d358cd76, and Julie Rovner, "Timeline: Despite GOP's Failure to Repeal Obamacare, the ACA Has Changed," Kaiser Health News, April 5, 2018, https://khn.org/ news/timeline-roadblocks-to-affordable-care-act-enrollment/.

37. Charles Gaba, "There Will Be Math: The Silver Switcharoo: How to Make Trump's CSR Sabotage Backfire," *Charles Gaba's Blog*, ACASignups .net, July 31, 2017, http://acasignups.net/17/10/12/there-will-be-math-silver -switcharoo-how-make-trumps-csr-sabotage-backfire.

38. Ben Casselman, Margot Sanger-Katz, and Jeanna Smialek, "Share of Americans with Health Insurance Declined in 2018," *New York Times*, September 10, 2019, https://www.nytimes.com/2019/09/10/business/economy /health-insurance-poverty-rate-census.html.

Chapter 7. The ACA and the Republican Alternative

1. Scott J. Anderson, "Tax Credits at Heart of McCain's Health Care Proposal," Politics, CNN, last modified April 29, 2008, http://www.cnn .com/2008/POLITICS/04/29/mccain.healthcare/.

2. Nina Owcharenko Schaefer and Robert Moffit, "The McCain Health Care Plan: More Power to Families," The Heritage Foundation, October 15, 2008, https://www.heritage.org/health-care-reform/report/the-mccain -health-care-plan-more-power-families, and Michael Tanner, "A Fork in the Road: Obama, McCain, and Health Care," CATO Institute Briefing Papers, no. 104, Washington, DC, July 29, 2008, https://www.cato.org/sites/cato.org /files/pubs/pdf/bp104.pdf.

3. "Obama Attacks McCain's Health Care Plan," *Denver Post*, October 4, 2008, https://www.denverpost.com/2008/10/04/obama-attacks-mccains -health-care-plan/, and Maeve Reston and Seema Mehta, "Obama Attacks Mc-Cain Health Plan on Trail, in Ads," *Los Angeles Times*, October 5, 2008, https:// www.latimes.com/archives/la-xpm-2008-oct-05-na-campaign5-story.html.

4. Quoted in Angie Drobnic Holan, "Obama's Plan Expands Existing System," Politifact, last modified October 9, 2008, https://www.politifact .com/truth-o-meter/statements/2008/oct/09/barack-obama/obamas-plan -expands-existing-system/.

5. Tom Rosentiel, "Inside Obama's Sweeping Victory," Pew Research Center, last modified November 5, 2008, https://www.pewresearch.org/2008 /11/05/inside-obamas-sweeping-victory/.

6. Middle Class Health Benefits Tax Repeal Act of 2019, H.R. 748, 116th Cong. (2019).

7. Jeff Zeleny and David M. Herszenhorn, "Obama Seeks Wide Support in Congress for Stimulus," *New York Times*, January 5, 2009, https://www .nytimes.com/2009/01/06/us/politics/06stimulus.html.

8. Quoted in Carol E. Lee and Jonathan Martin, "Obama to GOP: 'I Won'," *Politico*, last modified January 24, 2009, https://www.politico.com /story/2009/01/obama-to-gop-i-won-017862.

9. "White House Forum on Health Reform Attendees and Breakout Session Participants," Briefing Room, The White House, March 5, 2009, https://obamawhitehouse.archives.gov/the-press-office/white-house-forum -health-reform-attendees-and-breakout-session-participants.

10. Patrick O'Connor and Jonathan Martin, "Obama Makes Quiet Play for GOP Aid," Politico, May 18, 2009, https://www.politico.com/story/2009/05 /obama-makes-quiet-play-for-gop-aid-022625.

11. "What the 'Gang of Six' Wants from Health Care Bill," NPR, last modified September 9, 2009, https://www.npr.org/templates/story/story.php ?storyId=112222617?storyId=112222617.

12. Robert Pear and David M. Herszenhorn, "House Unveils Health Bill, Minus Key Details," *New York Times*, June 19, 2009, https://www.nytimes .com/2009/06/20/health/policy/20health.html.

13. "In Historic Vote, HELP Committee Approves the Affordable Health Choices Act," US Senate Committee on Health, Education, Labor and Pen-

sions, July 15, 2009, https://www.help.senate.gov/ranking/newsroom/press/in-historic-vote-help-committee-approves-the-affordable-health-choices-act.

14. Gail Russell Chaddock, "Town-Hall Meetings: Facing Voter Wrath on Healthcare," *Christian Science Monitor*, September 4, 2009, https://www.csmonitor.com/USA/Politics/2009/0904/town-hall-meetings-facing-voter-wrath-on-healthcare.

15. "Rep. Wilson Shouts, 'You Lie' to Obama During Speech," Politics, CNN, last modified September 10, 2009, https://www.cnn.com/2009/POLITICS/09/09/joe.wilson/.

16. Affordable Health Care for America Act, H.R. 3962, 111th Cong. (2009).

17. Quoted in Robert Pear, "Senate Passes Health Care Overhaul on Party-Line Vote," *New York Times*, December 24, 2009, https://www.nytimes.com/2009/12/25/health/policy/25health.html.

18. Nick Wing, "After Massachusetts Victory, Republicans Demand Concessions from Democrats," *HuffPost*, last modified May 25, 2011, https://www.huffpost.com/entry/after-massachusetts-victo_n_429911?guccounter=1.

19. "Obama Scolds Rep. Cantor at Summit for Paper Prop," Boston.com, last modified February 25, 2010, http://archive.boston.com/news/nation/washington/articles/2010/02/25/obama_scolds_rep_cantor_at_summit_for_paper_prop/.

20. "Bipartisanship Runs Aground at Health Care Summit," NPR, last modified February 25, 2010, https://www.npr.org/templates/story/story.php?storyId=124075675.

21. "Health Care Reform Anger Takes a Nasty, Violent Turn," CNN, last modified March 26, 2010, https://www.cnn.com/2010/POLITICS/03/25/congress.threats/index.html.

22. Gary Langer, "2010 Elections Exit Poll Analysis: The Political Price of Economic Pain," ABC News, https://abcnews.go.com/Politics/2010-midterms-political-price-economic-pain/story?id=12041739.

23. John Parkinson, "House Obamacare Repeal: Thirty-Third Time's the Charm?," ABC News, last modified July 11, 2012, https://abcnews.go.com/blogs/politics/2012/07/house-obamacare-repeal-thirty-third-times-the-charm.

24. Barack Obama, "President Barack Obama's State of the Union Address," The White House, January 28, 2014, https://obamawhitehouse.archives.gov/the-press-office/2014/01/28/president-barack-obamas-state-union-address.

25. Douglas W. Elmendorf, Director of the US Congressional Budget Office to House Minority Leader John A. Boehner, "Preliminary Estimate of the Effects on the Deficit of the Amendment in the Nature of a Substitute to H.R. 3962, Offered by Representative Boehner," Congressional

Budget Office, November 4, 2009, https://www.cbo.gov/sites/default/files/111th-congress-2009-2010/costestimate/hr3962amendmentboehner0.pdf.

26. Michael A. Memoli, "House GOP Will Offer Obamacare Alternative This Year," *Los Angeles Times*, January 30, 2014, https://www.latimes.com/politics/la-xpm-2014-jan-30-la-pn-house-gop-obamacare-alternative-20140130-story.html.

27. Jessica C. Barnett and Edward R. Berchick, *Health Insurance Coverage in the United States: 2016*, US Department of Commerce, Washington, DC, September 2017, https://www.census.gov/content/dam/Census/library/publications/2017/demo/p60-260.pdf.

28. Ashley Kirzinger et al., "KFF Election Tracking Poll: Health Care in the 2018 Midterms," Polling, Kaiser Family Foundation, last modified October 18, 2018, https://www.kff.org/health-reform/poll-finding/kff-election-tracking-poll-health-care-in-the-2018-midterms/.

29. Mark Moore, "Democrats Baffled as 2020 Candidates Go on the Attack—Against Obama," *New York Post*, August 1, 2019, https://nypost.com/2019/08/01/democrats-baffled-as-2020-candidates-go-on-the-attack-against-obama/.

30. Benjy Sarlin, "Democrats Duel over Health Care in New Campaign Dust-up," NBC News, last modified July 16, 2019, https://www.nbcnews.com/politics/2020-election/democrats-duel-over-health-care-new-campaign-dust-n1030171.

31. Max Nisen and Elaine He, "The Democrats Are Fighting for Your Health in 2020," *Bloomberg*, October 14, 2019, https://www.bloomberg.com/graphics/2019-opinion-democratic-presidential-medicare-debate/.

Chapter 8. The ACA and the Courts:
Two Perspectives, Part One

1. 567 U.S. 519 (2012).

2. 135 S. Ct. 2480 (2015).

3. I served as the solicitor general of the United States during the first 2 phases of this fight, from 2011 to 2016. The solicitor general, an officer in the Department of Justice, is responsible for representing the US government before the Supreme Court.

4. 317 U.S. 111 (1942).

5. Patient Protection and Affordable Care Act, 42 U.S.C. § 1396a(a)(10)(A)(i)(VIII).

6. *The Volokh Conspiracy* (blog), Reason, https://reason.com/volokh/.

7. Texas v. United States, 352 F. Supp. 3d 665 (N.D. Texas 2018).

8. Texas v. United States, 19-10011 (6th Cir., filed Jan. 7, 2019).

Chapter 9. The ACA and the Courts:
Two Perspectives, Part Two

1. See Neal Devins, "Why Congress Did Not Think About the Constitution When Enacting the Affordable Care Act," *Northwestern University Law Review Colloquy* 106 (2012): 261–282, at 275–276.

2. See, for example, City of Boerne v. Flores, 521 U.S. 507 (1997) (striking down application of the Religious Freedom Restoration Act to states, despite near-unanimous passage of the Act).

3. See Devins, "Why Congress Did Not Think," noting that just "[s]ix House Republicans and four Senate Republicans questioned the bill's constitutionality in floor debates" (276).

4. Joan Biskupic, "Insight: Behind the Healthcare-Law Case: The Challengers' Tale," Reuters, March 13, 2012, https://www.reuters.com/article/us-usa-healthcare-court/insight-behind-the-healthcare-law-case-the-challengers-tale-idUSBRE82C19J20120313.

5. Dellinger had suggested elsewhere that if the cases did reach the Court, the vote would be 8–1 in favor of the Act's constitutionality, with only Justice Thomas dissenting. Stuart Taylor Jr., "Will the Supreme Court Strike Down Health-Care Reform?," *Newsweek*, September 20, 2010, www.newsweek.com/will-supreme-court-strike-down-health-care-reform-71985.

6. 545 U.S. 1 (2005).

7. 547 U.S. 715 (2006).

8. See Art. I, sec. 8 of the Constitution.

9. Virginia ex rel. Cuccinelli v. Sebelius, 728 F. Supp. 2d 768 (E.D. Va. 2010).

10. Fla. ex rel. Bondi v. U.S. Department of Health and Human Services, 780 F. Supp. 2d 1256 (N.D. Fla. 2011).

11. Mead v. Holder, 766 F. Supp. 2d 16 (D.D.C. 2011).

12. Robert Barnes, "Supreme Court to Hear Challenge to Obama's Health-Care Overhaul," *Washington Post*, November 14, 2011, https://www.washingtonpost.com/politics/supreme-court-to-hear-challenge-to-obamas-health-care-overhaul/2011/11/11/gIQALTvrKN_story.html. See also Kevin Sack, "Judge Voids Key Element of Obama Health Care Law," *New York Times*, December 13, 2010, https://www.nytimes.com/2010/12/14/health/policy/14health.html.

13. Fla. ex rel. Atty. Gen., 648 F.3d, at 1327–1328.

14. Another obstacle to Supreme Court review was removed when the federal government ultimately decided to bypass its right to see review from the full 11th Circuit. (Had that court upheld the constitutionality of the mandate, there would have been no Circuit split.)

15. David Ingram, "CNN 'Train Wreck' Comment on Healthcare Case Leaves a Mark," Reuters, March 28, 2012, https://www.reuters.com/article/

us-usa-healthcare-court-toobin/cnn-train-wreck-comment-on-healthcare
-case-leaves-a-mark-idUSBRE82R0ZL20120328.

16. Tom Goldstein, interview by Wolf Blitzer and Ashleigh Banfield, CNN Newsroom, March 27, 2012, http://transcripts.cnn.com/TRAN SCRIPTS/1203/27/cnr.04.html.

17. South Dakota v. Dole, 483 U.S. 203 (1987).

18. Byron Tau, "Toobin: Individual Mandate Seems 'Doomed'," *Politico44* (blog), *Politico*, March 28, 2012, https://www.politico.com/blogs/politico44 /2012/03/toobin-individual-mandate-seems-doomed-118950.

19. 158 Cong. Rec. 4331 (2012) (statement of Sen. Leahy).

20. Jeff Mason, "Obama Takes a Shot at Supreme Court over Healthcare," Reuters, April 2, 2012, https://www.reuters.com/article/us-obama-healthcare /obama-takes-a-shot-at-supreme-court-over-healthcare-idUSBRE8310 WP20120402.

21. Joan Biskupic, *The Chief: The Life and Turbulent Times of Chief Justice John Roberts* (New York: Basic Books, 2019), 238–240.

22. Nancy Pelosi, "Pelosi Remarks at the 2010 Legislative Conference for National Association of Counties," press releases, Congresswoman Nancy Pelosi, March 9, 2010, https://pelosi.house.gov/news/press-releases/pelosi -remarks-at-the-2010-legislative-conference-for-national-association-of.

23. 135 S. Ct. 2480 (2015).

24. 26 U.S.C. § 36 B(b)(2)(A).

25. Texas v. United States, 352 F. Supp. 3d 665 (N.D. Texas 2018).

26. Burwell v. Hobby Lobby Stores, Inc., 573 U.S. 682 (2014).

27. See, for example, Joan Biskupic, "How John Roberts Controls the Supreme Court," Politics, CNN, July 2, 2019, https://www.cnn.com/2019/07/02/ politics/supreme-court-john-roberts-control/index.html?no-st=1570672666.

Chapter 10. Federalism under the ACA:
Implementation, Opposition, Entrenchment

1. We are grateful to Erica Turret, Yale Law School Class of 2020, for her excellent assistance.

2. This chapter is based on our study of the first 5 years of ACA implementation, which we detail in, "What Is Federalism in Health Care For?," *Stanford Law Review* 70, no. 6 (2018): 1689, https://www.stanfordlawreview.org/ print/article/what-is-federalism-in-healthcare-for/, and "The New Health Care Federalism on the Ground," *Indiana Health Law Review* 15, no. 1 (2018): 1–21, https://doi.org/10.18060/3911.0041.

3. National Federation of Independent Business v. Sebelius, 567 U.S. 519 (2012).

4. Richard Cauchi, "State Laws and Actions Challenging Certain Health Reforms," National Conference of State Legislatures, last modified December 17, 2018, http://www.ncsl.org/research/health/state-laws-and-actions-challenging-ppaca.aspx, Table 1: State Legislative Enactments and Ballot Results.

5. As part of our study, "What Is Federalism in Health Care For?," we interviewed more than 20 high-ranking former state and federal officials who were at the forefront of the first years of ACA implementation. See also "The New Health Care Federalism on the Ground" (detailing interviews).

6. Larissa Antonisse et al., "The Effects of Medicaid Expansion Under the ACA: Updated Findings from a Literature Review," Medicaid, Kaiser Family Foundation, August 15, 2019, https://www.kff.org/medicaid/issue-brief/the-effects-of-medicaid-expansion-under-the-aca-updated-findings-from-a-literature-review-august-2019/.

7. Naomi Zewde and Christopher Wimer, "Antipoverty Impact of Medicaid Growing with State Expansions over Time," *Health Affairs* 38, no. 1 (2019): 132–138, https://doi.org/10.1377/hlthaff.2018.05155; Luojia Hu et al., "The Effect of the Affordable Care Act Medicaid Expansions on Financial Wellbeing," *Journal of Public Economics* 163 (2018): 99–112, https://doi.org/10.1016/j.jpubeco.2018.04.009.

8. Lewin Group, "Healthy Indiana Plan 2.0: POWER Account Contribution Assessment," March 2017, https://www.medicaid.gov/Medicaid-CHIP-Program-Information/By-Topics/Waivers/1115/downloads/in/Healthy-Indiana-Plan-2/in-healthy-indiana-plan-support-20-POWER-acct-cont-assesmnt-03312017.pdf.

9. Benjamin D. Sommers et al., "Medicaid Work Requirements—Results from the First Year in Arkansas," *New England Journal of Medicine* 381 (2019): 1073–1082, https://doi.org/10.1056/NEJMsr1901772.

10. Nicole Huberfeld, "Rural Health, Universality, and Legislative Targeting," *Harvard Law and Policy Review* 13 (2018): 241–271, https://harvardlpr.com/wp-content/uploads/sites/20/2019/02/20180713-1_Huberfeld.pdf.

11. See Justin Giovannelli and Emily Curran, "How Did State-Run Health Insurance Marketplaces Fare in 2017?," Commonwealth Fund, March 2018, https://www.commonwealthfund.org/publications/issue-briefs/2018/mar/how-did-state-run-health-insurance-marketplaces-fare-2017 (reporting results of interviews of 17 states (either SBMs or state-based-federal-platform); Sara Collins and Jeanne Lambrew, "Federalism, the Affordable Care Act, and Health Reform in the 2020 Election," Commonwealth Fund, July 2019, https://www.commonwealthfund.org/publications/fund-reports/2019/jul/federalism-affordable-care-act-health-reform-2020-election.

12. Charles Gaba, "UPDATE x2: 2017 Rate Hikes: Yes, Medicaid Expansion Matters. So Do State-Based Exchanges and Transitional Policies," *Charles Gaba's Blog*, ACASignups.net, last modified October 27, 2016, http://

acasignups.net/16/11/01/update-x2-2017-rate-hikes-yes-medicaid-expansion
-matters-so-do-state-based-exchanges-and.

13. Jon R. Gabel et al., "Why Are the Health Insurance Marketplaces Thriving in Some States but Struggling in Others?," Commonwealth Fund, November 2018, https://www.commonwealthfund.org/publications/issue -briefs/2018/nov/marketplaces-thriving-some-states-struggling-others.

14. Sara Rosenbaum et al., "Streamlining Medicaid Enrollment: The Role of the Health Insurance Marketplaces and the Impact of State Policies," Commonwealth Fund, March 2016, https://www.commonwealthfund .org/publications/issue-briefs/2016/mar/streamlining-medicaid-enrollment -role-health-insurance.

15. States that have aggressively intervened to support their insurance markets are projected to see lower rates in 2020. See Dylan Scott, "2020 Obamacare Premiums Are on Track for Smallest Increases Ever," *Vox*, October 28, 2019, https://www.vox.com/policy-and-politics/2019/10/28/20936573/ obamacare-health-insurance-open-enrollment-2020 (also summarizing successful efforts to lower premiums through reinsurance programs and other efforts by states to keep rates down and increase enrollment).

16. Jeanne Lambrew, "No 'ObamaCare Implosion' from Trump Payment Freeze," The Century Foundation, last modified April 19, 2018, https://tcf. org/content/commentary/no-obamacare-implosion-trump-payment-freeze/ ?session=1; See also Robert I. Field, "Even After Political Assaults, Obamacare Is Looking Much Healthier," *Philadelphia Inquirer*, August 14, 2018, https:// www.inquirer.com/philly/health/health-cents/even-after-political-assaults -obamacare-is-looking-much-healthier-20180813.html.

17. Preethi Rao and Sarah A. Nowak, *Effects of Alternative Insurer Responses to Discontinued Federal Cost-Sharing Reduction Payments*, RAND Corporation, 2019, https://doi.org/10.7249/RR2963.

18. Stan Dorn, "Silver Linings for Silver Loading," *Health Affairs Blog*, June 3, 2019, https://www.healthaffairs.org/do/10.1377/hblog20190530.156527/full/.

19. Federal program design that relies on state implementation may be open to more constitutional challenges under the Court's murky conditional spending doctrine than straight nationalization would be; *NFIB* is a prime example of this.

Chapter 11. Executive Power and the ACA

1. Valerie Jarrett, "We're Listening to Businesses About the Health Care Law," blog, The White House, July 2, 2013, https://obamawhitehouse .archives.gov/blog/2013/07/02/we-re-listening-businesses-about-health-care -law.

2. D'Angelo Gore, FactCheck.org, "If You Like Your Health Plan, You Can Keep It," *USA Today*, November 11, 2013, https://www.usatoday.com/ story/news/politics/2013/11/11/fact-check-keeping-your-health-plan/3500187/.

3. Gary Cohen, Director for the Center for Consumer Information and Insurance Oversight to Insurance Commissioners, Washington, DC, November 14, 2013, https://www.cms.gov/cciio/resources/letters/downloads/ commissioner-letter-11-14-2013.pdf.

4. Louise Norris, "The State of Grandmothered and Grandfathered Plans," Healthinsurance.org, last modified June 8, 2019, https://www.health insurance.org/obamacare-enrollment-guide/should-i-keep-my-grandmothered -health-plan/.

5. Heckler v. Chaney, 470 U.S. 821, 831 (1985).

6. Crowley Caribbean Transport, Inc. v. Peña, 37 F.3d 671, 677 (DC Cir. 1994) (internal quotation omitted).

7. For an extended discussion of the delays, see Nicholas Bagley, "Legal Limits and the Implementation of the Affordable Care Act," *University of Pennsylvania Law Review* 164, no. 7 (2016): 1715–1752, https://scholarship.law .upenn.edu/penn_law_review/vol164/iss7/16/.

8. U.S. Constitution, Art. II, sec. 3.

9. Sarah Kliff, "Trump May Stop Enforcing the Individual Mandate, a Hugely Damaging Move for Obamacare," *Vox*, Jan. 23, 2017, https://www.vox .com/policy-and-politics/2017/1/23/14354106/trump-may-stop-enforcing -individual-mandate-obamacare.

10. "Cost-Sharing for Plans Offered in the Federal Marketplace for 2019," Kaiser Family Foundation, last modified October 7, 2019, https://www.kff .org/health-reform/fact-sheet/cost-sharing-for-plans-offered-in-the-federal -marketplace-for-2019/.

11. U.S. Constitution, Art. I, sec. 9.

12. 31 U.S.C. §1301(d).

13. House v. Burwell, 185 F.Supp.3d 165 (D.D.C. 2016).

14. Proclamation 9844 (February 15, 2019) (reprinted at 84 Fed. Reg. 4949).

15. E.O. 13765, reprinted at 82 Fed. Reg. 8351.

16. Curtis W. Copeland, *Rulemaking Requirements and Authorities in the Patient Protection and Affordable Care Act (PPACA)*, Congressional Research Service, Washington, DC, February 2011, https://healthcarereform.procon .org/sourcefiles/CRS_Rulemaking_Requirements_HR3590.pdf.

17. Noam M. Levey, "Trump's New Insurance Rules Are Panned by Nearly Every Healthcare Group That Submitted Formal Comments," *Los Angeles Times*, May 30, 2018, https://www.latimes.com/politics/la-na-pol-trump -insurance-opposition-20180530-story.html.

18. New York v. Department of Labor, No. 18-1747 (D.D.C. 2019).

19. Association for Community Health Plans, No. 18-2133 (D.D.C. 2019).

20. New Mexico Health Connections v. HHS, 16-878 (D.N.M. 2018).

21. Nicholas Bagley, "Taking a Dive on Risk Adjustment," *The Incidental Economist* (blog), July 9, 2018, https://theincidentaleconomist.com/wordpress /taking-a-dive-on-risk-adjustment/.

22. 84 Fed. Reg. 17454.

23. Peter Sullivan, "Top Trump Health Official Warned Against Controversial ObamaCare Changes in Private Memo," *The Hill*, last modified June 14, 2019, https://thehill.com/policy/healthcare/448576-top-trump-health -official-warned-against-controversial-obamacare-changes-in.

24. Charles Gaba, "The Chart That Shows the Price Tag for Trump's Obamacare Sabotage," *New York Times*, December 27, 2018, https://www.ny times.com/2018/12/27/opinion/trump-obamacare-sabotage-chart-cost.html.

25. Stewart v. Azar, 18-152 (D.D.C. 2019); Gresham v. Azar, 18-1900 (D.D.C. 2019); Philbrick v. Azar, 19-773 (D.D.C. 2019).

26. *Stewart v. Azar.*

27. Donald J. Trump (@realdonaldtrump), Twitter, December 24, 2017, 2:35 p.m., https://twitter.com/realdonaldtrump/status/945030174290186241 ?lang=en.

28. Daniel J. Meltzer, "Executive Defense of Congressional Acts," *Duke Law Journal* 61 (2012): 1183–1235, https://scholarship.law.duke.edu/cgi/view content.cgi?article=1530&context=dlj.

29. Texas v. United States, 18-167 (N.D. Tex. 2018).

Chapter 12. Insurance Access and Health Care Outcomes

1. Caren DeNavas-Walt, Bernadette D. Proctor, and Jessica C. Smith, "Income, Poverty, and Health Insurance Coverage in the United States: 2010," US Census Bureau, Washington, DC, September 2011, https://www.census .gov/prod/2011pubs/p60-239.pdf.

2. See Jonathan Gruber and Benjamin D. Sommers, "The Affordable Care Act's Effects on Patients, Providers and the Economy: What We've Learned So Far," *Journal of Policy Analysis and Management* 38, no. 4 (2019): 1028–1052, https://doi.org/10.1002/pam.22158; Larisa Antonisse et al., "The Effects of Medicaid Expansion Under the ACA: Updated Findings from a Literature Review," Medicaid, Kaiser Family Foundation, August 15, 2019, https:// www.kff.org/medicaid/issue-brief/the-effects-of-medicaid-expansion-under -the-aca-updated-findings-from-a-literature-review-august-2019/; Gerald F. Kominski, Narissa J. Nonzee, and Andrea Sorensen, "The Affordable Care Act's Impacts on Access to Insurance and Health Care for Low-Income Populations," *Annual Review of Public Health* 38 (2017): 489–505, https://

doi.org/10.1146/annurev-publhealth-031816-044555; Olena Mazurenko et al., "The Effects of Medicaid Expansion under the ACA: A Systematic Review," *Health Affairs* 37, no. 6 (June 2018): 944–950, https://doi.org/10.1377/hlthaff.2017.1491.

3. Based on a search of the term "Affordable Care Act" in PubMed, a widely used database of academic peer-reviewed publications.

4. John M. Eisenberg and Elaine J. Power, "Transforming Insurance Coverage into Quality Health Care: Voltage Drops from Potential to Delivered Quality," *JAMA* 284, no. 16 (2000): 2100–2107, https://doi.org/10.1001/jama.284.16.2100.

5. Abby Goodnough, Robert Pear, and Richard Pérez-Peña, "Opening Rush to Insurance Market Runs into Snags," *New York Times*, October 1, 2013, https://www.nytimes.com/2013/10/02/us/health-insurance-marketplaces-open.html.

6. Benjamin D. Sommers and Richard Kronick, "The Affordable Care Act and Insurance Coverage for Young Adults," *JAMA* 307, no. 9 (2012): 913–914, https://doi.org/10.1001/jama.307.9.913.

7. Ibid. See also Benjamin D. Sommers and Karyn Schwartz, "2.5 Million Young Adults Gain Health Insurance Due to the Affordable Care Act," Office of the Assistant Secretary for Planning and Evaluation, US Department of Health and Human Services, last modified December 14, 2011, https://aspe.hhs.gov/basic-report/25-million-young-adults-gain-health-insurance-due-affordable-care-act, and Yaa Akosa Antwi, Asako S. Moriya, and Kosali Simon, "Effects of Federal Policy to Insure Young Adults: Evidence from the 2010 Affordable Care Act's Dependent Coverage Mandate," *American Economic Journal: Economic Policy* 5, no. 4 (November 2013): 1–28, https://doi.org/10.1257/pol.5.4.1.

8. "Health Insurance Marketplace: Summary Enrollment Report for the Initial Annual Open Enrollment Period," Office of the Assistant Secretary for Planning and Evaluation, US Department of Health and Human Services, http://aspe.hhs.gov/health/reports/2014/MarketPlaceEnrollment/Apr2014/ib_2014Apr_enrollment.pdf, and "Health Insurance Marketplaces 2017 Open Enrollment Period: January Enrollment Report," Newsroom, CMS.gov, January 10, 2017, https://www.cms.gov/newsroom/fact-sheets/health-insurance-marketplaces-2017-open-enrollment-period-january-enrollment-report.

9. Benjamin D. Sommers, "Insurance Cancellations in Context: Stability of Coverage in the Nongroup Market prior to Health Reform," *Health Affairs* 33 no. 5 (2014): 887–894, https://doi.org/10.1377/hlthaff.2014.0005, and Lisa Clemans-Cope and Nathaniel Anderson, "How Many Nongroup Policies Were Canceled? Estimates from December 2013," *Health Affairs Blog*, March 3, 2014, https://www.healthaffairs.org/do/10.1377/hblog20140303.037517/full/.

10. "January Enrollment Report," and "Estimates for the Insurance Coverage Provisions of the Affordable Care Act Updated for the Recent Supreme Court Decision," Congressional Budget Office, Washington, DC, July 2012, https://www.cbo.gov/sites/default/files/112th-congress-2011-2012/reports/43472-07-24-2012-coverageestimates.pdf.

11. Jean Abraham, Anne B. Royalty, and Coleman Drake, "Employer-Sponsored Insurance Offers: Largely Stable in 2014 Following ACA Implementation," *Health Affairs* 35, no. 11 (2016): 2133–2137, https://doi.org/10.1377/hlthaff.2016.0631.

12. Henry J. Aaron et al., "Turmoil in the Individual Insurance Market—Where It Came From and How to Fix It," *New England Journal of Medicine* 377 (2017): 314–315, https://doi.org/10.1056/NEJMp1707593.

13. Matthew Fiedler et al., "Building on the ACA to Achieve Universal Coverage," *New England Journal of Medicine* 380 (2019): 1685–1688, https://doi.org/10.1056/NEJMp1901532.

14. Sara R. Collins et al., "To Enroll or Not to Enroll? Why Many Americans Have Gained Insurance Under the Affordable Care Act While Others Have Not," Commonwealth Fund, September 25, 2015, https://www.commonwealthfund.org/publications/issue-briefs/2015/sep/enroll-or-not-enroll-why-many-americans-have-gained-insurance.

15. "Health Insurance Marketplaces 2017 Open Enrollment Period Final Enrollment Report: November 1, 2016–January 31, 2017," Newsroom, CMS.gov, last modified March 15, 2017, https://www.cms.gov/newsroom/fact-sheets/health-insurance-marketplaces-2017-open-enrollment-period-final-enrollment-report-november-1-2016.

16. This figure comes from the authors' analysis of the 2017 American Community Survey.

17. Sara R. Collins, Munira Z. Gunja, and Michelle M. Doty, "Following the ACA Repeal-and-Replace Effort, Where Does the U.S. Stand on Insurance Coverage? Findings from the Commonwealth Fund Affordable Care Act Tracking Survey, March–June 2017," Commonwealth Fund, September 7, 2017, https://www.commonwealthfund.org/publications/issue-briefs/2017/sep/following-aca-repeal-and-replace-effort-where-does-us-stand.

18. Molly Frean, Jonathan Gruber, and Benjamin D. Sommers, "Premium Subsidies, the Mandate, and Medicaid Expansion: Coverage Effects of the Affordable Care Act," *Journal of Health Economics* 53 (2017): 72–86, https://doi.org/10.1016/j.jhealeco.2017.02.004.

19. Benjamin D. Sommers et al., "The Impact of State Policies on ACA Applications and Enrollment Among Low-Income Adults in Arkansas, Kentucky, and Texas," *Health Affairs* 34, no. 6 (2015): 1010–1018, https://doi.org/10.1377/hlthaff.2015.0215.

20. Pinar Karaca-Mandic et al., "The Volume of TV Advertisements During the ACA's First Enrollment Period Was Associated with Increased

Insurance Coverage," *Health Affairs* 36, no. 4 (2017): 747–754, https://doi.org /10.1377/hlthaff.2016.1440.

21. Robert Vargas, "How Health Navigators Legitimize the Affordable Care Act to the Uninsured Poor," *Social Science and Medicine* 165 (2016): 263– 270, https://doi.org/10.1016/j.socscimed.2016.01.012.

22. Samantha Artiga, "Where Are States Today? Medicaid and State-Funded Coverage Eligibility Levels for Low-Income Adults," Kaiser Family Foundation, December 2009, https://www.scha.org/tools/files/where -are-states-todaymedicaid-statefunded-coverage-eligibility-levels-for-low income-adultskff1209.pdf.

23. "Medicaid & CHIP: Preliminary August 2017 Applications, Eligibility, and Enrollment Data," Centers for Medicare and Medicaid Services, Baltimore, MD, 2017.

24. Benjamin D. Sommers et al., "Reasons for the Wide Variation in Medicaid Participation Rates Among States Hold Lessons for Coverage Expansion in 2014," *Health Affairs* 31, no. 5 (2012): 909–919, https://doi .org/10.1377/hlthaff.2011.0977, and Genevieve M. Kenney et al., "Variation in Medicaid Eligibility and Participation Among Adults: Implications for the Affordable Care Act," *INQUIRY: The Journal of Health Care Organization, Provision, and Financing* 49 (2012): 231–253, https://doi.org/10.5034/ inquiryjrnl_49.03.08.

25. Frean, Gruber, and Sommers, "Premium Subsidies," and Genevieve M. Kenney et al., "Children's Coverage Climb Continues: Uninsurance and Medicaid/CHIP Eligibility and Participation Under the ACA," Urban Institute and the Robert Wood Johnson Foundation, May 2016, http://www .urban.org/sites/default/files/publication/80536/2000787-Childrens-Cover age-Climb-Continues-Uninsurance-and-Medicaid-CHIP-Eligibility-and -Participation-Under-the-ACA.pdf.

26. Charles Courtemanche et al., "Early Impacts of the Affordable Care Act on Health Insurance Coverage in Medicaid Expansion and Non-Expansion States," *Journal of Policy Analysis and Management* 36, no. 1 (2016): 178–210, https://doi.org/10.1002/pam.21961; Robert Kaestner et al., "Effects of ACA Medicaid Expansions on Health Insurance Coverage and Labor Supply," *Journal of Policy Analysis and Management* 36, no. 3 (2017): 608–642, https://doi.org/10.1002/pam.21993; Benjamin D. Sommers et al., "Changes in Self-Reported Insurance Coverage, Access to Care, and Health Under the Affordable Care Act," *JAMA* 314, no. 4 (2015): 366–374, https://doi.org /10.1001/jama.2015.8421.

27. Jessica C. Barnett and Edward R. Berchick, *Health Insurance Coverage in the United States: 2016* (Washington, DC: US Census Bureau, 2017), https://www.census.gov/library/publications/2017/demo/p60-260.html.

28. Namrata Uberoi, Kenneth Finegold, and Emily Gee, "Health Insurance Coverage and the Affordable Care Act, 2010–2016," Office of the

Assistant Secretary for Planning and Evaluation, Health and Human Services, Washington, DC, March 2016, https://aspe.hhs.gov/system/files/pdf/187551/ACA2010-2016.pdf.

29. Frean, Gruber, and Sommers, "Premium Subsidies."

30. John E. McDonough et al., "The Third Wave of Massachusetts Health Care Access Reform," *Health Affairs* 25, no. Supplement 1 (2006): w420–431, https://doi.org/10.1377/hlthaff.25.w420.

31. Benjamin D. Sommers, Sharon K. Long, and Katherine Baicker, "Changes in Mortality After Massachusetts Health Care Reform: A Quasi-Experimental Study," *Annals of Internal Medicine* 160, no. 9 (2014): 585–593, https://doi.org/10.7326/m13-2275.

32. Alina S. Schnake-Mahl and Benjamin D. Sommers, "Health Care in the Suburbs: An Analysis of Suburban Poverty and Health Care Access," *Health Affairs* 36, no. 10 (2017): 1777–1785, https://doi.org/10.1377/hlthaff.2017.0545.

33. Brett O'Hara and Matthew W. Brault, "The Disparate Impact of the ACA-Dependent Expansion Across Population Subgroups," *Health Services Research* 48, no. 5 (2013): 1581–1592, https://doi.org/10.1111/1475-6773.12067.

34. Kevin Griffith, Leigh Evans, and Jacob Bor, "The Affordable Care Act Reduced Socioeconomic Disparities in Health Care Access," *Health Affairs* 36, no. 8 (2017): 1503–1510, https://doi.org/10.1377/hlthaff.2017.0083.

35. From author's analysis of survey data from the US Census Bureau of US residents ages 0 to 64.

36. Molly Frean et al., "Health Reform and Coverage Changes Among Native Americans," *JAMA Internal Medicine* 176, no. 6 (2016): 858–860, https://doi.org/10.1001/jamainternmed.2016.1695; John J. Park et al., "Health Insurance for Asian Americans, Native Hawaiians, and Pacific Islanders under the Affordable Care Act," *JAMA Internal Medicine* 178, no. 8 (2018): 1128–1129, https://doi.org/10.1001/jamainternmed.2018.1476; Sergio Gonzales and Benjamin D. Sommers, "Intra-Ethnic Coverage Disparities Among Latinos and the Effects of Health Reform," *Health Services Research* 53, no. 3 (2017): 1373–1386, https://doi.org/10.1111/1475-6773.12733; Thomas C. Buchmueller et al., "Effect of the Affordable Care Act on Racial and Ethnic Disparities in Health Insurance Coverage," *American Journal of Public Health* 106, no. 8 (2016): 1416–1421, https://doi.org/10.2105/ajph.2016.303155.

37. Abraham, Royalty, and Drake, "Employer-Sponsored Insurance Offers"; Angshuman Gooptu et al., "Medicaid Expansion Did Not Result in Significant Employment Changes or Job Reductions in 2014," *Health Affairs* 35, no. 1 (2016): 111–118, https://doi.org/10.1377/hlthaff.2015.0747; Asako S. Moriya, Thomas M. Selden, and Kosali I. Simon, "Little Change Seen in Part-Time Employment as a Result of the Affordable Care Act," *Health Affairs* 35, no. 1 (2016): 119–123, https://doi.org/10.1377/hlthaff.2015.0949; Benjamin D. Sommers, Mark Shepard, and Katherine Hempstead, "Why Did

Employer Coverage Fall in Massachusetts After the ACA? Potential Consequences of a Changing Employer Mandate," *Health Affairs* 37, no. 7 (2018): 1144–1152, https://doi.org/10.1377/hlthaff.2018.0220.

38. Sandra L. Decker, Asako S. Moriya, and Aparna Soni, "Coverage for Self-Employed and Others Without Employer Offers Increased After 2014," *Health Affairs* 37, no. 8 (2018): 1238–1242, https://doi.org/10.1377/hlthaff.2017.1663, and Sumit D. Agarwal, Anna L. Goldman, and Benjamin D. Sommers, "Blue-Collar Workers Had Greatest Insurance Gains After ACA Implementation," *Health Affairs* 38, no. 7 (2019): 1140–1144, https://doi.org/10.1377/hlthaff.2018.05454.

39. Benjamin D. Sommers, Kathryn L. Clark, and Arnold M. Epstein, "Early Changes in Health Insurance Coverage Under the Trump Administration," *New England Journal of Medicine* 378 (2018): 1061–1063, https://doi.org/10.1056/NEJMc1800106; Sara R. Collins et al., "First Look at Health Insurance Coverage in 2018 Finds ACA Gains Beginning to Reverse," *To the Point* (blog), Commonwealth Fund, last modified May 1, 2018, https://www.commonwealthfund.org/blog/2018/first-look-health-insurance-coverage-2018-finds-aca-gains-beginning-reverse; Robin A. Cohen, Michael E. Martinez, and Emily P. Zammitti, *Health Insurance Coverage: Early Release of Estimates from the National Health Interview Survey, January–June 2018* (National Center for Health Statistics, 2018), https://www.cdc.gov/nchs/data/nhis/earlyrelease/Insur201811.pdf; Edward R. Berchick, Jessica C. Barnett, and Rachel D. Upton, *Health Insurance Coverage in the United States: 2018* (Washington, DC: US Census Bureau, 2019), https://www.census.gov/library/publications/2019/demo/p60-267.html.

40. Aaron et al., "Turmoil."

41. Frean et al., "Health Reform and Coverage Changes," and Vicki Fung et al., "Potential Effects of Eliminating the Individual Mandate Penalty in California," *Health Affairs* 38, no. 1 (2019): 147–154, https://doi.org/10.1377/hlthaff.2018.05161.

42. J. Craig Wilson and Joseph Thompson, "Nation's First Medicaid Work Requirement Sheds Thousands from Rolls in Arkansas," *Health Affairs Blog*, October 2, 2018, https://www.healthaffairs.org/do/10.1377/hblog20181001.233969/full/, and Benjamin D. Sommers et al., "Medicaid Work Requirements—Results from the First Year in Arkansas," *New England Journal of Medicine* 381 (2019): 1073–1082, https://doi.org/10.1056/NEJMsr1901772.

43. Seema Verma, "Remarks by Administrator Seema Verma at the National Association of Medicaid Directors (NAMD) 2017 Fall Conference," Newsroom, CMS.gov, November 7, 2017, https://www.cms.gov/newsroom/fact-sheets/speech-remarks-administrator-seema-verma-national-association-medicaid-directors-namd-2017-fall.

44. Sandra L. Decker, "In 2011 Nearly One-Third of Physicians Said They Would Not Accept New Medicaid Patients, But Rising Fees May Help," *Health Affairs* 31, no. 8 (2012): 1673–1679, https://doi.org/10.1377/hlthaff.2012.0294.

45. Brendan Saloner, Lindsay Sabik, and Benjamin D. Sommers, "Pinching the Poor? Medicaid Cost Sharing Under the ACA," *New England Journal of Medicine* 370 (2014): 1177–1180, https://doi.org/10.1056/NEJMp1316370.

46. "January Enrollment Report."

47. Ibid.

48. Matthew Rae et al., "Patient Cost-Sharing in Marketplace Plans, 2016," Health Costs, Kaiser Family Foundation, November 13, 2015, https://www.kff.org/health-costs/issue-brief/patient-cost-sharing-in-marketplace-plans-2016/.

49. Sara R. Collins, Munira Z. Gunja, and Michelle M. Doty, "How Well Does Insurance Coverage Protect Consumers from Health Care Costs?," Commonwealth Fund, October 18, 2017, https://www.commonwealthfund.org/publications/issue-briefs/2017/oct/how-well-does-insurance-coverage-protect-consumers-health-care.

50. Douglas B. Jacobs and Benjamin D. Sommers, "Using Drugs to Discriminate—Adverse Selection in the Insurance Marketplace," *New England Journal of Medicine* 372 (2015): 399–402, https://doi.org/10.1056/NEJMp1411376.

51. Stephen C. Dorner, Douglas B. Jacobs, and Benjamin D. Sommers, "Adequacy of Outpatient Specialty Care Access in Marketplace Plans Under the Affordable Care Act," *JAMA* 314, no. 16 (2015): 1749–1750, https://doi.org/10.1001/jama.2015.9375.

52. Linda J. Blumberg, Matthew Buettgens, and Robin Wang, *The Potential Impact of Short-Term Limited-Duration Policies on Insurance Coverage, Premiums, and Federal Spending* (Washington, DC: Urban Institute, 2018), https://www.urban.org/sites/default/files/publication/96781/2001727_updated_finalized.pdf.

53. Benjamin D. Sommers et al., "The Affordable Care Act Has Led to Significant Gains in Health Insurance and Access to Care for Young Adults," *Health Affairs* 32, no. 1 (2013): 165–174, https://doi.org/10.1377/hlthaff.2012.0552, and Kao-Ping Chua and Benjamin D. Sommers, "Changes in Health and Medical Spending Among Young Adults Under Health Reform," *JAMA* 311, no. 23 (2014): 2437–2439, https://doi.org/10.1001/jama.2014.2202.

54. Andrew Mulcahy et al., "Insurance Coverage of Emergency Care for Young Adults Under Health Reform," *New England Journal of Medicine* 368 (2013): 2105–2112, https://doi.org/10.1056/NEJMsa1212779.

55. Antonisse et al., "The Effects of Medicaid Expansion"; Kominski, Nonzee, and Sorensen, "The Affordable Care Act's Impacts"; Mazurenko et al., "The Effects of Medicaid Expansion."

56. Stacey McMorrow et al., "Medicaid Expansion Increased Coverage, Improved Affordability, and Reduced Psychological Distress for Low-Income Parents," *Health Affairs* 36, no. 5 (2017): 808–818, https://doi.org/10.1377/hlthaff.2016.1650, and Miller and Wherry, "Health and Access to Care."

57. Kosali Simon, Aparna Soni, and John Cawley, "The Impact of Health Insurance on Preventive Care and Health Behaviors: Evidence from the First Two Years of the ACA Medicaid Expansions," *Journal of Policy Analysis and Management* 36, no. 2 (2017): 390–417, https://doi.org/10.1002/pam.21972; Benjamin D. Sommers et al., "Changes in Utilization and Health Among Low-Income Adults After Medicaid Expansion or Expanded Private Insurance," *JAMA Internal Medicine* 176, no. 10 (2016): 1501–1509, https://doi.org/10.1001/jamainternmed.2016.4419; Charles Courtemanche et al., "Effects of the Affordable Care Act on Health Behaviors after 3 Years," *Eastern Economic Journal* 45, no. 1 (2019): 7–33, https://doi.org/10.1057/s41302-018-0119-4; Sommers et al., "Three-Year Impacts."

58. Kamyar Nasseh and Marko Vujicic, "Early Impact of the Affordable Care Act's Medicaid Expansion on Dental Care Use," *Health Services Research* 52, no. 6 (2017): 2256–2268, https://doi.org/10.1111/1475-6773.12606.

59. Miller and Wherry, "Health and Access to Care"; Sommers et al., "Three-Year Impacts"; Laura R. Wherry and Sarah Miller, "Early Coverage, Access, Utilization, and Health Effects Associated with the Affordable Care Act Medicaid Expansions: A Quasi-Experimental Study," *Annals of Internal Medicine* 164, no. 12 (2016): 795–803, https://doi.org/10.7326/M15-2234.

60. Miller and Wherry, "Health and Access to Care."

61. Daniel Polsky et al., "Appointment Availability After Increases in Medicaid Payments for Primary Care," *New England Journal of Medicine* 372 (2015): 537–545, https://doi.org/10.1056/NEJMsa1413299, and Renuka Tipirneni et al., "Primary Care Appointment Availability for New Medicaid Patients Increased After Medicaid Expansion in Michigan," *Health Affairs* 34, no. 8 (2015): 1399–1406, https://doi.org/10.1377/hlthaff.2014.1425.

62. Miller and Wherry, "Health and Access to Care," and Sommers et al., "Three-Year Impacts."

63. Ausmita Ghosh, Kosali Simon, and Benjamin D. Sommers, "The Effect of Health Insurance on Prescription Drug Use Among Low-Income Adults: Evidence from Recent Medicaid Expansions," *Journal of Health Economics* 63 (2019): 64–80, https://doi.org/10.1016/j.jhealeco.2018.11.002.

64. Sommers et al., "Changes in Utilization," and Yaa Akosa Antwi et al., "Changes in Emergency Department Use Among Young Adults After the Patient Protection and Affordable Care Act's Dependent Coverage Provision," *Annals of Emergency Medicine* 65, no. 6 (2015): 664–672.e2, https://doi.org/10.1016/j.annemergmed.2015.01.010.

65. Eili Y. Klein et al., "The Effect of Medicaid Expansion on Utilization

in Maryland Emergency Departments," *Annals of Emergency Medicine* 70, no. 5 (2017): 607–614.e1, https://doi.org/10.1016/j.annemergmed.2017.06.021.

66. Sarah L. Taubman et al., "Medicaid Increases Emergency-Department Use: Evidence from Oregon's Health Insurance Experiment," *Science* 343, no. 6168 (2014): 263–268, https://doi.org/10.1126/science.1246183.

67. Anna L. Goldman et al., "Effects of the ACA's Health Insurance Marketplaces on the Previously Uninsured: A Quasi-Experimental Analysis," *Health Affairs* 37, no. 4 (2018): 591–599, https://doi.org/10.1377/hlthaff.2017.1390.

68. Emily Gallagher, Radhakrishnan Gopalan, and Michal Grinstein-Weiss, "The Effect of Health Insurance on Home Payment Delinquency: Evidence from ACA Marketplace Subsidies," *Journal of Public Economics* 172 (2018): 67–83, https://doi.org/10.1016/j.jpubeco.2018.12.007.

69. Sommers et al., "Changes in Self-Reported Insurance Coverage."

70. Sommers et al., "The Affordable Care Act Has Led to Significant Gains."

71. Chua and Sommers, "Changes in Health and Medical Spending," and Jacob Wallace and Benjamin D. Sommers, "Effect of Dependent Coverage Expansion of the Affordable Care Act on Health and Access to Care for Young Adults," *JAMA Pediatrics* 169, no. 5 (2015): 495–497, https://doi.org/10.1001/jamapediatrics.2014.3574.

72. John Scott et al., "Impact of ACA Insurance Coverage Expansion on Perforated Appendix Rates Among Young Adults," *Medical Care* 54, no. 9 (2016): 818–826, https://doi.org/10.1097/MLR.0000000000000586.

73. Jamie R. Daw and Benjamin D. Sommers, "Association of the Affordable Care Act Dependent Coverage Provision with Prenatal Care Use and Birth Outcomes," *JAMA* 319, no. 6 (2018): 579–587, https://doi.org/10.1001/jama.2018.0030.

74. Wherry and Miller, "Early Coverage, Access, Utilization," and Goldman et al., "Effects of the ACA's Health Insurance Marketplaces."

75. Gracie Himmelstein, "Effect of the Affordable Care Act's Medicaid Expansions on Food Security, 2010–2016," *American Journal of Public Health* 109, no. 9 (2019): 1243–1248, https://doi.org/10.2105/ajph.2019.305168, and Christian A. Gregory and Alisha Coleman-Jensen, *Food Insecurity, Chronic Disease, and Health Among Working-Age Adults* (Washington, DC: US Department of Agriculture, Economic Research Service, 2017), Economic Research Report Number 235, https://www.ers.usda.gov/webdocs/publications/84467/err-235.pdf?v=0.

76. Sommers et al., "Three-Year Impacts."

77. Megan B. Cole et al., "At Federally Funded Health Centers, Medicaid Expansion Was Associated with Improved Quality of Care," *Health Affairs* 36, no. 1 (2017): 40–48, https://doi.org/10.1377/hlthaff.2016.0804, and Shailender Swaminathan et al., "Association of Medicaid Expansion with

1-Year Mortality Among Patients with End-Stage Renal Disease," *JAMA* 320, no. 21 (2018): 2242–2250, https://doi.org/10.1001/jama.2018.16504.

78. Andrew P. Loehrer et al., "The Affordable Care Act Medicaid Expansion and Changes in the Care of Surgical Conditions," *JAMA Surgery* 153, no. 3 (2018): e175568, https://doi.org/10.1001/jamasurg.2017.5568.

79. Rishi K. Wadhera et al., "Association of the Affordable Care Act's Medicaid Expansion with Care Quality and Outcomes for Low-Income Patients Hospitalized with Heart Failure," *Circulation: Cardiovascular Quality and Outcomes* 11 (2018): e004729, https://doi.org/10.1161/CIRCOUTCOMES.118.004729, and Rishi K. Wadhera et al., "Association of State Medicaid Expansion with Quality of Care and Outcomes for Low-Income Patients Hospitalized with Acute Myocardial Infarction," *JAMA Cardiology* 4, no. 2 (2019): 120–127, https://doi.org/10.1001/jamacardio.2018.4577.

80. Katherine Baicker et al., "The Oregon Experiment—Effects of Medicaid on Clinical Outcomes," *New England Journal of Medicine* 368 (2013): 1713–1722, https://doi.org/10.1056/NEJMsa1212321, and Amy Finkelstein et al., "The Oregon Health Insurance Experiment: Evidence from the First Year," *Quarterly Journal of Economics* 127, no. 3 (2012): 1057–1106, https://doi.org/10.1093/qje/qjs020.

81. Sommers et al., "Changes in Self-Reported Insurance Coverage."

82. Patrick Flavin, "State Medicaid Expansion and Citizens' Quality of Life," *Social Science Quarterly* 99, no. 2 (2018): 616–625, https://doi.org/10.1111/ssqu.12452.

83. McMorrow et al., "Medicaid Expansion Increased Coverage."

84. Simon, Soni, and Cawley, "The Impact of Health Insurance"; Courtemanche et al., "Effects of the Affordable Care Act"; Sommers et al., "Three-Year Impacts"; Tyler N. A. Winkelman and Virginia W. Chang, "Medicaid Expansion, Mental Health, and Access to Care Among Childless Adults with and Without Chronic Conditions," *Journal of General Internal Medicine* 33, no. 3 (2018): 376–383, https://doi.org/10.1007/s11606-017-4217-5.

85. Miller and Wherry, "Health and Access to Care."

86. Wadhera et al., "Association of the Affordable Care Act's Medicaid Expansion," and Mark Duggan, Atul Gupta, and Emilie Jackson, "The Impact of the Affordable Care Act: Evidence from California's Hospital Sector," NBER Working Paper no. 25488, National Bureau of Economic Research, Cambridge, MA, January 2019, https://doi.org/10.3386/w25488.

87. Chandler McClellan, "The Affordable Care Act's Dependent Care Coverage and Mortality," *Medical Care* 55, no. 5 (2017): 514–519, https://doi.org/10.1097/MLR.0000000000000711.

88. Swaminathan et al., "Association of Medicaid Expansion with 1-Year Mortality."

89. Sommers, Long, and Baicker, "Changes in Mortality," and Benjamin D. Sommers, Katherine Baicker, and Arnold M. Epstein, "Mortality and Access to Care Among Adults After State Medicaid Expansions," *New England Journal of Medicine* 367 (2012): 1025–1034, https://doi.org/10.1056/NEJMsa1202099.

90. Bernard Black et al., "The Effect of Health Insurance on Mortality: Power Analysis and What We Can Learn from the Affordable Care Act Coverage Expansions," NBER Working Paper No. 25568, National Bureau of Economic Research, Cambridge, MA, February 2019, https://doi.org/10.3386/w25568.

91. Sameed Ahmed M. Khatana et al., "Association of Medicaid Expansion with Cardiovascular Mortality," *JAMA Cardiology* 4, no. 7 (2019): 671–679, https://doi.org/10.1001/jamacardio.2019.1651.

92. Sarah Miller et al., "Medicaid and Mortality: New Evidence from Linked Survey and Administrative Data," NBER Working Paper No. 26081, National Bureau of Economic Research, Cambridge, MA, rev. August 2019, https://doi.org/10.3386/w26081.

Chapter 13. Delivery-System Reforms: Evaluating the Effectiveness of the ACA's Delivery-System Reforms at Slowing Cost Growth and Improving Quality and Patient Experience

1. Zirui Song and Elliott S. Fisher, "The ACO Experiment in Infancy—Looking Back and Looking Forward," *JAMA* 316, no. 7 (2016): 705–706, https://doi.org/10.1001/jama.2016.9958, and J. Michael McWilliams et al., "Changes in Postacute Care in the Medicare Shared Savings Program," *JAMA Internal Medicine* 177, no. 4 (2017): 518–526, https://doi.org/10.1001/jamainternmed.2016.9115.

2. Jane M. Zhu et al., "Hospitals Using Bundled Payment Report Reducing Skilled Nursing Facility Use and Improving Care Integration," *Health Affairs* 37, no. 8 (2018): 1282–1289, https://doi.org/10.1377/hlthaff.2018.0257, and J. Michael McWilliams, Bruce E. Landon, and Michael E. Chernew, "Changes in Health Care Spending and Quality for Medicare Beneficiaries Associated with a Commercial ACO Contract," *JAMA* 310, no. 8 (2013): 829–836, https://doi.org/10.1001/jama.2013.276302.

3. Carrie H. Colla and Elliott S. Fisher, "Moving Forward with Accountable Care Organizations: Some Answers, More Questions," *JAMA Internal Medicine* 177, no. 4 (2017): 527–528, https://doi.org/10.1001/jamainternmed.2016.9122.

4. Anne B. Martin et al., "National Health Care Spending in 2017: Growth Slows to Post–Great Recession Rates; Share of GDP Stabilizes," *Health Af-*

fairs 38, no. 1 (2018): 96–106, https://doi.org/10.1377/hlthaff.2018.05085, and Office of the Actuary, *Estimated Financial Effects of the "Patient Protection and Affordable Care Act," as Amended* (Baltimore, MD: Centers for Medicare & Medicaid Services, 2010), https://www.cms.gov/Research-Statistics -Data-and-Systems/Research/ActuarialStudies/downloads/PPACA_2010-04 -22.pdf.

5. John P. Kotter, *Leading Change* (Boston: Harvard Business School Press, 2012).

6. Colleen K. McIlvennan, Zubin J. Eapen, and Larry A. Allen, "Hospital Readmissions Reduction Program," *Circulation* 131, no. 20 (2015): 1796–1803, https://doi.org/10.1161/CIRCULATIONAHA.114.010270.

7. Rachael B. Zuckerman et al., "Readmissions, Observation, and the Hospital Readmissions Reduction Program," *New England Journal of Medicine* 374, no. 16 (2016): 1543–1551, https://doi.org/10.1056/NEJMsa1513024.

8. Nihar R. Desai et al., "Association Between Hospital Penalty Status Under the Hospital Readmission Reduction Program and Readmission Rates for Target and Nontarget Conditions," *JAMA* 316, no. 24 (2016): 2647–2656, https://doi.org/10.1001/jama.2016.18533.

9. Kumar Dharmarajan et al., "Declining Admission Rates and Thirty-Day Readmission Rates Positively Associated Even Though Patients Grew Sicker over Time," *Health Affairs* 35, no. 7 (2016): 1294–1302, https://doi.org /10.1377/hlthaff.2015.1614.

10. Amber K. Sabbatini and Brad Wright, "Excluding Observation Stays from Readmission Rates—What Quality Measures Are Missing," *New England Journal of Medicine* 378, no. 22 (2018): 2062–2065, https://doi.org/10 .1056/NEJMp1800732.

11. Andrew M. Ibrahim et al., "Association of Coded Severity with Readmission Reduction After the Hospital Readmissions Reduction Program," *JAMA Internal Medicine* 178, no. 2 (2018): 290–292, https://doi.org/10.1001/ jamainternmed.2017.6148.

12. Kathleen Carey and Meng-Yun Lin, "Readmissions to New York Hospitals Fell for Three Target Conditions from 2008 to 2012, Consistent with Medicare Goals," *Health Affairs* 34, no. 6 (2015): 978–985, https://doi .org/10.1377/hlthaff.2014.1408, and Enrico G. Ferro et al., "Patient Readmission Rates for All Insurance Types After Implementation of the Hospital Readmissions Reduction Program," *Health Affairs* 38, no. 4 (2019): 585–593, https://doi.org/10.1377/hlthaff.2018.05412.

13. Eric T. Roberts et al., "Assessment of the Effect of Adjustment for Patient Characteristics on Hospital Readmission Rates: Implications for Pay for Performance," *JAMA Internal Medicine* 178, no. 11 (2018): 1498–1507, https://doi.org/10.1001/jamainternmed.2018.4481; Michael L. Barnett, John Hsu, and J. Michael McWilliams, "Patient Characteristics and Differences

in Hospital Readmission Rates," *JAMA Internal Medicine* 175, no. 11 (2015): 1803–1812, https://doi.org/10.1001/jamainternmed.2015.4660; Karen E. Joynt and Ashish K. Jha, "Characteristics of Hospitals Receiving Penalties Under the Hospital Readmissions Reduction Program," *JAMA* 309, no. 4 (2013): 342–343, https://doi.org/10.1001/jama.2012.94856; Michael P. Thompson et al., "Most Hospitals Received Annual Penalties for Excess Readmissions, but Some Fared Better Than Others," *Health Affairs* 36, no. 5 (2017): 893–901, https://doi.org/10.1377/hlthaff.2016.1204; Kathleen Carey and Meng-Yun Lin, "Hospital Readmissions Reduction Program: Safety-Net Hospitals Show Improvement, Modifications to Penalty Formula Still Needed," *Health Affairs* 35, no. 10 (2016): 1918–1923, https://doi.org/10.1377/hlthaff.2016.0537; Matlin Gilman et al., "California Safety-Net Hospitals Likely to Be Penalized by ACA Value, Readmission, and Meaningful-Use Programs," *Health Affairs* 33, no. 8 (2014): 1314–1322, https://doi.org/10.1377/hlthaff.2014.0138.

14. Susannah M. Bernheim et al., "Accounting for Patients' Socioeconomic Status Does Not Change Hospital Readmission Rates," *Health Affairs* 35, no. 8 (2016): 1461–1470, https://doi.org/10.1377/hlthaff.2015.0394.

15. Ankur Gupta et al., "Association of the Hospital Readmissions Reduction Program Implementation with Readmission and Mortality Outcomes in Heart Failure," *JAMA Cardiology* 3, no. 1 (2018): 44–53, https://doi.org/10.1001/jamacardio.2017.4265, and Rishi K. Wadhera et al., "Association of the Hospital Readmissions Reduction Program with Mortality Among Medicare Beneficiaries Hospitalized for Heart Failure, Acute Myocardial Infarction, and Pneumonia," *JAMA* 320, no. 24 (2018): 2542–2552, https://doi.org/10.1001/jama.2018.19232.

16. Rohan Khera et al., "Association of the Hospital Readmissions Reduction Program with Mortality During and After Hospitalization for Acute Myocardial Infarction, Heart Failure, and Pneumonia," *JAMA Network Open* 1, no. 5 (2018): e182777, https://doi.org/10.1001/jamanetworkopen.2018.2777.

17. Peter R. Orszag, "In Defense of the Federal Hospital Readmissions Reduction Program," *NEJM Catalyst*, January 24, 2019, https://catalyst.nejm.org/defense-hospital-readmissions-reduction-program/.

18. Khera et al., "Association of the Hospital Readmissions Reduction Program with Mortality," and Wadhera et al., "Association of the Hospital Readmissions Reduction Program with Mortality."

19. Khera et al., "Association of the Hospital Readmissions Reduction Program with Mortality."

20. Medicare Payment Advisory Commission, "Mandated Report: The Effects of the Hospital Readmissions Reduction Program," in *June 2018 Report to the Congress: Medicare and the Health Care Delivery System* (Washington, DC, 2018), 3–31, http://www.medpac.gov/docs/default-source/reports/jun18_ch1_medpacreport_sec.pdf.

21. Arkansas, Colorado, New Jersey, District-Hudson Valley Region of New York, Cincinnati-Dayton Region of Ohio and Kentucky, Greater Tulsa Region of Oklahoma, and Oregon.

22. Deborah Peikes et al., "The Comprehensive Primary Care Initiative: Effects on Spending, Quality, Patients, and Physicians," *Health Affairs* 37, no. 6 (2018): 890–899, https://doi.org/10.1377/hlthaff.2017.1678.

23. Stacy B. Dale et al., "Two-Year Costs and Quality in the Comprehensive Primary Care Initiative," *New England Journal of Medicine* 374, no. 24 (2016): 2345–2356, https://doi.org/10.1056/NEJMsa1414953.

24. Peikes et al., "The Comprehensive Primary Care Initiative."

25. Ann S. O'Malley et al., "Patient Dismissal by Primary Care Practices," *JAMA Internal Medicine* 177, no. 7 (2017): 1048–1050, https://doi.org/10.1001/jamainternmed.2017.1309.

26. Arkansas, Colorado, Hawaii, Greater Kansas City Region of Kansas and Missouri, Louisiana, Michigan, Montana, Nebraska, North Dakota, Greater Buffalo Region of New York, North Hudson-Capital Region of New York, New Jersey, Ohio and Northern Kentucky Region, Oklahoma, Oregon, Greater Philadelphia Region of Pennsylvania, Rhode Island, and Tennessee.

27. Leavitt Partners Insight, August 2019.

28. Taressa K. Fraze et al., "Comparison of Populations Served in Hospital Service Areas With and Without Comprehensive Primary Care Plus Medical Homes," *JAMA Network Open* 1, no. 5 (2018): e182169, https://doi.org/10.1001/jamanetworkopen.2018.2169.

29. Laura L. Sessums, "Payment and Care Delivery Improvements Could Benefit All Patients," *JAMA Network Open* 1, no. 5 (2018): e182883, https://doi.org/10.1001/jamanetworkopen.2018.2883.

30. J. Michael McWilliams et al., "Medicare Spending After 3 Years of the Medicare Shared Savings Program," *New England Journal of Medicine* 379, no. 12 (2018): 1139–1149, https://doi.org/10.1056/NEJMsa1803388.

31. Ibid.

32. Song and Fisher, "The ACO Experiment in Infancy."

33. J. Michael McWilliams, "Changes in Medicare Shared Savings Program Savings from 2013 to 2014," *JAMA* 316, no. 16 (2016): 1711–1713, https://doi.org/10.1001/jama.2016.12049.

34. Rachel M. Werner, Genevieve P. Kanter, and Daniel Polsky, "Association of Physician Group Participation in Accountable Care Organizations with Patient Social and Clinical Characteristics," *JAMA Network Open* 2, no. 1 (2019): e187220, https://doi.org/10.1001/jamanetworkopen.2018.7220.

35. Aaron L. Shwartz et al., "Changes in Low-Value Services in Year 1 of the Medicare Pioneer Accountable Care Organization Program," *JAMA Internal Medicine* 175, no. 11 (2015): 1815–1825, https://doi.org/10.1001/jamainternmed.2015.4525; J. Michael McWilliams et al., "Performance Differences in

Year 1 of Pioneer Accountable Care Organizations," *New England Journal of Medicine* 372, no. 20 (2015): 1927–1936, https://doi.org/10.1056/NEJM sa1414929; David J. Nyweide et al., "Association of Pioneer Accountable Care Organizations vs Traditional Medicare Fee for Service with Spending, Utilization, and Patient Experience," *JAMA* 313, no. 21 (2015): 2152–2161, https://doi.org/10.1001/jama.2015.4930.

36. Kristina Hanson Lowell et al., *Next Generation Accountable Care Organization (NGACO) Model Evaluation* (Bethesda, MD: University of Chicago, 2018), https://innovation.cms.gov/files/reports/nextgenaco-firstannrpt.pdf.

37. Medicare Acute Care Episode (ACE), Center for Medicare and Medicaid Services, https://innovation.cms.gov/initiatives/ACE/.

38. Zhu et al., "Hospitals Using Bundled Payment."

39. Laura A. Dummit et al., "Association Between Hospital Participation in a Medicare Bundled Payment Initiative and Payments and Quality Outcomes for Lower Extremity Joint Replacement Episodes," *JAMA* 316, no. 12 (2016): 1267–1278, https://doi.org/10.1001/jama.2016.12717.

40. Amol S. Navathe et al., "Spending and Quality After 3 Years of Medicare's Bundled Payments for Joint Replacement Surgery," *Health Affairs* (forthcoming).

41. Amol S. Navathe et al., "Cost of Joint Replacement Using Bundled Payment Models," *JAMA Internal Medicine* 177, no. 2 (2017): 214–222, https://doi.org/10.1001/jamainternmed.2016.8263.

42. Dummit et al. "Association Between Hospital Participation," and Lewin Group, *CMS Bundled Payments for Care Improvement Initiative Models 2–4: Year 5 Evaluation & Monitoring Annual Report* (Falls Church, VA, October 2018), https://downloads.cms.gov/files/cmmi/bpci-models2-4-yr5evalrpt.pdf.

43. Amol S. Navathe et al., "Association of Hospital Participation in a Medicare Bundled Payment Program with Volume and Case Mix of Lower Extremity Joint Replacement Episodes," *JAMA* 320, no. 9 (2018): 901–910, https://doi.org/10.1001/jama.2018.12345.

44. Karen E. Joynt Maddox et al., "Evaluation of Medicare's Bundled Payments Initiative for Medical Conditions," *New England Journal of Medicine* 379, no. 3 (2018): 260–269, https://doi.org/10.1056/NEJMsa1801569.

45. "National Summary of Inpatient Charge Data by Medicare Severity Diagnosis Related Group (MS-DRG), FY2017," Data.CMS.gov, August 20, 2019, https://data.cms.gov/Medicare-Inpatient/National-Summary-of-Inpatient-Charge-Data-by-Medic/ijhk-r7bw.

46. Amy Finkelstein et al., "Mandatory Medicare Bundled Payment Program for Lower Extremity Joint Replacement and Discharge to Institutional Postacute Care: Interim Analysis of the First Year of a 5-Year Randomized Trial," *JAMA* 320, no. 9 (2018): 892–900, https://doi.org/10.1001/jama.2018.12346.

47. Michael L. Barnett et al., "Two-Year Evaluation of Mandatory Bundled Payments for Joint Replacement," *New England Journal of Medicine* 380, no. 3 (2019): 252–262, https://doi.org/10.1056/NEJMsa1809010.

48. Zhu et al., "Hospitals Using Bundled Payment."

49. Daniel M. Blumenthal, "Making It Easier for Hospitals to Participate in, and Succeed Under, Bundled Payments," *JAMA Internal Medicine* 178, no. 12 (2018): 1717–1719, https://doi.org/10.1001/jamainternmed.2018.4739.

50. Caroline P. Thirukumaran et al., "Performance of Safety-Net Hospitals in Year 1 of the Comprehensive Care for Joint Replacement Model," *Health Affairs* 38, no. 2 (2019): 190–196, https://doi.org/10.1377/hlthaff.2018.05264.

51. Amol S. Navathe et al., "Characteristics of Hospitals Earning Savings in the First Year of Mandatory Bundled Payment for Hip and Knee Surgery," *JAMA* 319, no. 9 (2018): 930–932, https://doi.org/10.1001/jama.2018.0678.

52. Joshua M. Liao et al., "National Representativeness of Hospitals and Markets in Medicare's Mandatory Bundled Payment Program," *Health Affairs* 38, no. 1 (2019): 44–53, https://doi.org/10.1377/hlthaff.2018.05177.

53. Abt Associates, "Evaluation of the Oncology Care Model: Performance Period One," for the Center for Medicare and Medicaid Innovation, December 2018, https://innovation.cms.gov/Files/reports/ocm-secondannual eval-pp1.pdf.

Chapter 14. Has the ACA Made Health Care More Affordable?

1. We are grateful to Victor Fuchs and Ezekiel Emanuel for very helpful suggestions, Alexander Mainor for outstanding assistance, and to Paul Hughes-Cromwick and the Altarum Institute for providing invaluable data.

2. That is, providing subsidized insurance coverage makes health care more affordable to the enrollee but does not make health care more affordable for society as a whole because someone—most likely the taxpayer—is paying for the subsidy.

3. Cathy Schoen, "The Affordable Care Act and the U.S. Economy: A Five-Year Perspective," Commonwealth Fund, February 2016, https://www .commonwealthfund.org/publications/fund-reports/2016/feb/affordable-care -act-and-us-economy.

4. Ezekiel J. Emanuel, "Name the Much-Criticized Federal Program That Has Saved the U.S. $2.3 Trillion. Hint: It Starts with Affordable," STAT, March 22, 2019, https://www.statnews.com/2019/03/22/affordable-care-act -controls-costs/.

5. J. Michael McWilliams et al., "Early Performance of Accountable Care Organizations in Medicare," *New England Journal of Medicine* 374, no. 24 (2016): 2357–2366, https://doi.org/10.1056/NEJMsa1600142; J. Michael

McWilliams et al., "Performance Differences in Year 1 of Pioneer Accountable Care Organizations," *New England Journal of Medicine* 372, no. 20 (2015): 1927–1936, https://doi.org/10.1056/NEJMsa1414929; J. Michael Williams et al., "Medicare Spending After 3 Years of the Medicare Shared Savings Program," *New England Journal of Medicine* 379, no. 12 (2018): 1139–1149, https://doi.org/10.1056/NEJMsa1803388.

6. Sherry Glied and Thomas H. Lee, "Is CBO Forecasting Good Enough for Government Work?," *New England Journal of Medicine* 380, no. 23 (2019): 2187–2189, https://doi.org/10.1056/NEJMp1817536.

7. Bloomberg, "Since Obamacare Became Law, 20 Million More Americans Have Gained Health Insurance," *Fortune*, November 15, 2018, http://fortune.com/2018/11/15/obamacare-americans-with-health-insurance-uninsured/.

8. Amitabh Chandra, Jonathan Holmes, and Jonathan Skinner, "Is This Time Different? The Slowdown in Health Care Spending," *Brookings Papers on Economic Activity* 47, no. 2 (2013): 261–302, https://www.brookings.edu/wp-content/uploads/2016/07/2013b_chandra_healthcare_spending.pdf.

9. Ani Turner, George Miller, and Matt Daly, "Health Sector Economic Indicators: Insights from Monthly Employment Data through April 2019," Altarum Center for Value in Health Care, May 2019, https://altarum.org/sites/default/files/uploaded-publication-files/SHSS%20Labor-Brief_May_2019.pdf.

10. "Economic News Release: Employment Situation Summary, August 2019," Bureau of Labor Statistics, October 4, 2019, https://www.bls.gov/news.release/empsit.nro.htm.

11. Jonathan Skinner and Amitabh Chandra, "The Past and Future of the Affordable Care Act," *JAMA* 316, no. 5 (2016): 497–499, https://doi.org/10.1001/jama.2016.10158.

12. Jon D. Lurie et al., "Long-Term Outcomes of Lumbar Spinal Stenosis: Eight-Year Results of the Spine Patient Outcomes Research Trial (SPORT)," *Spine* 40, no. 2 (2015): 63–76, https://doi.org/10.1097/BRS.0000000000000731.

13. *CBO's August 2010 Baseline: Medicare*, Congressional Budget Office, August 25, 2010, https://www.cbo.gov/sites/default/files/recurringdata/51302-2010-08-medicare.pdf, and *Medicare—CBO's May 2019 Baseline*, Congressional Budget Office, May 2, 2019, https://www.cbo.gov/system/files?file=2019-05/51302-2019-05-medicare.pdf.

14. "Chapter 3: The Medicare Advantage Program," in *Report to the Congress: Medicare Payment Policy*, Medicare Payment Advisory Commission, March 2009, 251–269, http://www.medpac.gov/docs/default-source/reports/march-2009-report-to-congress-medicare-payment-policy.pdf.

15. Schoen, "The Affordable Care Act."

16. Douglas W. Elmendorf, Director of the US Congressional Budget Office to Speaker Nancy Pelosi, "Estimate of Changes in Direct Spending and Revenue Effects of the Reconciliation Proposal Combined with H.R. 3590 as Passed by the Senate," Congressional Budget Office, Washington, DC, March 20, 2010, https://www.cbo.gov/sites/default/files/111th-congress-2009-2010/costestimate/amendreconprop.pdf.

17. Philip Ellis et al., *Budgetary and Economic Effects of Repealing the Affordable Care Act* (Washington, DC: Congressional Budget Office, 2015), https://www.cbo.gov/sites/default/files/114th-congress-2015-2016/reports/50252-effectsofacarepeal.pdf.

18. Elmendorf to Pelosi, "Estimate of Changes."

19. "Medicare's DMEPOS Competitive Bidding Program: Frequently Asked Questions," CMS.gov, https://www.cms.gov/outreach-and-education/outreach/partnerships/downloads/dmepospartnerfaqsrevised4813508.pdf.

20. Ellis et al., *Budgetary and Economic Effects*.

21. Juliette Cubanski et al., "What Are the Implications of Repealing the Affordable Care Act for Medicare Spending and Beneficiaries?," Health Reform, Kaiser Family Foundation, December 13, 2016, https://www.kff.org/health-reform/issue-brief/what-are-the-implications-of-repealing-the-afford able-care-act-for-medicare-spending-and-beneficiaries/.

22. Joshua Cohen, "What's Holding Back Market Uptake of Biosimilars?," *Forbes*, June 20, 2018, https://www.forbes.com/sites/joshuacohen/2018/06/20/whats-holding-back-market-uptake-of-biosimilars/#495e2db1691a.

23. Andrew W. Mulcahy, Jakub P. Hlavka, and Spencer R. Case, "Biosimilar Cost Savings in the United States: Initial Experience and Future Potential," *Rand Health Quarterly* 7, no. 4 (2018): 3, https://www.rand.org/pubs/perspectives/PE264.html.

24. Leemore Dafny, Jonathan Gruber, and Christopher Ody, "More Insurers Lower Premiums: Evidence from Initial Pricing in the Health Insurance Marketplaces," *American Journal of Health Economics* 1, no. 1 (2015): 53–81, https://doi.org/10.1162/AJHE_a_00003, and Edmund Haislmaier, *2018 Obamacare Health Insurance Exchanges: Competition and Choice Continue to Shrink*, The Heritage Foundation, January 25, 2018, https://www.heritage.org/health-care-reform/report/2018-obamacare-health-insurance-exchanges-competition-and-choice-continue.

25. McWilliams et al, "Early Performance of Accountable Care Organizations," and Carrie H. Colla et al., "Association Between Medicare Accountable Care Organization Implementation and Spending Among Clinically Vulnerable Beneficiaries," *JAMA Internal Medicine* 176, no. 8 (2016): 1167–1175, https://doi.org/10.1001/jamainternmed.2016.2827.

26. A recent study by Zirui Song et al. considered a precursor to ACOs, the Alternative Quality Contract initiated by Blue Cross Blue Shield (BCBS)

of Massachusetts, which was launched in 2009, prior to the ACA. For 3 cohorts—those starting in 2010, 2011, and 2012, they found overall reductions in costs of 12%, 7%, and 2%, respectively. These cost savings were attenuated substantially by the bonus payments made by BCBS, however, although the authors still found some savings for the early cohorts. Thus, future savings from ACOs could be larger, especially if there were spillover effects from ACOs to non-ACO health systems. Zirui Song et al., "Health Care Spending, Utilization, and Quality 8 Years into Global Payment," *New England Journal of Medicine* 381, no. 3 (2019): 252–263, https://doi.org/10.1056/NEJMsa1813621. See also McWilliams et al., "Medicare Spending After 3 Years," and J. Michael McWilliams, "Changes in Medicare Shared Savings Program Savings from 2013 to 2014," *JAMA* 316, no. 16 (2016): 1711–1713, https://doi.org/10.1001/jama.2016.12049.

27. Winta Mehtsun et al., "National Trends in Readmission Following Inpatient Surgery in the Hospital Readmissions Reduction Program Era," *Annals of Surgery* 267, no. 4 (2018): 599–605, https://doi.org/10.1097/SLA.0000000000002350; Rachael B. Zuckerman et al. "Readmissions, Observation, and the Hospital Readmissions Reduction Program," *New England Journal of Medicine* 374, no. 16 (2016): 1543–1551, https://doi.org/10.1056/NEJMsa1513024; Kathleen Carey and Meng-Yun Lin, "Readmissions to New York Hospitals Fell for Three Target Conditions from 2008 to 2012, Consistent with Medicare Goals," *Health Affairs* 34, no. 6 (2015): 978–985, https://doi.org/10.1377/hlthaff.2014.1408.

28. Christopher Ody et al., "Decreases in Readmissions Credited to Medicare's Program to Reduce Hospital Readmissions Have Been Overstated," *Health Affairs* 38, no. 1 (2019): 36–43, https://doi.org/10.1377/hlthaff.2018.05178.

29. Sushant Joshi et al., "Regression to the Mean in the Medicare Hospital Readmissions Reduction Program," *JAMA Internal Medicine* 179, no. 9 (2019): 1167–1173, https://doi.org/10.1001/jamainternmed.2019.1004.

30. Amy Finkelstein et al., "Mandatory Medicare Bundled Payment Program for Lower Extremity Joint Replacement and Discharge to Institutional Postacute Care: Interim Analysis of the First Year of a 5-Year Randomized Trial," *JAMA* 320, no. 9 (2018): 892–900, https://doi.org/10.1001/jama.2018.12346; Michael L. Barnett et al., "Two-Year Evaluation of Mandatory Bundled Payments for Joint Replacement," *New England Journal of Medicine* 380, no. 3 (2019): 252–262, https://doi.org/10.1056/NEJMsa1809010; Derek A. Haas et al., "Evaluation of Economic and Clinical Outcomes Under Centers for Medicare & Medicaid Services Mandatory Bundled Payments for Joint Replacements," *JAMA Internal Medicine* 179, no. 7 (2019): 924–931, https://doi.org/10.1001/jamainternmed.2019.0480.

31. Peter R. Orszag and Ezekiel J. Emanuel, "Health Care Reform and Cost Control," *New England Journal of Medicine* 363 (2010): 601–603, https://doi.org/10.1056/NEJMp1006571.

32. Talesha Reynolds and Lisa Myers, "Large Employers Cite Obamacare 'Cadillac' Tax in Reducing Benefits," NBC News, last modified November 25, 2013, https://www.nbcnews.com/news/world/large-employers-cite-obama care-cadillac-tax-reducing-benefits-flna2D11655467; William H. Frist, "Obamacare's 'Cadillac Tax' Could Help Reduce the Cost of Health Care," *Forbes*, February 26, 2014, https://www.forbes.com/sites/theapoth ecary/2014/02/26/obamacares-cadillac-tax-could-help-reduce-the-cost-of -health-care/#2c6cd0343989; Reed Abelson, "High-End Health Plans Scale Back to Avoid 'Cadillac Tax'," *New York Times*, May 28, 2013, https://www .nytimes.com/2013/05/28/business/cadillac-tax-health-insurance.html.

33. For the first half of the time period, we use the original CBO estimates, dated March 20, 2010 (Elmendorf to Pelosi, "Estimate of Changes"). At that time the CBO estimated $196 billion in savings from Medicare FFS payment reductions and $136 billion in savings from MA changes. We used half of this 10-year number for the time period 2010–2015 ($166 billion). For the second half of the time period we use the CBO's July 2015 10-year estimate of $715 billion, which they attribute to FFS reimbursement changes and MA payment methodology changes, and divide by half to represent the included time period ($358 billion, per Ellis et al., *Budgetary and Economic Effects*).

34. If the cost savings are back-loaded, as one might expect when MA enrollment continues to grow and payment cuts compound, the reduction in growth rates would be greater in later years. Bending the cost curve requires reducing the *growth rate* of spending, not just a one-time cost reduction.

35. We adjust by the GDP deflator rather than a health care price index because our primary interest is in spending on health care relative to other goods and services.

36. See the Dartmouth Atlas (www.dartmouthatlas.org); rates of major surgical procedures in the United States declined from 103.1 per 1,000 Medicare enrollees in 2006 to 71.2 in 2015, with medical admissions declining by similar amounts. (We are grateful to Laura Yasaitis for pointing this out to us.) Some of this decline may also reflect a shift to outpatient procedures, which tend to be less costly; Cutler et al. suggest that the decline is because of an increase in prescription drugs that thereby keep patients out of the hospital. David M. Cutler et al., "Explaining the Slowdown in Medical Spending Growth among the Elderly, 1999–2012," *Health Affairs* 38, no. 2 (2019): 222–229, https://doi.org/10.1377/hlthaff.2018.05372.

37. Michael Levine and Melinda Buntin, "Why Has Growth in Spending for Fee-for-Service Medicare Slowed?," Working Paper 2013.03, Congressional

Budget Office, Washington DC, August 2013, https://www.cbo.gov/sites/default/files/44513_MedicareSpendingGrowth-8-22.pdf.

38. Len M. Nichols, "Containing Health Care Costs: Recent Progress and Remaining Challenges," testimony for the Committee on the Budget, Washington, DC, July 30, 2013, https://www.budget.senate.gov/imo/media/doc/Nichols_Senate%20Budget%20July%2030%202013%20Testimony.pdf.

39. McWilliams et al., "Early Performance of Accountable Care Organizations," and Sean Lowry, "The Excise Tax on High-Cost Employer-Sponsored Health Coverage: Background and Economic Analysis," Congressional Research Service, August 20, 2015, https://fas.org/sgp/crs/misc/R44160.pdf.

40. Gary Claxton et al., "Health Benefits in 2018: Modest Growth in Premiums, Higher Worker Contributions at Firms with More Low-Wage Workers," *Health Affairs* 37, no. 11 (2018): 1892–1900, https://doi.org/10.1377/hlthaff.2018.1001; Rajender Agarwal, Olena Mazurenko, and Nir Menachemi, "High-Deductible Health Plans Reduce Health Care Cost and Utilization, Including Use of Needed Preventive Services," *Health Affairs* 36, no. 10 (2017): 1762–1768, https:/doi.org/10.1377/hlthaff.2017.0610; Amelia M. Haviland et al., "Do 'Consumer-Directed' Health Plans Bend the Cost Curve over Time?," *Journal of Health Economics* 46 (2016): 33–51, https://doi.org/10.1016/j.jhealeco.2016.01.001.

41. Gary Claxton et al., "Employer Health Benefits: 2018 Annual Survey,", Kaiser Family Foundation, 2018, http://files.kff.org/attachment/Report-Employer-Health-Benefits-Annual-Survey-2018.

42. "Assessing the Effects of the Economy on the Recent Slowdown in Health Spending," Health Costs, Kaiser Family Foundation, April 22, 2013, https://www.kff.org/health-costs/issue-brief/assessing-the-effects-of-the-economy-on-the-recent-slowdown-in-health-spending-2/.

43. David Dranove, Craig Garthwaite, and Christopher Ody, "Health Spending Slowdown Is Mostly Due to Economic Factors, Not Structural Change in the Health Care Sector," *Health Affairs* 33, no. 8 (2014): 1399–1406, https://doi.org/10.1377/hlthaff.2013.1416.

44. David M. Cutler and Nikhil R. Sahni, "If Slow Rate of Health Care Spending Growth Persists, Projections May Be Off by $770 Billion," *Health Affairs* 32, no. 5 (2013): 841–850, https://doi.org/10.1377/hlthaff.2012.0289.

45. As determined by the National Bureau of Economic Research.

46. Cutler and Sahni, "If Slow Rate of Health Care Spending Growth Persists," and Alexander J. Ryu et al., "The Slowdown in Health Care Spending in 2009–11 Reflected Factors Other Than the Weak Economy and Thus May Persist," *Health Affairs* 32, no. 5 (2013), 835–840, https://doi.org/10.1377/hlthaff.2012.1297.

47. George Miller et al., "Health Sector Economic Indicators: Insights from Monthly National Health Spending Data Through March 2019," Alta-

rum Center for Value in Health Care, May 16, 2019, https://altarum.org/sites/default/files/uploaded-publication-files/SHSS-Spending-Brief_May_2019.pdf, and Zack Cooper et al., "Hospital Prices Grew Substantially Faster Than Physician Prices for Hospital-Based Care in 2007–14," *Health Affairs* 38, no. 1 (2019): 184–189, https://doi.org/10.1377/hlthaff.2018.05424.

48. David Blumenthal, Melinda Abrams, and Rachel Nuzum, "The Affordable Care Act at 5 Years," *New England Journal of Medicine* 372 (2015): 2451–2458, https://doi.org/10.1056/NEJMhpr1503614.

49. Sally Kraft et al., "A Simple Framework for Complex System Improvement," *American Journal of Medical Quality* 30, no. 3 (2015): 223–231, https://doi.org/10.1177/1062860614530184.

50. Office of the Actuary, *Estimated Financial Effects of the "Patient Protection and Affordable Care Act," as Amended* (Baltimore, MD: Centers for Medicare and Medicaid Services, 2010), https://www.cms.gov/Research-Statistics-Data-and-Systems/Research/ActuarialStudies/downloads/PPACA_2010-04-22.pdf.

51. Anne B. Martin et al., "National Health Care Spending in 2017: Growth Slows to Post-Great Recession Rates; Share of GDP Stabilizes," *Health Affairs* 38, no. 1 (2018): 96–106, https://doi.org/10.1377/hlthaff.2018.05085.

52. Emanuel, "Name the Much-Criticized Federal Program."

53. Note that during the "great pause" period, health care spending still grew at 1.1% in real per-capita terms, most likely because of the expansion of insurance coverage and the gradual aging of the US population. For Figure 14.4, we interpolate the annual population (from the Federal Reserve Bank of St. Louis's FRED database) to monthly populations, and project 2019 population using the annual 2017 population growth rate.

54. Turner, Miller, and Daly, "Health Sector Economic Indicators."

55. Cooper et al., "Hospital Prices Grew."

56. Sarah Kliff, "Surprise Medical Bills, the High Cost of Emergency Department Care, and the Effects on Patients," *JAMA Internal Medicine* (August 2019), https://doi.org/10.1001/jamainternmed.2019.3448.

57. Jim Norman, "Healthcare Once Again Tops List of Americans' Worries," Gallup, https://news.gallup.com/poll/248159/healthcare-once-again-tops-list-americans-worries.aspx.

58. Renuka Rayasam, "Poll: Americans Blame Pharma, Insurers and Providers for High Health Costs," *Politico*, March 29, 2019, https://www.politico.com/story/2019/03/29/poll-pharma-insurers-providers-health-costs-1302986.

59. Sherry Glied, Stephanie Ma, and Claudia Solis-Roman, "Where the Money Goes: The Evolving Expenses of the US Health Care System," *Health Affairs* 35, no. 7 (2016): 1197–1203, https://doi.org/10.1377/hlthaff.2015.1356.

60. M. Edmunds and F. A. Sloan, eds., *Geographic Adjustment in Medicare Payment, Phase I: Improving Accuracy* (Washington, DC: National Academies

Press, 2011), and Jonathan Skinner and Amitabh Chandra, "Health Care Employment Growth and the Future of US Cost Containment," *JAMA* 319, no. 18 (2018): 1861–1862, https://doi.org/10.1001/jama.2018.2078.

61. Derek Thompson, "Health Care Just Became the U.S.'s Largest Employer," *The Atlantic*, January 9, 2018, https://www.theatlantic.com/business /archive/2018/01/health-care-america-jobs/550079/.

62. Edward Salsberg and Robert Martiniano, "Health Care Jobs Projected to Continue to Grow Far Faster Than Jobs in the General Economy," *Health Affairs Blog*, May 9, 2018, https://www.healthaffairs.org/do/10.1377 /hblog20180502.984593/full/; Robert Martiniano and J. Moore, "Health Care Employment Projections, 2016–2026: An Analysis of Bureau of Labor Statistics Projections by Setting and by Occupation," Center for Health Workforce Studies, School of Public Health, SUNY Albany, Rensselaer, NY, February 2018, http://www.chwsny.org/wp-content/uploads/2018/02/BLS-Projections -2_26_18.pdf; T. Alan Lacey et al., "Projections Overview and Highlights, 2016–26," *Monthly Labor Review*, US Bureau of Labor Statistics, October 2017, https://doi.org/10.21916/mlr.2017.29.

63. Chandra, Holmes, and Skinner, "Is This Time Different?"

64. Theodore Marmor and Jonathan Oberlander, "From HMOs to ACOs: The Quest for the Holy Grail in U.S. Health Policy," *Journal of General Internal Medicine* 27, no. 9 (2012): 1215–1218, https://doi.org/10.1007/s11606-012 -2024-6, and Jonathan Oberlander, "The Politics of Health Reform: Why Do Bad Things Happen to Good Plans?," *Health Affairs* 22, no. Supplement 1 (2003): w3-391–404, https://doi.org/10.1377/hlthaff.w3.391.

65. Jill Quadagno, *One Nation, Uninsured: Why the U.S. Has No National Health Insurance* (Oxford: Oxford University Press, 2005), and Theodore R. Marmor, *Political Analysis and American Medical Care* (Cambridge: Cambridge University Press, 1983).

66. *2019 Annual Report of the Boards of Trustees of the Federal Hospital Insurance Trust Fund and Federal Supplementary Medical Insurance Trust Funds*, Washington, DC, April 22, 2019, https://www.cms.gov/Research-Statistics -Data-and-Systems/Statistics-Trends-and-Reports/ReportsTrustFunds /Downloads/TR2019.pdf.

67. Chapin White, "Contrary to Cost-Shift Theory, Lower Medicare Hospital Payment Rates for Inpatient Care Lead to Lower Private Payment Rates," *Health Affairs* 32, no. 5 (2013): 935–943, https://doi.org/10.1377/hlth aff.2012.0332, and Jeffrey Clemens and Joshua D. Gottlieb, "In the Shadow of a Giant: Medicare's Influence on Private Physician Payments," *Journal of Political Economy* 125, no. 1 (2017): 1–39, https://doi.org/10.1086/689772.

68. Laurence Baker et al., "The Relationship Between Technology Availability and Health Care Spending," *Health Affairs* 22, Supplement 1 (2003): w3-537–551, https://doi.org/10.1377/hlthaff.w3.537.

69. Kimon Bekelis et al., "De-Adoption and Exnovation in the Use of Carotid Revascularization: Retrospective Cohort Study," *BMJ* 359, no. 8129 (2017): j4695, https://doi.org/10.1136/bmj.j4695.

Chapter 15. Health Care Markets a Decade after the ACA: Bigger, but Probably Not Better

1. Harvard University and NBER. During 2012–2013, I served as the deputy director for Healthcare and Antitrust in the Bureau of Economics at the Federal Trade Commission. I thank Abbe R. Gluck for her thoughtful editing, Cory Capps and Thomas Lee for valuable comments, and Steven Lee for research assistance.

2. National Health Expenditures Data Historical, CMS.gov, last modified December 11, 2018, https://www.cms.gov/Research-Statistics-Data-and -Systems/Statistics-Trends-and-Reports/NationalHealthExpendData /NationalHealthAccountsHistorical.html.

3. National Health Expenditures Data Projected, CMS.gov, last modified February 26, 2019, https://www.cms.gov/Research-Statistics-Data-and -Systems/Statistics-Trends-and-Reports/NationalHealthExpendData /NationalHealthAccountsProjected.html.

4. Author's calculations and comparisons of monthly returns for the following stock indices: S&P 500 Health Care, S&P 500, S&P 500 Financials, S&P 500 Industrials, and S&P 500 Information Technology. Stock market data from Investing.com.

5. See Chapters 4 and 5.

6. Author's analysis of public data from the Center for Consumer Information and Insurance Oversight. The unit of observation is the state-year. Each observation is weighted by the number of covered lives.

7. Anna W. Mathews and Brent Kendall, "Antitrust Rulings Put Chill on Health-Insurance Mergers," Business, *Wall Street Journal*, February 15, 2017, https://www.wsj.com/articles/cigna-calls-off-merger-with-anthem-1487 104016.

8. José R. Guardado, David W. Emmons, and Carol K. Kane, "The Price Effects of a Large Merger of Health Insurers: A Case Study of United Health-Sierra," *Health Management, Policy and Innovation* 1, no. 3 (2013): 16–35, https://hmpi.org/wp-content/uploads/2017/02/HMPI-Guardado-Emmons -Kane-Price-Effects-of-a-Larger-Merger-of-Health-Insurers.pdf, and Leemore S. Dafny, Mark Duggan, and Subramaniam Ramanarayanan, "Paying a Premium on Your Premium? Consolidation in the US Health Insurance Industry," *American Economic Review* 102, no. 2 (2012): 1161–1185, https://doi .org/10.1257/aer.102.2.1161.

9. Leemore S. Dafny, Jonathan Gruber, and Christopher Ody, "More Insurers, Lower Premiums: Evidence from Initial Pricing in the Health Insurance Marketplaces," *American Journal of Health Economics* 1, no. 1 (2015): 53–81, https://doi.org/10.1162/AJHE_a_00003.

10. Zirui Song, Mary Beth Landrum, and Michael E. Chernew, "Competitive Bidding in Medicare: Who Benefits from Competition?," *American Journal of Managed Care* 18, no. 9 (2012): 546–552, https://www.ajmc.com/journals/issue/2012/2012-9-vol18-n9/competitive-bidding-in-medicare-who-benefits-from-competition.

11. Bob Herman, "Potential Insurance Mergers Could Spur More Provider Consolidation," *Modern Healthcare*, June 20, 2015, https://www.modernhealthcare.com/article/20150620/MAGAZINE/306209961/potential-insurance-mergers-could-spur-more-provider-consolidation.

12. American Hospital Association, "Chart 2.9: Announced Hospital Mergers and Acquisitions, 2005–2017," in *Trendwatch Chartbook 2018*, American Hospital Association, May 2018, https://www.aha.org/system/files/2018-05/2018-chartbook-chart-2-9.pdf.

13. Thomas L. Greaney, "The State of Competition in the Health Care Marketplace: The Patient Protection and Affordable Care Act's Impact on Competition," September 10, 2015, https://docs.house.gov/meetings/JU/JU05/20150910/103924/HHRG-114-JU05-Wstate-GreaneyT-20150910.pdf, original emphasis.

14. American Hospital Association, "Chart 2.9."

15. American Hospital Association, "Chart 2.9: Announced Hospital Mergers and Acquisitions, 1998–2015," in *Trendwatch Chartbook 2016*, American Hospital Association, 2016, https://www.aha.org/system/files/research/reports/tw/chartbook/2016/chart2-9.pdf.

16. Cory Capps, David Dranove, and Christopher Ody, "Physician Practice Consolidation Driven by Small Acquisitions, So Antitrust Agencies Have Few Tools to Intervene," *Health Affairs* 36, no. 9 (2017): 1556–1563, https://doi.org/10.1377/hlthaff.2017.0054.

17. David B. Muhlestein and Nathan J. Smith, "Physician Consolidation: Rapid Movement from Small to Large Group Practices," *Health Affairs* 35, no. 9 (2016): 1638–1642, https://doi.org/10.1377/hlthaff.2016.0130.

18. Brent D. Fulton, "Health Care Market Concentration Trends in the United States: Evidence and Policy Responses," *Health Affairs* 36, no. 9 (2017): 1530–1538, https://doi.org/10.1377/hlthaff.2017.0556.

19. Carol K. Kane, *2018 Benchmark Survey: For the First Time, Fewer Physicians Are Owners Than Employees*, American Medical Association, 2019, https://www.ama-assn.org/system/files/2019-07/prp-fewer-owners-benchmark-survey-2018.pdf.

20. Hannah T. Neprash, Michael E. Chernew, and J. Michael McWilliams, "Little Evidence Exists to Support the Expectation That Providers

Would Consolidate to Enter New Payment Models," *Health Affairs* 36, no. 2 (2017): 346–354, https://doi.org/10.1377/hlthaff.2016.0840.

21. Kenneth L. Davis, "Hospital Mergers Can Lower Costs and Improve Medical Care," Opinion, *Wall Street Journal*, September 15, 2014, https://www.wsj.com/articles/kenneth-l-davis-hospital-mergers-can-lower-costs-and-improve-medical-care-1410823048.

22. Leemore S. Dafny and Thomas H. Lee, "The Good Merger," *New England Journal of Medicine* 372 (2015): 2077–2079, https://doi.org/10.1056/NEJMp1502338.

23. "Table 4.4: Aggregate Hospital Payment-to-Cost Ratios for Private Payers, Medicare, and Medicaid, 1995–2016," in *Trendwatch Chartbook 2018*, American Hospital Association, May 2018, https://www.aha.org/system/files/2018-05/2018-chartbook-table-4-4.pdf.

24. Leemore S. Dafny, "Estimation and Identification of Merger Effects: An Application to Hospital Mergers," *Journal of Law and Economics* 52, no. 3 (2009): 523–550, https://doi.org/10.1086/600079; Martin Gaynor and Robert Town, *The Impact of Hospital Consolidation—Update*, The Synthesis Project, Robert Wood Johnson Foundation, June 2012, https://www.rwjf.org/en/library/research/2012/06/the-impact-of-hospital-consolidation.html; Zack Cooper et al., "The Price Ain't Right? Hospital Prices and Health Spending on the Privately Insured," *Quarterly Journal of Economics* 134, no. 1 (2019): 51–107, https://doi.org/10.1093/qje/qjy020.

25. Cooper et al., "The Price Ain't Right?"

26. Leemore Dafny, Kate Ho, and Robin S. Lee, "The Price Effects of Cross-Market Mergers: Theory and Evidence from the Hospital Industry," *RAND Journal of Economics* 50, no. 2 (2019): 286–325, https://doi.org/10.1111/1756-2171.12270, and Matthew S. Lewis and Keven E. Pflum, "Hospital Systems and Bargaining Power: Evidence from Out-of-Market Acquisitions," *RAND Journal of Economics* 48, no. 3 (2017): 579–610, https://doi.org/10.1111/1756-2171.12186.

27. Matt Schmitt, "Do Hospital Mergers Reduce Costs?," *Journal of Health Economics* 52 (2017): 74–94, https://doi.org/10.1016/j.jhealeco.2017.01.007.

28. Elena Prager and Matt Schmitt, "Employer Consolidation and Wages: Evidence from Hospitals," working paper, Washington Center for Equitable Growth, February 2019, https://equitablegrowth.org/working-papers/employer-consolidation-and-wages-evidence-from-hospitals/. A comprehensive discussion of the provider merger literature is available in the March 2019 testimony of Professor Martin Gaynor before a House subcommittee exploring the implications of consolidation and anticompetitive conduct in the health care sector: Martin Gaynor, "Examining the Impact of Health Care Consolidation," February 14, 2018, https://docs.house.gov/meetings/IF/IF02/20180214/106855/HHRG-115-IF02-Wstate-GaynorM-20180214.pdf.

29. On orthopedics, see Thomas Koch and Shawn W. Ulrick, "Price Effects of a Merger: Evidence from a Physicians' Market," Working Paper No. 333, Federal Trade Commission, Washington, DC, August 2017, https://www.ftc.gov/reports/price-effects-merger-evidence-physicians-market; on all physicians, see Cory Capps, David Dranove, and Christopher Ody, "The Effect of Hospital Acquisitions of Physician Practices on Prices and Spending," *Journal of Health Economics* 59, no. 5 (2018): 139–152, https://doi.org/10.1016/j.jhealeco.2018.04.001.

30. Capps, Dranove, and Ody, "The Effect of Hospital Acquisitions"; Hanna T. Neprash et al., "Association of Financial Integration Between Physicians and Hospitals with Commercial Health Care Prices," *JAMA Internal Medicine* 175, no. 12 (2015): 1932–1939, https://doi.org/10.1001/jamainternmed.2015.4610; Laurence C. Baker et al., "Physician Practice Competition and Prices Paid by Private Insurers for Office Visits," *JAMA* 312, no. 16 (2014): 1653–1662, https://doi.org/10.1001/jama.2014.10921.

31. Thomas Koch, Brett Wendling, and Nathan E. Wilson, "Physician Market Structure, Patient Outcomes, and Spending: An Examination of Medicare Beneficiaries," *Health Services Research* 53, no. 5 (2018): 3549–3568, https://doi.org/10.1111/1475-6773.12825.

32. Top 25 lists for 2009 and 2019 were obtained from "Global 500 2009," *Financial Times*, https://www.ft.com/content/ef628996-4c52-11de-a6c5-00144feabdc0, and "The World's Largest Public Companies," *Forbes*, https://www.forbes.com/global2000/list/.

33. USN&WR ranks the top 20 but had ties in both years. Avery Comarow, "America's Best Hospitals: the 2009–10 Honor Roll," *US News and World Report*, July 15, 2009, https://health.usnews.com/health-news/best-hospitals/articles/2009/07/15/americas-best-hospitals-the-2009-2010-honor-roll; Ben Harder, "2019–20 Best Hospitals Honor Roll and Medical Specialties Rankings," *US News and World Report*, July 29, 2019, https://health.usnews.com/health-care/best-hospitals/articles/best-hospitals-honor-roll-and-overview.

34. Richard Rubin and Stephanie Armour, "Bipartisan House Coalition Votes to Repeal Health Law's Cadillac Tax," Politics, *Wall Street Journal*, last modified July 17, 2019, https://www.wsj.com/articles/bipartisan-house-coalition-strikes-against-health-laws-cadillac-tax-11563357600.

35. Real wages have increased since 2014Q2, shortly after the full implementation of the ACA. "Employed Full Time: Median Usual Weekly Real Earnings; Wage and Salary Workers: 16 Years and Over [LES1252881600Q]," FRED, Federal Reserve Bank of St. Louis, https://fred.stlouisfed.org/series/LES1252881600Q.

36. Active co-ops exist in Maine, Montana/Idaho, New Mexico, and Wisconsin; "Health Co-Op," Center for Insurance Policy and Research, National Association of Insurance Commissioners, last modified April 18, 2019, https://www.naic.org/cipr_topics/topic_health_co-op.htm. Enrollment data

were obtained from NCQA's Health Plan Report Cards, https://reportcards.ncqa.org/#/health-plans/list.

37. Per the Annual Competition Reports from the FTC (https://www.ftc.gov/policy/reports/policy-reports/annual-competition-reports) and DOJ appropriation figures for the Antitrust Division (last modified September 2019, https://www.justice.gov/atr/appropriation-figures-antitrust-division).

38. Author's tabulations using annual reports available at https://www.ftc.gov/policy/reports/policy-reports/annual-competition-reports. Healthcare transactions are defined as those where the acquired entity is classified under NAICS codes 621–624.

39. John Kwoka, "U.S. Antitrust and Competition Policy Amid the New Merger Wave," Washington Center for Equitable Growth, last modified July 27, 2017, https://equitablegrowth.org/research-paper/u-s-merger-policy-amid-the-new-merger-wave/.

40. Thomas G. Wollmann, "Stealth Consolidation: Evidence from an Amendment to the Hart-Scott-Rodino Act," *American Economic Review: Insight* 1, no. 1 (2019): 77–94, https://doi.org/10.1257/aeri.20180137, and Diana L. Moss, "The Record of Weak U.S. Merger Enforcement in Big Tech," last modified July 8, 2019, https://papers.ssrn.com/sol3/papers.cfm?abstract_id=3417978.

41. Gaynor, "Examining the Impact."

42. Dafny, Ho, and Lee, 2019, "The Price Effects."

43. See, for example, Leemore S. Dafny et al., "Narrow Networks on the Health Insurance Marketplaces: Prevalence, Pricing, and the Cost of Network Breadth," *Health Affairs* 36, no. 9 (2017): 1606–1614, https://doi.org/10.1377/hlthaff.2016.1669; Daniel Polsky, Zuleyha Cidav, and Ashley Swanson, "Marketplace Plans with Narrow Physician Networks Feature Lower Monthly Premiums Than Plans with Larger Networks," *Health Affairs* 35, no. 10 (2016): 1842–1848, https://www.healthaffairs.org/doi/10.1377/hlthaff.2016.0693.

Chapter 16. The ACA's Effects on Medical Practice

1. "Key Facts About the Uninsured Population," Kaiser Family Foundation, December 7, 2018, https://www.kff.org/uninsured/fact-sheet/key-facts-about-the-uninsured-population/#footnote-198942-20.

2. "Primary Care Incentive Payment Program (PCIP)," Center for Medicare and Medicaid Services, https://www.cms.gov/Medicare/Medicare-Fee-for-Service-Payment/PhysicianFeeSched/Downloads/ PCIP-2012-Payments.pdf.

3. Daniel Polsky et al., "Appointment Availability After Increases in Medicaid Payments for Primary Care," *New England Journal of Medicine* 372 (2015): 537–545, https://doi.org/10.1056/NEJMsa1413299.

4. Sandra L. Decker, "No Association Found Between the Medicaid Primary Care Fee Bump and Physician-Reported Participation in Medicaid," *Health Affairs* 37, no. 7 (2018): 1092–1098, https://doi.org/10.1377/hlthaff .2018.0078.

5. "National Health Service Corps Site Reference Guide," US Department of Health and Human Services, April 2019, https://nhsc.hrsa.gov/sites /default/files/NHSC/nhsc-sites/nhsc-site-reference-guide.pdf.

6. Sanjay Basu et al., "Association of Primary Care Physician Supply with Population Mortality in the United States, 2005–2015," *JAMA Internal Medicine* 179, no. 4 (2019): 506–514, https://doi.org/10.1001/jamaintern med.2018.7624.

7. David Muhlestein et al, "Recent Progress in the Value Journey: Growth of ACOs and Value-Based Payment Models in 2018," *Health Affairs Blog*, August 14, 2018, https://www.healthaffairs.org/do/10.1377/hblog20180810.481968 /full/.

8. Lisa S. Rotenstein et al., "Prevalence of Burnout Among Physicians: A Systematic Review," *JAMA* 320, no. 11 (2018): 1131–1150, https://doi.org/10.1001 /jama.2018.12777.

9. "Non-Federal Acute Care Hospital Electronic Health Record Adoption," Office of the National Coordinator for Health Information Technology, September 2017, dashboard.healthit.gov/quickstats/pages/FIG -Hospital-EHR-Adoption.php.

10. Richard M. Scheffler et al, "Consolidation in California's Health System Leads to Higher Prices and Premiums," Commonwealth Fund, September 6, 2018, https://www.commonwealthfund.org/publications/journal -article/2018/sep/consolidation-california-health-system-higher-prices.

Chapter 17. The Impact of the ACA on the Debate
over Drug Pricing Regulation

1. Brett Norman and Sarah Karlin-Smith, "The One That Got Away: Obamacare and the Drug Industry," *Politico*, last modified July 13, 2016, https://www.politico.com/story/2016/07/obamacare-prescription-drugs -pharma-225444; Ryan Grim, "Internal Memo Confirms Big Giveaways in White House Deal with Big Pharma," Politics, *HuffPost*, last modified December 6, 2017, http://www.huffingtonpost.com/2009/08/13/internal-memo -confirms-bi_n_258285.html.

2. Norman and Karlin-Smith, "The One That Got Away."

3. "Key Facts About the Uninsured Population," Uninsured, Kaiser Family Foundation, last modified December 7, 2018, https://www.kff.org/unin sured/fact-sheet/key-facts-about-the-uninsured-population/.

4. Patient Protection and Affordable Care Act, 42 U.S.C. § 18022(b)(1).

5. Christopher Weaver, "Closing Medicare Drug Gap Helps Democrats Sell Reform," Kaiser Health News, last modified March 29, 2010, https://khn.org/news/health-reform-doughnut-hole/.

6. Dena Bunis, "Medicare 'Doughnut Hole' Will Close in 2019," *AARP*, February 9, 2018, https://www.aarp.org/health/medicare-insurance/info-2018/part-d-donut-hole-closes-fd.html.

7. Patient Protection and Affordable Care Act, 42 U.S.C. § 1396r-8(c)(1)(B)(i)(VI) and (c)(3)(B)(iii).

8. Ibid., § 256(b)(a)(4)(M)–(O).

9. "Drug Discount Program: Characteristics of Hospitals Participating and Not Participating in the 340B Program," Government Accountability Office, Washington, DC, June 2018, https://www.gao.gov/assets/700/692587.pdf.

10. Biologics Price Competition and Innovation Act of 2009, 42 U.S.C. § 262(k)(7)(A).

11. W. Nicholson Price II and Arti K. Rai, "Manufacturing Barriers to Biologics Competition and Innovation," *Iowa Law Review* 101, no. 3 (2016): 1023–1064, https://ilr.law.uiowa.edu/print/volume-101-issue-3/manufacturing-barriers-to-biologics-competition-and-innovation/.

12. Ned Pagliarulo, "Humira Biosimilars Launch in Europe, Testing AbbVie," BioPharmaDive, last modified October 19, 2018, https://www.biopharmadive.com/news/abbvie-humira-biosimilars-launch-europe/539938/.

13. Gail R Wilensky, "Developing a Center for Comparative Effectiveness Information," *Health Affairs* 25, Supplement 1 (2006): w572–585, https://doi.org/10.1377/hlthaff.25.w572, and American Academy of Family Physicians, American College of Physicians, and Society of General Internal Medicine to 111th Congress, July 13, 2009, http://www.acponline.org/advocacy/where_we_stand/access/cer_draft09.pdf.

14. Kalipso Chalkidou et al., "Comparative Effectiveness Research and Evidence-Based Health Policy: Experience from Four Countries," *Milbank Quarterly* 87, no. 2 (2009): 339–367, https://doi.org/10.1111/j.1468-0009.2009.00560.x.

15. Betsy McCaughey, "GovernmentCare's Assault on Seniors," Opinion, *Wall Street Journal*, last modified July 23, 2009, http://online.wsj.com/article/SB10001424052970203517304574303903498159292.html.

16. Alan M. Garber, "A Menu Without Prices," *Annals of Internal Medicine* 148, no. 12 (2008): 964–966, https://doi.org/10.7326/0003-4819-148-12-200806170-00223, and American College of Physicians, "Information on Cost-Effectiveness: An Essential Product of a National Comparative Effectiveness Program," *Annals of Internal Medicine* 148, no. 12 (2008): 956–961, https://doi.org/10.7326/0003-4819-148-12-200806170-00222.

17. Patient Protection and Affordable Care Act, 42 U.S.C. § 1320e-1(e).

18. Norman and Karlin-Smith, "The One That Got Away."

19. Eric M. Patashnik, Alan S. Gerber, and Conor M. Dowling, *Unhealthy Politics: The Battle over Evidence-Based Medicine* (Princeton, NJ: Princeton University Press, 2017), 162.

20. Rachel E. Sachs, "Delinking Reimbursement," *Minnesota Law Review* 102 (2018): 2307–2356, https://www.minnesotalawreview.org/wp-content /uploads/2018/07/Sachs_MLR.pdf.

21. Gary Claxton et al., "Increases in Cost-Sharing Payments Continue to Outpace Wage Growth," Access and Affordability, Peterson-Kaiser Health System Tracker, last modified June 15, 2018, https://www.healthsystemtracker.org /brief/increases-in-cost-sharing-payments-have-far-outpaced-wage-growth/.

22. Stacie B. Dusetzina et al., "Association of Prescription Drug Price Rebates in Medicare Part D with Patient Out-of-Pocket and Federal Spending," *JAMA Internal Medicine* 177, no. 8 (2017): 1185–1188, https://doi.org/10.1001 /jamainternmed.2017.1885.

23. Rabah Kamal, Cynthia Cox, and Daniel McDermott, "What Are the Recent and Forecasted Trends in Prescription Drug Spending?," Health Spending, Peterson-Kaiser Health System Tracker, last modified February 20, 2019, https://www.healthsystemtracker.org/chart-collection/recent-forecasted -trends-prescription-drug-spending/.

24. Robin A. Cohen and Maria A. Villarroel, "Strategies Used by Adults to Reduce Their Prescription Drug Costs: United States, 2013," NCHS Data Brief No. 184, Department of Health and Human Services, Washington, DC, January 2015, https://www.cdc.gov/nchs/data/databriefs/db184.pdf.

25. "Offsetting Effects of Prescription Drug Use on Medicare's Spending for Medical Services," Congressional Budget Office, Washington, DC, November 2012, https://www.cbo.gov/sites/default/files/112th-congress-2011-2012 /reports/MedicalOffsets_One-col.pdf.

26. Bram Sable-Smith, "Insulin's High Cost Leads to Lethal Rationing," NPR, last modified September 1, 2018, https://www.npr.org/sections/health -shots/2018/09/01/641615877/insulins-high-cost-leads-to-lethal-rationing.

27. Ashley Kirzinger, Bryan Wu, and Mollyann Brodie, "Kaiser Health Tracking Poll—March 2018: Views on Prescription Drug Pricing and Medicare-for-All Proposals," Polling, Kaiser Family Foundation, last modified March 23, 2018, https://www.kff.org/health-costs/poll-findingkaiser-health -tracking-poll-march-2018-prescription-drug-pricing-medicare-for-all -proposals/.

28. Medicare Payment Advisory Commission (hereafter MedPAC), *Report to the Congress: Medicare and the Health Care Delivery System*, Washington, DC, June 2016, http://www.medpac.gov/docs/default-source/reports/june

-2016-report-to-the-congress-medicare-and-the-health-care-delivery-system
.pdf?sfvrsn=0.

29. *2017 Annual Report of the Boards of Trustees of the Federal Hospital Insur-
ance and Federal Supplementary Medical Insurance Trust Funds*, Washington,
DC, July 2017, https://www.cms.gov/Research-Statistics-Data-and-Systems
/Statistics-Trends-and-Reports/ReportsTrustFunds/Downloads/TR2017.pdf.

30. MedPAC, *A Data Book: Health Care Spending and the Medicare Program*, Washington, DC, June 2018, http://www.medpac.gov/docs/default
-source/data-book/jun18_databookentirereport_sec.pdf?sfvrsn=0.

31. MedPAC, *Report to the Congress*, xi.

32. "Observations on Trends in Prescription Drug Spending," Office
of the Assistant Secretary for Planning and Evaluation, US Department of
Health and Human Services, Washington, DC, March 2016, https://aspe
.hhs.gov/system/files/pdf/187586/Drugspending.pdf.

33. Kamal, Cox, and McDermott, "What Are the Recent and Forecasted
Trends."

34. Peter Sullivan, "Grassley, Wyden Working on Plan to Cap Seniors' Drug
Costs in Medicare," *The Hill*, last modified May 8, 2019, https://thehill.com
/policy/healthcare/442776-grassley-wyden-working-on-plan-to-cap-seniors
-drug-costs-in-medicare.

35. Juliette Cubanski et al., "No Limit: Medicare Part D Enrollees Ex-
posed to High Out-of-Pocket Drug Costs Without a Hard Cap on Spending,"
Kaiser Family Foundation, November 2017, http://files.kff.org/attachment
/Issue-Brief-No-Limit-Medicare-Part-D-Enrollees-Exposed-to-High-Out-of
-Pocket-Drug-Costs-Without-a-Hard-Cap-on-Spending.

36. Improving Access to Affordable Prescription Drugs Act, H.R. 1776,
115th Cong. (2017), https://www.congress.gov/bill/115th-congress/house-bill
/1776/cosponsors.

37. Rachel Sachs, "Trump Administration Releases Long-Awaited Drug
Rebate Proposal," *Health Affairs Blog*, February 1, 2019, https://www.health
affairs.org/do/10.1377/hblog20190201.545950/full/.

38. Gerard F. Anderson, "What We Know and Don't Know About Drug
Pricing," in *Examining the Actions of Drug Companies in Raising Prescription
Drug Prices: Hearings Before the United States House of Representatives Com-
mittee on Oversight and Government Reform*, 116th Cong., January 29, 2019,
https://docs.house.gov/meetings/GO/GO00/20190129/108817/HHRG-116
-GO00-Wstate-AndersonG-20190129.pdf.

39. MedPAC, *Report to the Congress*, 118.

40. Dana O. Sarnak, David Squires, and Shawn Bishop, "Paying for Prescription Drugs Around the World: Why Is the U.S. an Outlier?," Commonwealth Fund, October 5, 2017, https://www.commonwealthfund.org

/publications/issue-briefs/2017/oct/paying-prescription-drugs-around-world
-why-us-outlier.

41. Steven Pearson, Len Nichols, and Amitabh Chandra, "Policy Strategies for Aligning Price and Value for Brand-Name Pharmaceuticals," Policy Options Paper, Health Affairs, March 15, 2018, https://doi.org/10.1377/hpb20180216.92303.

42. Rachel E. Sachs and Austin B. Frakt, "Innovation—Innovation Tradeoffs in Drug Pricing," *Annals of Internal Medicine* 165, no. 12 (2016): 871–872, https://doi.org/10.7326/M16-2167.

Chapter 18. Toward Equality and the Right to Health Care

1. Abbe R. Gluck and Thomas Scott-Railton, "Affordable Care Act Entrenchment," *Georgetown Law Journal* 108 (forthcoming 2020).

2. "Data Note: 10 Charts About Public Opinion on Medicaid," Polling, Kaiser Family Foundation, last modified June 27, 2017, https://www.kff.org/medicaid/poll-finding/data-note-10-charts-about-public-opinion-on-medicaid/.

3. Daniel Greenberg et al., "America's Growing Support for Transgender Rights," PRRI, last modified June 11, 2019, https://www.prri.org/research/americas-growing-support-for-transgender-rights/.

4. Tricia Brooks, "The Family Glitch," Briefs, Health Affairs, last modified November 10, 2014, https://www.healthaffairs.org/do/10.1377/hpb2014
1110.62257/full/.

5. 567 U.S. 519 (2012)

6. "Medicaid Enrollment Changes Following the ACA," Medicaid and CHIP Payment and Access Commission (MACPAC), https://www.macpac.gov/subtopic/medicaid-enrollment-changes-following-the-aca/.

7. Sara Rosenbaum et al., "Community Health Centers: Growing Importance in a Changing Health Care System," Kaiser Family Foundation, March 2018, http://files.kff.org/attachment/Issue-Brief-Community-Health-Centers-Growing-Importance-in-a-Changing-Health-Care-System.

8. "Health Center Program: Impact and Growth," Health Resources and Services Administration (HRSA), last modified August 2019, https://bphc.hrsa.gov/about/healthcenterprogram/index.html.

9. Katie Keith, "More Courts Rule on Section 1557 as HHS Reconsiders Regulation," *Health Affairs Blog*, October 2, 2018, https://www.healthaffairs.org/do/10.1377/hblog20181002.142178/full/.

10. Sara Rosenbaum, "The Myths We Tell Ourselves About the Poor: From the English Poor Law to the Council of Economic Advisers," *The Mil-*

bank Quarterly 96 (2018): 12 paragraphs, https://www.milbank.org/quarterly /articles/the-myths-we-tell-ourselves-about-the-poor-from-the-english-poor -law-to-the-council-of-economic-advisers/.

11. David Smith and Judith Moore, *Medicaid Politics and Policy*, 2nd ed. (New Brunswick, NJ: Transaction Publishers, 2015).

12. Sara Rosenbaum, "A Program for All Seasons," *St. Louis University Journal of Health Law and Policy* (forthcoming 2020).

13. Smith and Moore, *Medicaid Policy and Politics*.

14. *NIFB v. Sebelius* 567 U.S. 519 (2012).

15. Rachel Garfield, Kendal Orgera, and Anthony Damico, "The Coverage Gap: Uninsured Poor Adults in States That Do Not Expand Medicaid," Medicaid, Kaiser Family Foundation, March 21, 2019, https://www.kff.org /medicaid/issue-brief/the-coverage-gap-uninsured-poor-adults-in-states-that -do-not-expand-medicaid/.

16. Michael F. Cannon, "50 Vetoes: How States Can Stop the Obama Health Care Law" (white paper, CATO Institute, March 21, 2013), https:// www.cato.org/publications/white-paper/50-vetoes-how-states-can-stop -obama-health-care-law.

17. American Health Care Act of 2017, H.R. 1628, 115th Congress (2017), https://www.congress.gov/bill/115th-congress/house-bill/1628, Title I § 111 and 112.

18. Tom Price, secretary of Health and Human Services, and Seema Verma, Centers for Medicare and Medicaid Services to US Governors, March 14, 2017, https://www.hhs.gov/sites/default/files/sec-price-admin-verma-ltr .pdf.

19. Sara Rosenbaum et al., "Will Evaluations of Medicaid 1115 Demonstrations That Restrict Eligibility Tell Policymakers What They Need to Know?," Commonwealth Fund, December 12, 2018, https://www.commonwealth fund.org/publications/issue-briefs/2018/dec/evaluations-medicaid-1115 -restrict-eligibility.

20. See Sara Rosenbaum and Alexander Somodevilla, "Inside the Latest Medicaid Work Experiment Decisions: Stewart v Azar and Gresham v Azar," *Health Affairs Blog*, April 2, 2019, https://www.healthaffairs.org/do/10.1377 /hblog20190402.282257/full/.

21. Benjamin D. Sommers et al., "Medicaid Work Requirements—Results from the First Year in Arkansas," *New England Journal of Medicine* 381 (2019): 1073–1082, https://doi.org/10.1056/NEJMsr1901772.

22. Wendy E. Parmet, "The Trump Administration's New Public Charge Rule: Implications for Health Care & Public Health," *Health Affairs Blog*, August 13, 2019, https://www.healthaffairs.org/do/10.1377/hblog20190813.84831 /full/.

23. La Clinica de la Raza et al. v. Donald Trump et al. (N.D. Ca, 2019), Case No. 4:19-cv-4980-PJH (filed September 4, 2019), Declaration of Leighton Ku PH.D., MPH in Support of Plaintiffs' Motion for a Preliminary Injunction.

24. Debra Cassens Weiss, "4 Federal Judges Rule Against Trump on Immigration Issues in 1 Day," *ABA Journal*, October 15, 2019, http://www.aba journal.com/news/article/4-federal-judges-rule-against-trump-on-immigra tion-issues-in-1-day.

25. "Medicaid Enrollment Changes Following the ACA."

26. Edward R. Berchick, Emily Hood, and Jessica C. Barnett, *Health Insurance Coverage in the United States: 2017*, US Census Bureau, Washington, DC, September 2018, https://www.census.gov/content/dam/Census/library /publications/2018/demo/p60-264.pdf, Figure 5.

27. Larisa Antonisse et al., "The Effects of Medicaid Expansion Under the ACA: Updated Findings from a Literature Review," Medicaid, Kaiser Family Foundation, August 15, 2019, https://www.kff.org/medicaid/issue-brief/the -effects-of-medicaid-expansion-under-the-aca-updated-findings-from-a-liter ature-review-march-2018/.

28. Stacey McMorrow et al., "Medicaid Expansion Increased Coverage, Improved Affordability, and Reduced Psychological Distress for Low-Income Parents," *Health Affairs* 36, no. 5 (2017): 808–818, https://doi.org/10.1377 /hlthaff.2016.1650.

29. Benjamin D. Sommers, "State Medicaid Expansions and Mortality, Revisited: A Cost-Benefit Analysis," *American Journal of Health Economics* 3, no. 3 (2017): 392–421, https://doi.org/10.1162/ajhe_a_00080.

30. Sara Rosenbaum et al., "Community Health Center Financing: The Role of Medicaid and Section 330 Grant Funding Explained," Medicaid, Kaiser Family Foundation, March 26, 2019, https://www.kff.org/medicaid /issue-brief/community-health-center-financing-the-role-of-medicaid-and -section-330-grant-funding-explained/.

31. Julia Paradise et al., "Community Health Centers: Recent Growth and the Role of the ACA," Medicaid, Kaiser Family Foundation, January 18, 2017, https://www.kff.org/report-section/community-health-centers-recent -growth-and-the-role-of-the-aca-issue-brief/.

32. Berchick, Hood, and Barnett, *Health Insurance Coverage*.

33. Jessica Sharac et al., "Community Health Centers Continue Steady Growth, but Challenges Loom," Milken Institute School of Public Health, George Washington University, Washington, DC, September 2019, https:// www.rchnfoundation.org/wp-content/uploads/2019/09/FINAL-GG-Brief -60_2018-UDS-Update.pdf.

34. Sara Rosenbaum et al., "Community Health Centers and Medicaid Delivery and Payment Reform: A Closer Look at Massachusetts and New York," Milken Institute School of Public Health, George Washington Uni-

versity, Washington, DC, March 2019, https://www.rchnfoundation.org/wp-content/uploads/2019/03/Final-GG-RCHN-IB-57-DSRIP_3.4.pdf.

35. Thomas J. Ward and H. Jack Geiger, *Out in the Rural: A Mississippi Health Center and Its War on Poverty* (New York: Oxford University Press, 2017).

36. Candice Chen et al., "Teaching Health Centers: A New Paradigm in Graduate Medical Education," *Academic Medicine* 87, no. 12 (2012): 1752–1756, https://doi.org/10.1097/ACM.0b013e3182720f4d.

37. David Barton Smith, *Health Care Divided: Race and Healing a Nation* (Ann Arbor: University of Michigan Press, 1999).

38. 81 Fed. Reg. 31376–31473 (May 18, 2016).

39. Edward R. Berchick, Jessica C. Barnett, and Rachel D. Upton, *Health Insurance Coverage in the United States: 2018* (Washington, DC: US Census Bureau, September 2019), https://www.census.gov/content/dam/Census/library/publications/2019/demo/p60-267.pdf.

40. *NFIB v. Sebelius*, 567 U.S. 519 at 602.

41. Franciscan Alliance v. Burwell, 227 F. Supp. 3d 660 (N.D. Texas, 2016).

42. Katie Keith, "Provider Conscience Rule Delayed Due to Lawsuits," *Health Affairs Blog*, July 2, 2019, https://www.healthaffairs.org/do/10.1377/hblog20190702.497856/full/.

43. Katie Keith, "Court Issues New Nationwide Injunction on Contraceptive Mandate," *Health Affairs Blog*, June 10, 2019, https://www.healthaffairs.org/do/10.1377/hblog20190610.936407/full/.

44. Katie Keith, "HHS Proposes to Strip Gender Identity, Language Access Protections from ACA Anti-Discrimination Rule," *Health Affairs Blog*, May 25, 2019, https://www.healthaffairs.org/do/10.1377/hblog20190525.831858/full/.

Chapter 20. From the ACA to Medicare for All?

1. Medicare for All Act of 2017, S. 1804, 116th Cong. (2019), "Cosponsors," Congress.gov, https://www.congress.gov/bill/115th-congress/senate-bill/1804/cosponsors.

2. Jacob S. Hacker, "Medicare Expansion as a Path as Well as a Destination: Achieving Universal Insurance Through a New Politics of Medicare," *ANNALS of the American Academy of Political and Social Science* 685, no. 1 (2019): 135–153, https://doi.org/10.1177/0002716219871017.

3. Peter A. Corning, *The Evolution of Medicare: From Idea to Law*, Washington, DC, US Social Security Administration, Office of Research and Statistics, 1969, 23–52.

4. Jacob S. Hacker, *The Divided Welfare State: The Battle over Public and Private Social Benefits in the United States* (New York: Cambridge University Press, 2002).

5. Jacob S. Hacker and Paul Pierson, "Policy Feedback in an Age of Polarization," *ANNALS of the American Academy of Political and Social Science* 685, no. 1 (2019): 8–28, https://doi.org/10.1177/0002716219871222.

6. Paul Starr, *Remedy and Reaction: The Peculiar American Struggle over Health Care Reform* (New Haven, CT: Yale University Press, 2011).

7. Hacker, "Medicare Expansion as a Path."

8. Jacob S. Hacker, "The Road to Medicare for Everyone," Health and Social Policy, American Prospect, last modified January 3, 2018, https://prospect.org/health/road-medicare-everyone/.

9. Frank Newport, "In U.S., Support for Government-Run Health System Edges Up," Gallup, last modified December 1, 2017, https://news.gallup.com/poll/223031/americans-support-government-run-health-system-edges.aspx.

10. Ibid.

11. Frank Newport, "Majority in U.S. Support Idea of Fed-Funded Healthcare System," Gallup, last modified May 16, 2016, https://news.gallup.com/poll/191504/majority-support-idea-fed-funded-healthcare-system.aspx.

12. Gretchen Jacobson et al., "A Dozen Facts About Medicare Advantage in 2019," Medicare, Kaiser Family Foundation, June 6, 2019, https://www.kff.org/medicare/issue-brief/a-dozen-facts-about-medicare-advantage-in-2019/.

13. Josh Bivens, "The Unfinished Business of Health Reform," Economic Policy Institute, Washington, DC, October 2018, https://www.epi.org/files/pdf/152676.pdf.

14. Josh Katz, Kevin Quealy, and Margot Sanger-Katz, "Would 'Medicare for All' Save Billions or Cost Billions?" The Upshot, *New York Times*, April 10, 2019, https://www.nytimes.com/interactive/2019/04/10/upshot/medicare-for-all-bernie-sanders-cost-estimates.html.

15. "Is Clinton's Tax Increase One of the Largest in History?" blog, Committee for a Responsible Federal Budget, last modified October 6, 2016, http://www.crfb.org/blogs/clintons-tax-increase-one-largest-history.

16. "Meet the Press—September 17, 2017 (Transcript)," Meet the Press, *NBC News*, September 17, 2017, https://www.nbcnews.com/meet-the-press/meet-press-september-17-2017-n802121.

17. Jacob S. Hacker, *Road to Nowhere: The Genesis of President Clinton's Plan for Health Security* (Princeton, NJ: Princeton University Press, 1997).

18. Theda Skocpol, "The Rise and Resounding Demise of the Clinton Plan," *Health Affairs* 14, no. 1 (1995): 66–85, https://doi.org/10.1377/hlthaff.14.1.66.

19. Hacker, "The Road to Medicare."

20. Personal communication with the author.

21. Hacker, "Medicare Expansion as a Path."

22. Paul Starr, "The Next Progressive Health Agenda," Health and Social Policy, American Prospect, last modified March 23, 2017, https://prospect .org/health/next-progressive-health-agenda/.

23. Brian Abel-Smith, *The Hospitals: 1800–1948* (London: Heinemann, 1964), 480.

INDEX

ABOUT THE EDITORS

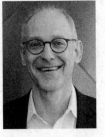

Stephen Zipp

Ezekiel J. Emanuel, MD, PhD, is the vice provost for Global Initiatives, Diane and Robert Levy University Professor, and codirector of the Healthcare Transformation Institute at the University of Pennsylvania. From 2009 to 2011 he was a special assistant in the Office of Management and Budget in the Obama administration. He has written *Reinventing American Health Care* and *Prescription for the Future* and in June 2020 will publish *Which Country Has the World's Best Health Care?* One component of his research focuses on designing and evaluating alternative payment models, especially bundled payment and capitation models.

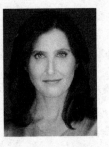

Peter Hurley

Abbe R. Gluck, JD, is professor of law and founding faculty director of the Solomon Center for Health Law and Policy at Yale Law School and professor of internal medicine at Yale Medical School. She has written extensively on the political and legal challenges to the ACA and coauthored US Supreme Court briefs in both major cases. She is a former law clerk to US Supreme Court Justice Ruth Bader Ginsburg and currently chairs the Uniform Law Commission's Health Care Committee and is an elected member of the leadership body of the American Law Institute.

PublicAffairs is a publishing house founded in 1997. It is a tribute to the standards, values, and flair of three persons who have served as mentors to countless reporters, writers, editors, and book people of all kinds, including me.

I. F. STONE, proprietor of *I. F. Stone's Weekly*, combined a commitment to the First Amendment with entrepreneurial zeal and reporting skill and became one of the great independent journalists in American history. At the age of eighty, Izzy published *The Trial of Socrates*, which was a national bestseller. He wrote the book after he taught himself ancient Greek.

BENJAMIN C. BRADLEE was for nearly thirty years the charismatic editorial leader of *The Washington Post*. It was Ben who gave the *Post* the range and courage to pursue such historic issues as Watergate. He supported his reporters with a tenacity that made them fearless and it is no accident that so many became authors of influential, best-selling books.

ROBERT L. BERNSTEIN, the chief executive of Random House for more than a quarter century, guided one of the nation's premier publishing houses. Bob was personally responsible for many books of political dissent and argument that challenged tyranny around the globe. He is also the founder and longtime chair of Human Rights Watch, one of the most respected human rights organizations in the world.

. . .

For fifty years, the banner of Public Affairs Press was carried by its owner Morris B. Schnapper, who published Gandhi, Nasser, Toynbee, Truman, and about 1,500 other authors. In 1983, Schnapper was described by *The Washington Post* as "a redoubtable gadfly." His legacy will endure in the books to come.

Peter Osnos, *Founder*